Topics in Arrhythmias and Ischemic Heart Disease

Emerging Concepts in Cardiology

Topics in Arrhythmias and Ischemic Heart Disease

Bruce B. Lerman, MD

H. Altschul Master Professor of Medicine
Chief, Division of Cardiology
Department of Medicine
Weill Medical College of Cornell University
New York Presbyterian Hospital
New York, New York

Craig T. Basson, MD, PhD

Gladys and Roland Harriman Professor of Medicine
Director, Cardiovascular Research
Division of Cardiology
Department of Medicine
Weill Medical College of Cornell University
New York Presbyterian Hospital
New York, New York

demosMEDICAL
New York

Acquisitions Editor: Richard Winters
Cover Design: Joe Tenerelli
Compositor: NewGen North America
Printer: King Printing

Visit our website at www.demosmedpub.com

Library of Congress Cataloging-in-Publication Data

Topics in Arrhythmias and Ischemic Heart Disease / [edited by] Bruce B. Lerman, Craig T. Basson.
p.; cm.
Includes bibliographical references and index.
ISBN 978-1-933864-58-7
1. Coronary heart disease. 2. Arrhythmia. I. Lerman, Bruce B. II. Basson, Craig T.
[DNLM: 1. Myocardial Ischemia. 2. Arrhythmias, Cardiac. WG 300 I77335 2010]
RC685.C6I5895 2010
616.1'23—dc22 2009034461

Medicine is an ever-changing science. Research and clinical experience are continually expanding our knowledge, in particular our understanding of proper treatment and drug therapy. The authors, editors, and publisher have made every effort to ensure that all information in this book is in accordance with the state of knowledge at the time of production of the book.

Nevertheless, the authors, editors, and publisher are not responsible for errors or omissions or for any consequences from application of the information in this book and make no warranty, express or implied, with respect to the contents of the publication. Every reader should examine carefully the package inserts accompanying each drug and should carefully check whether the dosage schedules mentioned therein or the contraindications stated by the manufacturer differ from the statements made in this book. Such examination is particularly important with drugs that are either rarely used or have been newly released on the market.

Special discounts on bulk quantities of Demos Medical Publishing books are available to corporations, professional associations, pharmaceutical companies, health care organizations, and other qualifying groups. For details, please contact:

Special Sales Department
Demos Medical Publishing
11 W. 42nd Street, 15th Floor
New York, NY 10036
Phone: 800-532-8663 or 212-683-0072
Fax: 212-941-7842
E-mail: rsanta@demosmedpub.com

Made in the United States of America

09 10 11 12 13 5 4 3 2 1

To my wife, Karen,
my children, Josh, Jessica, Rachel and Jennifer,
and my parents, Lillian and Philip Lerman.

—Bruce B. Lerman

Contents

Preface

Cardiology continues to be a dynamic field, one fueled in part by innovation in mechanical and cell-based therapies. This makes the field fascinating to observe but challenges one to remain au courant. Therefore, the task before the editors is to strike a balance in a single source that is authoritative, current, and readily absorbed. This is the goal of the current volume. We have organized this text to reflect the most current thinking in the field. To accomplish this mission, we have solicited the efforts of recognized authorities in ischemic heart disease and cardiac arrhythmias from the Weill Medical College of Cornell University, Division of Cardiology.

Although this volume, *Topics in Arrhythmias and Ischemic Heart Disease*, emphasizes state-of-the-art modalities in the treatment of coronary artery disease and arrhythmias, we are mindful that any coherent and integrated approach to the treatment of such patients must incorporate the impressive advances made in risk stratification. To that end, we have included a chapter that deciphers the myriad and sometimes contradictory data regarding biomarkers and their prognostic significance in ischemic heart disease. Prognostication for sudden cardiac death has become more sophisticated with the completion of several large randomized studies. The chapter dealing with this subject guides the reader through the nuances of the data, allowing one to incorporate the information into sound clinical decisions.

Impressive advancements in the treatment of acute coronary syndromes and congestive heart failure have been introduced in recent years. This has relied on a better understanding of the underlying pathogenesis and the introduction of novel therapeutic approaches. Pulmonary hypertension is an area that was relatively dormant until recent advances promoted new approaches to patients with this disorder. The chapter on this topic synthesizes the striking developments in this area. Likewise, cardiac resynchronization therapy has provided dramatic symptomatic relief for appropriately screened patients. Familiarity with understanding who benefits from such therapy and the determinants of such an outcome are essential for the clinician.

Interventional cardiology no longer refers to just percutaneous coronary procedures. Peripheral vascular procedures are now a well-established part of the armamentarium. Perhaps the most exciting innovation in the interventional domain is percutaneous valvular repair for treatment of aortic stenosis and mitral regurgitation. This area has the potential to be transformative. Finally, in the field of electrophysiology, percutaneous ablation to isolate the pulmonary veins in patients with atrial fibrillation achieves success in the majority of patients. Whether this procedure will replace antiarrhythmic therapy as a first-line approach remains to be seen, but for time being this approach at the very least can offer dramatic symptomatic relief for debilitated patients.

We wish to express appreciation to Demos Medical Publishing for their professionalism and expertise. It is our hope that this book serves as a useful guide and supplement for clinicians treating patients with ischemic heart disease and cardiac arrhythmias.

Bruce B. Lerman, MD
Craig T. Basson, MD, PhD

Contributors

Hasan A. Ahmad, MD
Fellow in Medicine
Division of Cardiology
Department of Medicine
Weill Medical College of Cornell University
New York Presbyterian Hospital
New York, New York

Eric Au, MD
Fellow in Medicine
Division of Cardiology
Department of Medicine
Weill Medical College of Cornell University
New York Presbyterian Hospital
New York, New York

Dmitriy N. Feldman, MD
Assistant Professor of Medicine
Division of Cardiology
Department of Medicine
Weill Medical College of Cornell University
New York Presbyterian Hospital
New York, New York

Evelyn M. Horn, MD
Professor of Clinical Medicine
Director, Heart Failure and Pulmonary Hypertension
Division of Cardiology
Department of Medicine
Weill Medical College of Cornell University
New York Presbyterian Hospital
New York, New York

Sei Iwai, MD
Professor of Clinical Medicine
Director, Complex Arrhythmia Ablation Program
Division of Cardiology
Department of Medicine
Stony Brook University Medical Center
Stony Brook, New York

Luke K. Kim, MD
Fellow in Medicine
Division of Cardiology
Department of Medicine
Weill Medical College of Cornell University
New York Presbyterian Hospital
New York, New York

Robert J. Kim, MD
Assistant Professor
Department of Medicine
Division of Cardiology
Department of Medicine
Weill Medical College of Cornell University
New York Presbyterian Hospital
New York, New York

Andy Lin, MD
Fellow in Medicine
Division of Cardiology
Department of Medicine
Weill Medical College of Cornell University
New York Presbyterian Hospital
New York, New York

Christopher F. Liu, MD
Assistant Professor of Medicine
Division of Cardiology
Department of Medicine
Weill Medical College of Cornell University
New York Presbyterian Hospital
New York, New York

Steven M. Markowitz, MD
Associate Professor of Medicine
Division of Cardiology
Department of Medicine
Weill Medical College of Cornell University
New York Presbyterian Hospital
New York, New York

Robert M. Minutello, MD
Associate Professor of Medicine
Director, Interventional Cardiology Fellowship
Division of Cardiology
Department of Medicine
Weill Medical College of Cornell University
New York Presbyterian Hospital
New York, New York

Issam D. Moussa, MD
Associate Professor of Medicine
Director, Endovascular Services
Division of Cardiology
Department of Medicine
Weill Medical College of Cornell University
New York Presbyterian Hospital
New York, New York

Apoor Patel, MD
Fellow in Medicine
Division of Cardiology
Department of Medicine
Weill Medical College of Cornell University
New York Presbyterian Hospital
New York, New York

Irina Sobol, MD
Assistant Professor of Medicine
Division of Cardiology
Department of Medicine
Weill Medical College of Cornell University
New York Presbyterian Hospital
New York, New York

Kenneth M. Stein, MD
Division of Cardiology
Department of Medicine
Weill Medical College of Cornell University
New York Presbyterian Hospital
New York, New York

S. Chiu Wong, MD
Professor of Medicine
Director, Cardiac Catheterization Laboratory
Division of Cardiology
Department of Medicine
Weill Medical College of Cornell University
New York Presbyterian Hospital
New York, New York

Suzanne Zentko, MD
Fellow in Medicine
Division of Cardiology
Department of Medicine
Weill Medical College of Cornell University
New York Presbyterian Hospital
New York, New York

I Risk Stratification of Sudden Cardiac Death

APOOR PATEL
SEI IWAI

OUTLINE

EPIDEMIOLOGY OF SUDDEN CARDIAC DEATH

Heart disease is the leading cause of death in the United States and is responsible for approximately 870,000 deaths per year (1). Sudden cardiac death (SCD) is responsible for almost half of these deaths, claiming 350,000 to 400,000 lives per year (2). SCD is defined by the World Health Organization as death due to any cardiac disease that occurs out of hospital, in an emergency room, or a patient who is dead on arrival to a care facility. Of note, the death must occur within one hour after the onset of symptoms. The majority of SCD is likely arrhythmic in etiology. In women, up to 88% of sudden cardiac arrests may be due to arrhythmic causes (3). Of SCD due to cardiac arrhythmias, greater than 80% of events are due to ventricular tachycardia (VT) and ventricular fibrillation (VF), with the remainder due to bradyarrhythmias and asystole (4). Coronary artery disease (CAD), manifesting acutely as ischemic ventricular arrhythmias or chronically as scar-mediated arrhythmias, is responsible for 80% of SCD. Idiopathic dilated cardiomyopathies and hypertrophic cardiomyopathy are the next most common causes (5). While certain inherited ion channel disorders and acquired forms of structural heart disease are important etiologies of SCD, these entities are beyond the scope of this chapter, which will focus on risk stratification in patients with ischemic heart disease and nonischemic cardiomyopathies.

While medical therapy and the advent of the implantable cardioverter-defibrillator (ICD) have conferred a survival benefit to high-risk patients for SCD, there remains a substantial portion of the population at risk who do not meet current guidelines for ICD implantation. High-risk subgroups have a higher incidence of SCD but a lower absolute number of deaths, while low-risk subgroups have a low incidence of SCD but contribute a higher absolute number of deaths, as they represent a larger proportion of the overall population (Figure 1.1) (6). Liberalizing ICD implantation criteria to all patients in lower risk subgroups would, by definition, lead to an increase in the number needed to treat to save one life. Even utilizing current ICD implant criteria, most patients considered high risk do not benefit from defibrillator therapy and are exposed to the possibility of experiencing inappropriate ICD shocks as well as other device complications. Thus, identification of markers with better sensitivity and specificity for patients who would benefit from ICDs is critical.

A number of potential methods for risk stratification exist, including use of clinical parameters such as left ventricular ejection fraction (LVEF), electrophysiologic markers, imaging assessments, biochemical and genetic markers, and functional assessments (Table 1.1). A number of these methods will be discussed below. Some of the initial lessons were learned from ICD trials involving secondary prevention of SCD; that is, trials in patients

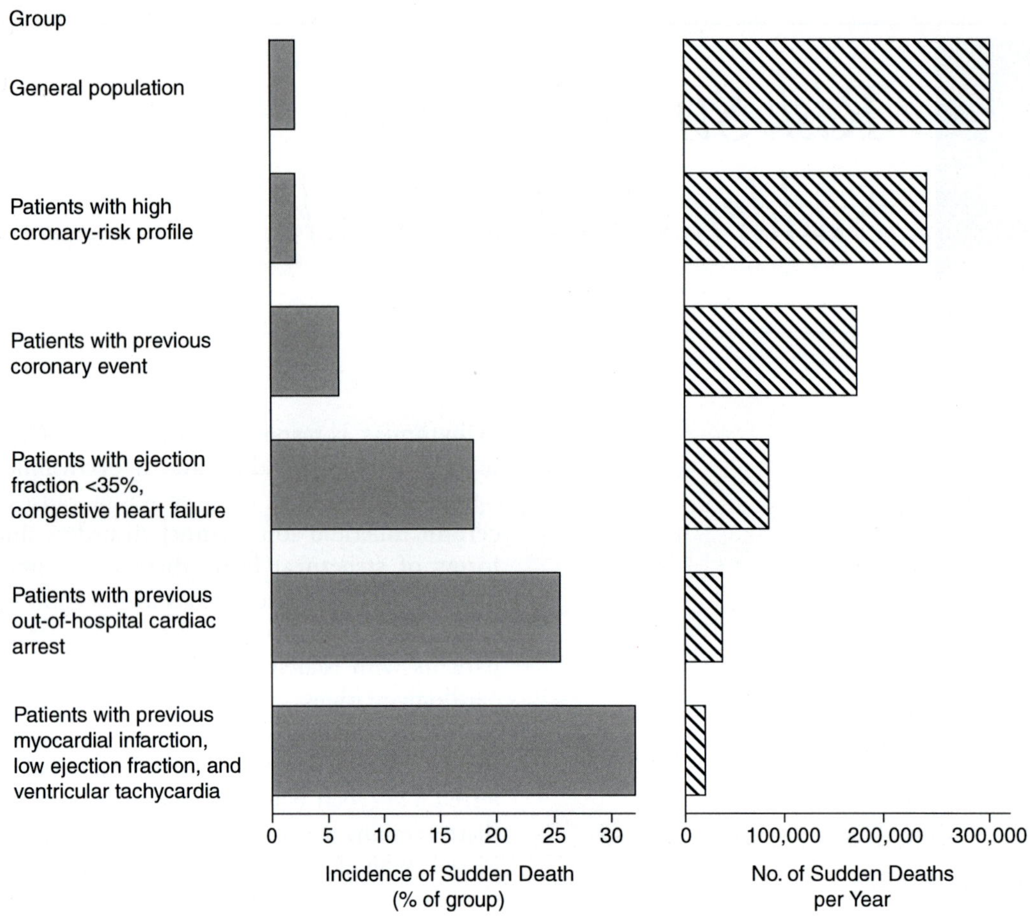

FIGURE 1.1 The incidence of sudden death in specific populations and the annual number of deaths in those populations. (Adapted from Ref. 6, with permission.)

Table 1.1 Methods of risk stratification for sudden cardiac death

Electrophysiologic markers	Anatomic markers
Electrophysiologic study	Left ventricular ejection fraction
T wave alternans	MRI for scar burden
Signal averaged ECG	Genetic markers
QRS duration	Functional markers
Measures of autonomic tone	Exercise testing
	Biochemical markers

EF, ejection fraction; MRI, magnetic resonance imaging; SCD, sudden cardiac death.

who had already survived cardiac arrest and were therefore identified to be in a high-risk subgroup. We will discuss these trials before continuing on to the utility of risk stratification tools in primary prevention of SCD.

SUDDEN CARDIAC DEATH SURVIVORS

Secondary Prevention ICD Trials

The Antiarrhythmics versus Implantable Defibrillators (AVID) trial (7) was the largest secondary prevention trial, and helped define ICD implant indications for patients with a history of ventricular arrhythmias. In AVID, 1013 patients who presented with VF, sustained VT with syncope, or sustained VT with a LVEF of ≤40% were randomized to either an ICD or antiarrhythmic therapy. The antiarrhythmic therapy was predominantly amiodarone (97%). Importantly, patients with VT/VF deemed to be due to reversible causes, VT/VF within five days of a myocardial infarction (MI) or revascularization, and with class IV heart failure (HF) were excluded from the trial. Over a mean follow-up of 18 months, the unadjusted total mortality for the ICD group and the antiarrhythmic drug group was 16% and 24%, respectively (Figure 1.2). Furthermore, the ICD group had better survival throughout the course of the study. As expected, the ICD reduced total mortality mainly via prevention of arrhythmic death, which was 4.7% in the ICD group and 10.8% in the antiarrhythmic group. Subgroup analysis of AVID based on LVEF demonstrated that patients with an LVEF of 20% to 34% had a survival benefit from ICD implantation compared to antiarrhythmic therapy (8). In patients with an LVEF of ≥35% there was no significant mortality difference between the ICD group and the antiarrhythmic group, and in patients with an LVEF of <20% there was only a trend towards benefit with an ICD. While some have used this data to question the benefit of an ICD in patients with an LVEF <20% or LVEF ≥35%, subgroup analysis should be interpreted with caution. Thus, current guidelines (9) call for ICD implantation in all survivors of SCD with a life expectancy of more than one year.

The Cardiac Arrest Study Hamburg (CASH) randomized 349 cardiac arrest survivors due to documented

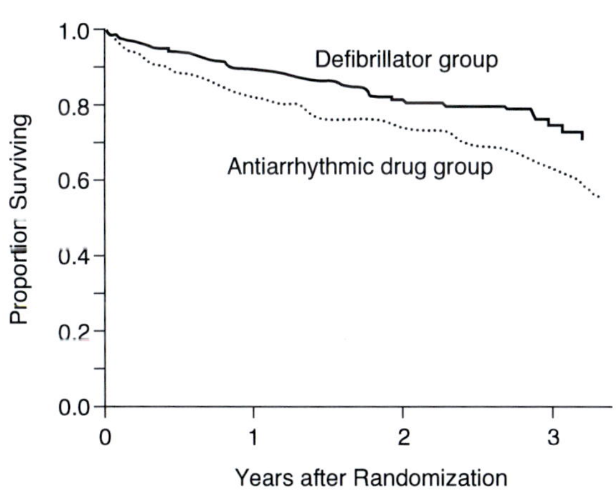

Patients at risk	1016	644	333	104
Percent surviving				
Defibrillator group		89.3	81.6	75.4
Antiarrhythmic-drug group		82.3	74.7	64.1

FIGURE 1.2 Overall survival in AVID. Unadjusted for baseline characteristics. (From Ref. 7, with permission.)

ventricular arrhythmias to an ICD, amiodarone, propafenone, or metoprolol (10). Propafenone was discontinued early when an interim analysis showed a 61% higher mortality in this group compared to the ICD group. ICD patients had a nonsignificant 23% reduction in all-cause mortality at a mean follow-up of 57 months, with the most benefit derived in the first five years. Of note, there was no significant difference in mortality between the patients assigned to metoprolol versus amiodarone, questioning the utility of amiodarone therapy for SCD prevention. Similar to CASH, the Canadian Implantable Defibrillator Study (CIDS) randomized 659 patients with resuscitated VT/VF or unmonitored syncope to an ICD or amiodarone (11). After a five-year follow-up, a nonsignificant decrease in risk of total mortality and arrhythmic death was observed in the ICD group versus the amiodarone group.

While AVID was the largest of these trials, it was stopped early (because the difference in the primary outcome variable between the two groups had crossed the statistical boundary for early termination). CASH and CIDS had fewer patients but longer follow-up, and thus a meta-analysis that was performed of the three trials is instructive (12). It demonstrated that ICD implantation resulted in a significant 27% reduction in total mortality driven by a 50% reduction in arrhythmic mortality. The analysis showed that the ICD was beneficial mainly in low LVEF (<35%) patients and those with advanced HF. Based on the demonstration of significant risk of recurrent SCD in patients in these secondary prevention trials, the ACC/AHA/HRS 2008 guidelines for device-based therapy of cardiac rhythm abnormalities assign a class I indication for ICD implantation in cardiac arrest survivors of VF or hemodynamically unstable VT not felt to be due to reversible causes (9). Patients with structural heart disease and sustained VT, whether hemodynamically stable or unstable, and patients with syncope of unknown origin with hemodynamically significant sustained VT or VF induced at electrophysiologic study (EPS) also meet class I indications for ICD therapy (9).

■ PRIMARY PREVENTION OF SUDDEN CARDIAC DEATH

Since SCD can be the first manifestation of heart disease in 50% of men and 63% of women (1), relying solely on a strategy of secondary prevention of SCD would be ineffective in substantially reducing the event rates. In addition, the median reported survival to hospital discharge after out-of-hospital cardiac arrest with any first recorded rhythm is 7.9% (13). Therefore, it is important to identify patients at risk prior to their first episode in order to have the biggest impact on reducing the number of SCDs that occur.

Ejection Fraction, Nonsustained VT, and Inducibility of Sustained VT

ICD Trials in Ischemic Cardiomyopathy

Primary prevention ICD trials initially focused on patients post-MI with significantly reduced LVEF, due to the high mortality rates in this population (14). Early primary prevention trials also utilized arrhythmic markers of nonsustained ventricular tachycardia (NSVT) and inducibility of sustained VT/VF at EPS as inclusion criteria in an attempt to identify the highest risk patients, based on prior studies (15). After these initial trials demonstrated mortality benefit to ICD implantation, subsequent studies evaluated patients post-MI with a low LVEF alone; presence of NSVT and inducibility at EPS were no longer utilized as inclusion criteria. These later trials also showed survival benefit, leading to current guidelines for ICD implantation in primary prevention candidates.

The Multicenter Automatic Defibrillator Trial (MADIT) randomized 196 patients with prior MI, class I–III congestive HF, a LVEF ≤35%, NSVT, and inducible VT on EP study that was not suppressible with procainamide, to an ICD or conventional therapy (16). Most patients in the conventional therapy arm received amiodarone. The trial was stopped early as it demonstrated a statistically significant, and impressive, 54% reduction in total mortality in the ICD arm at 27 months (16% and 39% in the ICD and conventional therapy groups, respectively). MADIT is notable in that it only enrolled a small number of patients and did not have a control group. In addition, more patients in the ICD group received beta-blockers.

The Multicenter Unsustained Tachycardia Trial (MUSTT) was not designed as an ICD trial per se, but rather to test whether EP-guided antiarrhythmic therapy would decrease the risk of SCD (17). The trial enrolled patients with CAD, LVEF 40% or less, NSVT, HF class I–III, and inducible VT during EP study. NSVT had to occur four days or more post-MI or revascularization. 704 inducible patients were randomized to EP-guided therapy (351 patients) or no therapy (353 patients). Of the patients randomized to EP-guided therapy, 29% received antiarrhythmic drugs and 58% received an ICD. Patients only qualified for an ICD if they failed one antiarrhythmic agent and remained inducible for VT/VF at repeat EP testing. MUSTT showed a decrease in the combined endpoint of cardiac arrest or death from arrhythmia at five years with EP-guided therapy compared to no antiarrhythmic therapy (25% versus 32%, respectively). Overall mortality was also reduced from 48% to 42% among patients receiving EP guided therapy (Figure 1.3). Subgroup analysis revealed that the benefit from EP-guided therapy was entirely due to the survival benefit of the ICD group. The ICD arm demonstrated a 31% reduction in mortality compared with those receiving antiarrhythmic therapy and a 24% mortality reduction compared to those receiving no therapy. Together, MADIT and MUSTT clearly demonstrated the benefit of ICD therapy in patients with a low LVEF, NSVT, and inducible ventricular arrhythmias on EP study.

The MUSTT trial also created a registry of the 1435 patients who had a low LVEF and NSVT, but were not inducible for VT/VF at EP study (18). They compared these patients with the 353 patients who received no antiarrhythmic therapy. Although, overall mortality at five years was significantly lower at 44% in the noninducible registry patients compared with 48% in the inducible patients not receiving antiarrhythmic therapy, it was still quite high overall. In addition, it was significantly higher than the 24% mortality in the ICD treated arm. Thus, results from the MUSTT registry suggested that even noninducible patients were at high risk and may benefit from ICD therapy.

Of the 2202 patients screened in the MUSTT trial, only 35% were inducible. Inducibility in the MUSTT trial was defined as monomorphic VT with up to three extrastimuli or burst pacing, or polymorphic VT or VF with up to two extrastimuli. The negative predictive value of an EP study was only 88% at two years and 76% at five years for cardiac arrest or death due to arrhythmia among the registry patients. Thus, while the EP study provides some utility in risk stratification, it appears to be inadequate in isolation to classify patients with CAD and LV dysfunction into a sufficiently low-risk category. Another substudy of the MUSTT trial examined the relationship between LVEF and inducibility to the risk of cardiac arrest or arrhythmic death (19). It found that patients with a

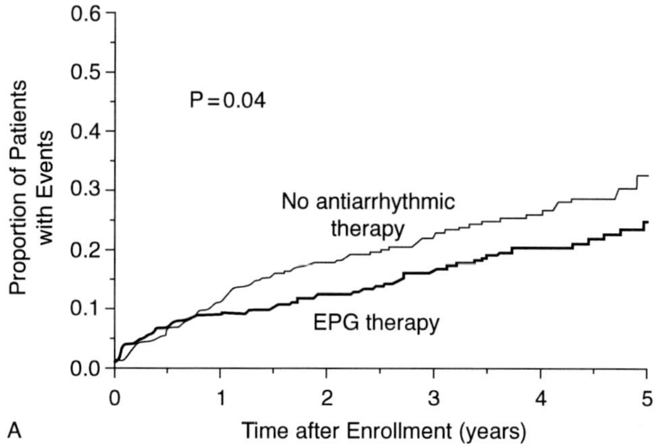

No. at Risk

	0	1	2	3	4	5
No antiarrhythmic therapy	353	290	242	178	118	67
EPG therapy	351	301	265	199	119	68

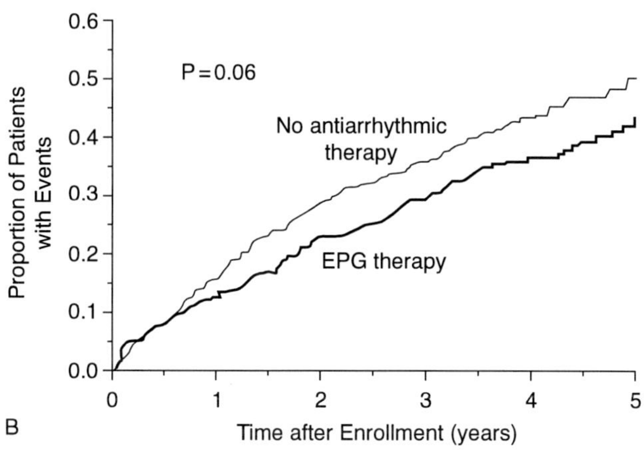

No. at Risk

	0	1	2	3	4	5
No antiarrhythmic therapy	353	296	248	185	122	71
EPG therapy	351	306	270	203	121	70

FIGURE 1.3 A: Kaplan–Meier estimates of the rates of cardiac arrest or death from arrhythmia. B: Death from all causes from the MUSTT trial. EPG notes electrophysiologically guided therapy. (From Ref. 17, with permission.)

LVEF <30% who were noninducible had the same rate of arrhythmic death or cardiac arrest as patients with a LVEF of 30% to 40% who were inducible. The only patients with a low event rate were those with an LVEF >30% who were noninducible. This implies that EPS may be of limited utility in higher risk patients—that is, those with severely decreased LVEF. The lower predictive power of EPS in patients with a lower LVEF might be due to these patients having more severe HF. Severe HF predisposes patients to having hormonal and electrolyte abnormalities, myocardial stretch, and repolarization abnormalities, all of which may predispose to arrhythmias (20,21). These conditions are dynamic, and thus may not be accurately assessed by an EP study that occurs at one point in time.

The MADIT-II trial addressed the possibility raised from the MUSTT registry data that patients with CAD and a low LVEF were at sufficiently high risk of SCD, and thus would benefit from an ICD (22), regardless of inducibility at EPS. In MADIT-II, 1232 patients with prior MI, LVEF ≤30%, and NYHA class I–III HF were randomly assigned in a 3:2 ratio to receive an ICD or conventional therapy. Patients were excluded if they had an MI within the past month, or if they were revascularized via percutaneous coronary intervention (PCI) or coronary artery bypass graft surgery (CABG) in the past three months. The mean time from MI to enrollment in the trial was 6.5 years. During an average follow-up of 20 months, the mortality rates were 19.8% in the conventional therapy group and 14.2% in the ICD group, representing a 31% relative risk reduction for death with ICD therapy (Figure 1.4). The mortality benefit was due to a reduction in sudden death (3.8% versus 10.0% in the ICD and conventional therapy arms, respectively). Interestingly, there was a higher rate of hospitalization for HF in the ICD group (20%) than in the conventional therapy group (15%). Potential explanations for this include the ICD preventing arrhythmic death thus leading to more HF, or the effects of right ventricular pacing leading to ventricular dyssynchrony.

While MADIT-II excluded patients who were less than 30 days post-MI, data from a substudy of the Valsartan in Acute Myocardial Infarction Trial (VALIANT) showed that the risk of sudden death was highest in the first 30 days post-MI (23). VALIANT was a trial of 14,609 patients with an ejection fraction of <40% or HF post-MI who were randomized to an angiotensin converting enzyme inhibitor, an angiotensin receptor blocker, or both (24). The trial also examined SCD rates and found that patients had a 1.4% event rate in the first month post-MI, which then diminished over time (23). The event rate was higher in the patients with an ejection fraction of <30%, with an event rate of 2.3% in the first month. Each decrease of LVEF by 5% was associated with a 21% increase in the risk of sudden death in the first month. At one year, the rates of SCD merged, regardless of LVEF, suggesting that the

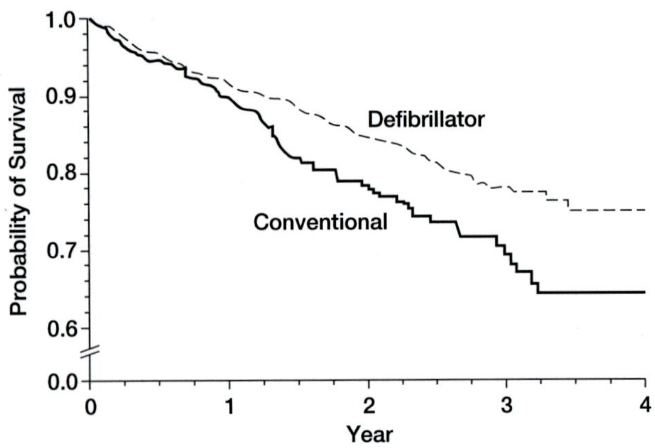

No. at Risk

Defibrillator	742	503 (0.91)	274 (0.84)	110 (0.78)	9
Conventional	490	329 (0.90)	170 (0.78)	65 (0.69)	3

FIGURE 1.4 Kaplan–Meier estimates of the probability of survival in the group assigned to receive an implantable defibrillator and the group assigned to receive conventional therapy in MADIT-II. (From Ref. 22, with permission.)

discriminatory effect of LVEF to distinguish patients at risk for SCD declines over time.

Further evidence of the dynamic temporal relationship of SCD and MI was presented in a surveillance study of 2997 post-MI patients (25). They reported an incidence of SCD of 1.2% in the 30 days posthospital discharge, and a subsequent 1.2% per year, with a five-year rate of 6.9%.

Contrasting evidence was found by the Defibrillation in Acute Myocardial Infarction Trial (DINAMIT) investigators, who assessed the utility of ICD implantation after recent MI (26). In their study, 674 patients with an MI within 6 to 40 days, LVEF ≤35%, and impaired cardiac autonomic function (manifest as either depressed heart rate variability or an elevated average 24-hour heart rate on Holter monitoring) were randomized to either medical therapy or an ICD. During a mean follow-up of 30 months, there was no difference in overall mortality between the two groups. While the ICD was effective in reducing death from arrhythmia by 58%, a prespecified secondary outcome, this was offset by a 75% increase in nonarrhythmic death in this group. Most of the nonarrhythmic deaths in the ICD group were due to cardiac causes, suggesting that ICD implantation shifted the mode of death from arrhythmia to HF in this population. As only 10% of patients were revascularized in the ICD group, recurrent ischemia leading to VT/VF—which would have normally led to cardiac arrest—was prevented by the ICD, but infarction and pump failure was not. However, the trial had a low event rate overall, which may have prevented detection of a difference between the control group and ICD group. It is also possible that the use of impaired autonomic tone as an inclusion criterion may have somehow selected for patients that had a higher propensity to die from HF and not sudden death. Ultimately, the results of DINAMIT suggest that immediate risk stratification of post-MI patients by LVEF and impaired autonomic tone may not be helpful, as the LVEF can recover over time, or scar formation may occur, thus changing the risk of SCD as time progresses.

In addition to DINAMIT, the Coronary Artery Bypass Graft (CABG)-Patch Trial failed to show the utility of ICD in primary prophylaxis (27). In CABG-Patch, 900 patients scheduled for a CABG with an LVEF ≤35% and a positive signal average electrocardiogram (SAECG) were randomized to CABG and an epicardial ICD or CABG and conventional therapy. There was no reduction in total mortality with the ICD after an average follow-up of 32 months, but the ICD group did have a reduction in arrhythmic death (4% versus 6.9% in the control group). Since the majority of the deaths were nonarrhythmic, the reduction in arrhythmic death did not affect total mortality. Reasons proposed for the lack of benefit include the beneficial effects of revascularization, including protection against arrhythmia and possible improvement of postoperative LVEF, thereby creating a lower risk patient population for SCD.

Given the results of MADIT-II, the Sudden Cardiac Death in Heart Failure Trial (SCD-HeFT), MUSTT, as well as DINAMIT and CABG-Patch, current guidelines for patients post-MI with a LVEF ≤35% with class II–III HF advocate waiting 40 days post-MI before ICD implantation, and waiting three months postrevascularization before ICD implantation (Figure 1.5a) (9). Post-MI patients with class I HF must have an LVEF ≤30% as only MADIT-II specifically included this group of patients. Based on MUSTT, patients with an LVEF ≤40% and NSVT may undergo EPS and receive an ICD if inducible for VF or sustained VT.

ICD Trials in Nonischemic Cardiomyopathy

Risk stratification of patients with nonischemic cardiomyopathy has proven to be more challenging than in their counterparts with CAD. The Defibrillators in Non-Ischemic Cardiomyopathy Treatment Evaluation

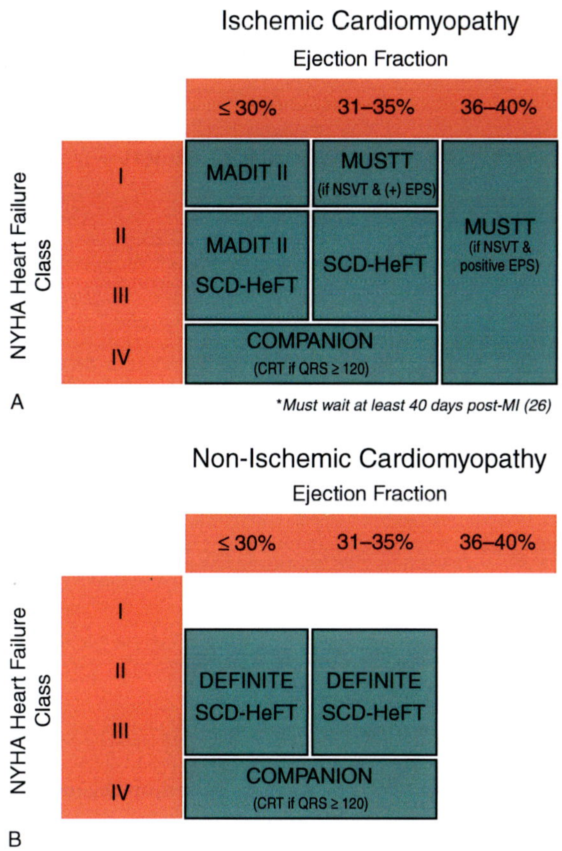

FIGURE 1.5 Summary of evidence supporting defibrillator implantation as stratified by ejection fraction and heart failure class in patients with ischemic cardiomyopathy (A) and nonischemic cardiomyopathy (B). For details of COMPANION trial, see Chapter 5. (CRT, cardiac resynchronization therapy; EPS, electrophysiology study; NYHA,New York Heart Association.)

(DEFINITE) Trial (28) randomized 458 patients with nonischemic dilated cardiomyopathy, LVEF <36%, and premature ventricular complexes or NSVT to standard medical therapy or standard medical therapy plus a single-chamber ICD. Of these patients, 86% were on an ACE inhibitor and 85% were on a beta-blocker. The ICD group had a significant reduction in arrhythmic death, but a nonsignificant reduction in total mortality. The trial was underpowered as the mortality rate in the medical therapy arm was lower than what the trial design had anticipated, and thus the primary endpoint may have reached statistical significance if there were a larger number of study subjects.

SCD-HeFT enrolled 2521 patients with ischemic or nonischemic cardiomyopathy with class II or III HF and an LVEF ≤35% (29). Patients were randomized to conventional therapy plus placebo, conventional therapy plus amiodarone, or conventional therapy plus a single-lead ICD. Placebo and amiodarone were administered in double-blind fashion. Amiodarone had no effect on the risk of death (28%) compared to placebo (29%). In contrast, ICD therapy was associated with an absolute decrease in mortality of 7.2% over amiodarone and medical therapy with ACE inhibitors and beta-blockers (Figure 1.6). These results held true for patients with both ischemic and nonischemic cardiomyopathies, a prespecified subgroup analysis. While MADIT-II had a follow-up period of 20 months, SCD-HeFT bolstered the MADIT-II findings with a follow-up of up to five years, demonstrating that beneficial effects of ICD implantation were not short-lived.

Subgroup analysis by HF class demonstrated that patients with class II HF derived benefit with ICD therapy, but not those with class III HF. Given that MADIT-II showed a greater benefit of ICD therapy the lower the LVEF, and that DEFINITE showed a greater benefit in class III patients, it is unlikely that this post-hoc subgroup analysis of SCD-HeFT represents a valid finding.

The results of these primary prevention trials in nonischemic cardiomyopathy patients led to an indication for ICD implantation in patients with a nonischemic cardiomyopathy, LVEF ≤35%, and class II or III HF (Figure 1.5b) (9). Importantly in SCD-HeFT, patients had to have a diagnosis of HF for at least three months and be on appropriate medical therapy.

■ OTHER METHODS OF RISK STRATIFICATION

Limitations of the LVEF in Risk Stratification

Based on data including the ICD trials described above, LVEF is the most well-established method for risk stratification for SCD. Furthermore, its accessibility and ease of measurement offers advantages over other risk stratification methods. The prognostic value of LVEF has remained strong despite improvements in treatments for acute MI, including beta-blocker therapy (30,31). However, while LVEF predicts both total mortality and arrhythmic death, it is poor at discriminating between the two (19). The results of DINAMIT and CABG-Patch also suggest that LVEF may be as much a

	Hazard Ratio (97.5% CI)	P Value
Amiodarone vs. placebo	1.06 (0.86–1.30)	0.53
ICD therapy vs. placebo	0.77 (0.62–1.96)	0.007

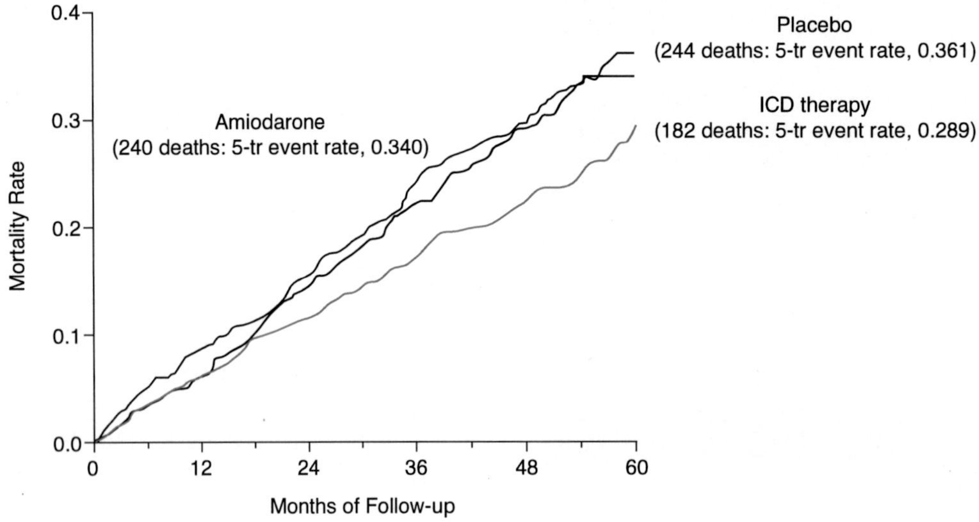

No. at Risk						
Amiodarone	845	772	715	484	280	97
Placebo	847	797	724	505	303	89
ICD therapy	829	778	733	501	304	103

FIGURE 1.6 Kaplan–Meier estimates of death from any cause in patients with both ischemic and nonischemic cardiomyopathy randomized to amiodarone, placebo, or implantable cardioverter-defibrillator therapy in SCD-HeFT. (From Ref. 29, with permission.)

marker for progressive pump failure as it is for arrhythmic death. While an LVEF of 35% to 40% has been identified as a cutoff for identifying high-risk patients (32,33), its specificity for prediction of SCD is poor, as the absolute number of SCD is higher in people with a more preserved LVEF. This is because the subgroup of patients with a moderately reduced or preserved LVEF is much larger than the population with an LVEF under the range of 35% to 40%.

When the primary prevention trials started using LVEF as essentially the sole criterion for ICD implantation (i.e., not requiring inducibility of VT/VF at EPS), the absolute reduction in mortality decreased with a corresponding increase in the number needed to treat to save one life. For instance, in MUSTT the absolute reduction in mortality was 31% and the number needed to treat was three at five years, and in MADIT the absolute reduction in mortality was 19% with a number needed to treat of four at two years. However, in MADIT-II and SCD-HeFT the absolute mortality reduction was 6% and 7% respectively, with a number needed to treat of 11 and 17 at three years, respectively. Neither MADIT-II nor SCD-HeFT used the EP study to risk stratify patients, as was the case in MADIT and MUSTT. As discussed earlier, while the MUSTT registry showed that EPS has a low negative predictive value at two years it clearly offered some enhancement of risk stratification, although this may be limited to lower risk, higher LVEF patients (19).

Better risk-stratifying tools, ideally with both higher sensitivity and specificity, are needed to avoid unnecessary ICD implantation in patients who will never benefit from them, and to identify those patients in traditionally "low-risk" populations who are actually at high risk. It is important to remember that most patients with an LVEF under the range of 30% to 35% that meet MADIT-II or SCD-HeFT criteria will not experience SCD and are subject to untoward complications of ICDs, including inappropriate shocks and device infections. In MADIT II, the rate of inappropriate shocks was 11.5% of patients (34) while in SCD-HeFT the rate of inappropriate shocks was 37%

of patients with AF versus 14% of patients in sinus rhythm (35).

Clinical Parameters in Risk Stratification

Analysis of clinical variables may enhance risk stratification. That is, a reduced LVEF may be a more potent risk factor in combination with other risk factors than in isolation (36). A substudy of MUSTT examined the subset of patients who were inducible but did not receive antiarrhythmic therapy (37). The authors evaluated 25 clinical variables and their relationship to total mortality and arrhythmic death. They then constructed a risk stratification algorithm to weight the impact of each variable and found that HF class, history of HF, NSVT not related to bypass surgery, LVEF, age, left ventricular conduction abnormalities, inducible sustained VT, inpatient enrollment in the trial, and atrial fibrillation had the greatest prognostic impact in the multivariate analysis. In this model, a patient age 60, with a LVEF < 30% and no other significant clinical risk factors, would have a risk of arrhythmic death of 2% and a total mortality of 5% at two years. In contrast, a patient with a LVEF >30%, of age 65, who had no prior CABG, a history of HF, inducible VT, and NSVT not within 10 days of their CABG, had an arrhythmic death risk of 11% and a total mortality of 19% at two years. The latter patient, despite having a higher LVEF, is at greater risk for SCD when other clinical variables are taken into account. Thus, evaluation of clinical risk factors may be able to better risk stratify patients beyond the discriminatory capability of LVEF alone.

In a MADIT-II substudy, a regression analysis was performed to determine clinical risk factors that would predict SCD using the patients that were assigned to the medical therapy arm of the trial (38). The study hypothesized that some patients with a low LVEF may be at low enough risk for SCD that ICD implantation could be withheld, while some patients would have such a high rate of nonarrhythmic death they would also not benefit from an ICD. After excluding a group of very high-risk patients based on a blood urea nitrogen (BUN) ≥50 and/or a creatinine ≥2.5, they made a risk score model based on HF class, age >70, BUN >26, (QRS) >120 msec, and presence of atrial fibrillation (AF), with one point being assigned to each of the five risk factors. Crude two-year mortality rates were 8% in the patients with zero risk factors, and 28% in patients with at least one risk factor. Mortality was 43% at two years in patients in the very high-risk group. As hypothesized, ICD therapy was of no benefit in patients with risk score of zero, or patients in the very high-risk group category. It was helpful in the intermediate risk group, thus generating a U-shaped curve.

The above studies imply that clinical risk models may be of great utility for further risk stratification in MUSTT and MADIT-II type patients, but need to be prospectively validated over longer follow-up periods.

Microvolt T-Wave Alternans Testing

T-wave alternans (TWA) measures beat-to-beat alternation in the T wave on ECG, specifically in its shape, amplitude, or timing. This alternation is a marker for cellular repolarization abnormalities, which can cause instability in cardiac repolarization and predispose to VF (39). Specifically, there is spatial or temporal dispersion of repolarization within the myocardium, which may be the result of alterations in calcium handling (40,41). Macroscopic TWA was originally described in the early 1900s and has been associated with myocardial ischemia, electrolyte abnormalities, and the long QT syndrome (39). Modern use relies on computer filtering and analysis (fast Fourier transform) to detect *microvolt* fluctuations that cannot otherwise be seen. The test is performed with exercise or atrial pacing during EP study and relies on gradual rate acceleration. While many normal patients will have TWA at an elevated heart rate, it occurs at a lower threshold in patients at risk for SCD, and use of a lower rate helps eliminate false positives. A positive test is considered to be sustained TWA of at least one minute duration, at a heart rate ≤110 bpm, and a voltage of ≥1.9 microvolts in a defined number of leads. A negative test is the absence of TWA (i.e., ≤1.9 microvolts) at a heart rate ≥105 bpm; an indeterminate test is any other result. Automated test results are available and simplify interpretation. Importantly, TWA evaluation cannot be performed in patients with atrial fibrillation, as the variation in heart rate prevents accurate analysis. Finally, due to the observation that patients with indeterminate TWA results have similar prognosis as those with a positive TWA, these two groups are often categorized together as "nonnegative" (42).

The utility of microvolt TWA to aid in risk stratification has been studied in numerous trials in patients with both ischemic and nonischemic heart disease. Selected illustrative studies will be presented below.

Microvolt TWA in Risk Stratification for Patients With Ischemic Heart Disease

In the Alternans Before Cardioverter Defibrillator (ABCD) Trial, TWA was compared to EP study in predicting VT/VF (43). The population consisted of 566 patients with CAD, LVEF ≤40%, NSVT, and class I–III HF. All patients underwent EP study and TWA testing. The patients had a mean LVEF of 28% and the median follow-up was 1.9 years. If either EP study or TWA was positive an ICD was mandated. An ICD was encouraged if both tests were negative, and ultimately >90% of patients in the trial received an ICD. The primary outcome was arrhythmic events which were determined from the ICD. The results showed that the positive predictive value (PPV) and negative predictive value (NPV) was similar for EP study and TWA (PPV 11% and 9% and NPV 96% and 95%, respectively). The highest arrhythmic event rate (12.6%) was in patients with both a positive TWA and EP study and the lowest rate (2.3%) was in TWA and EP study negative patients (Figure 1.7). Thus TWA was as effective as EP study for identifying patients most likely to have an arrhythmic event, and importantly, the two studies provide additional prognostic information together. The study also showed that neither EP study nor TWA by themselves has a sufficient NPV to withhold ICD implantation in patients with ischemic LV dysfunction.

TWA alternans was also assessed in a mixed population of 286 patient with ischemic (75% of patients) and nonischemic (25% of patients) cardiomyopathy (44). These patients had an LVEF ≤35%, class I–IV HF, and either NSVT (84%), syncope (8%), or both (8%). EP study and TWA was performed in all patients. The mean follow-up was 38 months and the mean LVEF was 26%. The primary endpoint was arrhythmia-free survival and the secondary endpoint was all-cause mortality. The study found that the NPV of TWA was better than that of EP study, but as seen in ABCD, the best NPV (85% at two years) was when both tests were negative. TWA was equally predictive in ischemic and nonischemic patients. The two-year event rate of 19% for TWA-negative patients was higher than that seen in other studies, suggesting that inclusion of patients in the study with NSVT, syncope, and class IV HF may have created a higher risk patient population. Thus, while TWA is predictive of arrhythmia-free survival, the high event rate in TWA-negative patients suggests that a negative TWA alone is not capable of identifying a low enough risk population to withhold ICD implantation. Even patients with both a negative TWA and EP study had a NPV of 85% at two years, arguably too low to prevent ICD implantation. It may be that in a lower risk population, the NPV of TWA or the combination of TWA and EP study may be sufficiently high to obviate the need for ICD implantation.

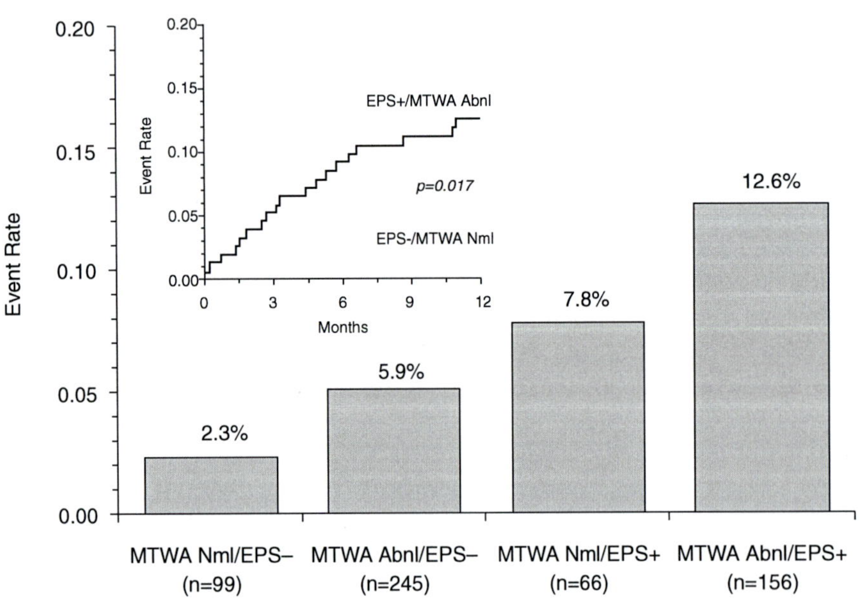

FIGURE 1.7 Combined effect of MTWA and EPS risk stratification on one-year actuarial event rates in the ABCD Trial. Patients having both normal MTWA tests and negative EPS (MTWA Nml/EPS–) exhibited lowest event rate, whereas patients having both positive EPS and abnormal MTWA tests (MTWA Abnl/EPS+) exhibited the highest event rate. Patients with discordant risk stratification testing (either MTWA Abnl/EPS– or MTWA Nml/EPS+) exhibited intermediate event rates, indicating a synergistic progression of risk with combined risk stratification. The inset compares Kaplan–Meier event rates between the groups with two negative versus two positive risk stratification tests. (Abnl, abnormal; EPS, electrophysiologic study; MTWA, microvolt T-wave alternans; Nml, normal.) (From Ref. 43, with permission.)

Conflicting data exist about the utility of TWA in patients with a LVEF ≤30% (i.e., a higher risk population than in ABCD). In a study of 177 MADIT II-like patients, Bloomfield et al. found that a negative TWA predicted lower mortality than an abnormal TWA with a hazard ratio of 4.8 over an average follow-up of 20 ± 6 months (45). The mortality rate for patients with a negative TWA test was 3.8% at two years. TWA was better than QRS duration at identifying both high- and low-risk groups for SCD. If MADIT II patients with a normal TWA did not undergo ICD implantation based on these results, the number needed to treat to save one life would fall from 18 to 7 at two years.

The Microvolt T-Wave Alternans Testing for Risk Stratification of Post-MI Patients (MASTER) trial (46) also evaluated TWA in a MADIT II-like population with contrasting results to those of the study by Bloomfield et al. MASTER enrolled 575 patients with an LVEF ≤ 30% and prior MI. Patients were classified by TWA as negative (37%) or nonnegative (63%). All patients underwent ICD implantation. The primary endpoint was arrhythmic death or ICD discharge and the secondary endpoint was total and cause-specific mortality. There was no difference in the primary endpoint between TWA-negative (10.3%) and TWA nonnegative (13.3%) patients (hazard ratio 1.26, 95% confidence interval [CI] 0.76–2.09, P = 0.37). However, total mortality was significantly lower in the TWA-negative cohort compared with the nonnegative cohort due to a decrease in noncardiac deaths. It is unclear why the nonnegative patients would have higher rates of noncardiac death, but this may possibly be due to statistical aberration or misclassification of deaths. Based on the inability of TWA to predict VT/VF in MASTER, at this point in time, patients with a prior MI and EF ≤30%, should not have ICD withheld due to a negative TWA test.

The discordant results of the various TWA trials may have to do with the risk level of the populations being studied. As per Bayes' theorem, it is more difficult to maintain a high NPV in a high-risk population. It is possible that TWA may be a more useful in intermediate risk populations. The upcoming Master II trial (47) will specifically study patients with a LVEF between 30% and 40%. It is also possible that the predictive accuracy of TWA, as with any other risk stratification tool, may be improved by combining tests in either intermediate or high-risk populations.

TWA for Risk Stratification in Patients With Nonischemic Cardiomyopathy

Risk stratification in patients with nonischemic cardiomyopathy is particularly difficult, as the utility of EP study in these patients has been shown to be limited (48). The absence of inducible monomorphic VT has not been found to be a reliable negative predictor for subsequent arrhythmic events. The presence of NSVT in addition to clinical variables is also not predictive of SCD in patients with moderate to severe HF (49). The TWA in patients with HF due to nonischemic cardiomyopathy (ALPHA) trial assessed the prognostic valued of TWA in 446 patients with nonischemic cardiomyopathy, class II and III HF, and LVEF ≤40% (50). All patients underwent TWA testing and the mean follow-up was 18 to 24months. The rates of cardiac death plus life threatening arrhythmias for TWA-abnormal and TWA-normal patients were 6.5% (95% CI 4.5–9.4%) and 1.6% (95% CI 0.6–4.4%), respectively. The adjusted hazard ratio was 3.2 (P = 0.013). Hazard ratios for secondary endpoints of total mortality and the combination of arrhythmic death or life threatening arrhythmia were 4.6 (P = 0.002) and 5.5 (P = 0.004), respectively. Thus, an abnormal TWA carried a fourfold higher risk cardiac death and life threatening arrhythmias. A negative TWA was found to have an excellent NPV in patients with nonischemic cardiomyopathy for both arrhythmic death and total mortality, suggesting that TWA may be used to identify patients who are likely to have little benefit from ICD therapy.

The ALPHA results contrast results of a SCD-HeFT substudy which investigated TWA in 490 patients with LVEF ≤35% and class II-III HF (51). In SCD-HeFT, TWA was unable to predict SCD or sustained ventricular arrhythmias. However, in SCD-HeFT the patients had a lower LVEF, a mix of ischemic and nonischemic cardiomyopathy, and a 41% indeterminate rate compared to a 20.6% rate in ALPHA, potentially lowering the predictive value of TWA.

TWA for Risk Stratification in Patients Immediately Post-MI

As demonstrated by the results of CABG-PATCH and DINAMIT, risk stratification immediately post-MI remains challenging and TWA may have a role in this setting. In a study of 1041 patients post-MI with an LVEF ≥40% (average 55 ± 10%), TWA was measured 48 ± 66 days post-MI (52). An abnormal TWA had a hazard ratio of 19.7 for subsequent SCD or life threatening arrhythmic events, but a PPV of only 9% at 32 ± 14 months. While the NPV of a normal TWA was 99.6%, as these patients were low risk to begin with given their preserved LVEF, it is unclear what additional information a normal TWA adds. Ideally a test with a higher PPV could help risk stratify post-MI patients. The Risk Estimation Following Infarction—Noninvasive Evaluation (REFINE) trial evaluated TWA along with markers of cardiac autonomic tone at different time points post-MI (53). While discussed in further detail below, the study found that a normal TWA combined with normal tests of autonomic tone had a 95% NPV for SCD at four years. However, even when both tests were abnormal and the LVEF was less than 50%, the PPV was still low at 23% at 4 years.

Conclusions Regarding TWA

To date, the most promising role of TWA appears to be in the risk stratification of patients with ischemic cardiomyopathy with a moderately reduced LVEF, especially in conjunction with another marker of risk stratification such as the EP study, as demonstrated in the ABCD trial. TWA is mainly useful for its high NPV in this population, as it is in patients with nonischemic cardiomopathy and in patients with a relatively preserved LVEF soon after a MI. Its NPV does not appear to be sufficient to withhold ICD placement in higher risk (lower LVEF) patients, and its PPV value is not sufficient in any of the studied populations to recommend ICD implantation, even when combined with other risk markers.

Signal Averaged ECG

Late potentials are low amplitude signals that occur after the end of the QRS complex. These potentials correspond to late, fragmented electrograms arising from scar and are related to the total mass of slowly activated cardiac tissue (54). Late potentials may represent a substrate for reentry which is thought to underlie most ventricular arrhythmias in patient with structural heart disease (55). These potentials are often detected during EP study and correspond to areas of delayed conduction in the myocardium which form the substrate for VT (55). By use of high-gain amplification and filtering to reduce noise, the signal averaged ECG (SAECG) averages hundreds of QRS complexes to noninvasively detect late potentials. Three parameters are usually assessed: filtered QRS duration, the duration of any low amplitude signal (LAS), and the root-mean-square voltage (RMS) in the last 40 msec of the QRS complex. The SAECG is considered to be abnormal if any two of the three parameters are abnormal. However, given the high correlation between the RMS and LAS, some data suggest that SAECG should only be considered abnormal only if the filtered QRS is prolonged, in addition to either the RMS or the LAS (56). In general, the SAECG is not useful in patients with a right or left bundle branch block (57), as the delayed potential is often obscured within the QRS instead of occurring at the end of it. SAECG is also less sensitive for arrhythmic events in the setting of an anterior MI and less specific in the setting of an inferior MI (58).

Early trials of SAECG showed that an abnormal test was associated with an increased risk of VT, SCD, and total mortality (59). SAECG had a low PPV in these trials, but a high NPV of between 81 and 89%. However, few of these patients were treated with contemporary therapy, making their relevance in current risk stratification paradigms less clear. A more recent trial of 1925 patients with ischemic cardiomyopathy and NSVT found that a filtered QRS duration >114 msec independently predicted the primary end point of arrhythmic death or cardiac arrest (58). However, the five-year rate of the primary end point was 28% versus 17% in patients with an abnormal test versus a normal test (P = 0.0001), revealing the limited PPV and NPV of SAECG to risk stratify these patients. The predictive value of the test was enhanced when it was combined with a low LVEF.

In a post-MI population of 700 patients in which 97% took beta-blockers, SAECG was found to have a low PPV of 13% but a NPV of 97% for SCD (60). However, these results were not reproduced in another trial of patients also on contemporary therapy, including statins and angiotensin-converting enzyme inhibitors, where SAECG did not predict arrhythmic events or death (61).

As with other risk stratification tests, the utility of SAECG may be enhanced by the presence of another test. In a post-MI population comparing TWA and SAECG, SAECG was more specific, but less sensitive than TWA (62). The highest positive predictive value (50%) was obtained when TWA and SAECG were combined.

SAECG was evaluated in the CABG-Patch trial, which, as discussed earlier, showed no benefit to ICD implantation at the time of CABG surgery. It is difficult to draw conclusions about the utility of SAECG from this trial, as revascularization may have reduced the risk of SCD.

In patients with nonischemic cardiomyopathy, SAECG has not been shown to be predictive of sustained VT, VF, or SCD (63).

In conclusion, the high NPV of SAECG in patients with ischemic LV dysfunction may help decide which patients do not need an ICD, but the results need to be reliably reproduced. Although the data are limited, there appears to be less of a role for SAECG in patients with nonischemic cardiomyopathy.

Measures of Autonomic Tone

Heart rate variability (HRV), heart rate turbulence (HRT), and baroreceptor reflex sensitivity (BRS) comprise the three currently used measures of autonomic tone. Autonomic tone is implicated in the pathogenesis of VT/VF, mainly as a result of enhanced sympathetic tone and diminished parasympathetic tone (64). Thus, analysis of autonomic tone may correlate with arrhythmic events or total mortality.

HRV assesses the modulation of autonomic tone on the sinus node, or simply put, the irregularity of sinus rhythm. Methods of measuring HRV fall under broad categories of being either time domain or frequency domain analyses. Time domain measurements involve statistical analyses of the variability in the R-R interval, while frequency domain measurements use spectral analysis of a series of R-R intervals to classify HRV into ultra-low frequency, very low frequency, low frequency, high frequency, and total power. One method is not better than another as there is no gold standard (65).

High frequency oscillations correspond well with vagal tone, and respiratory sinus arrhythmia is a large determinant of the high frequency component (59). Sympathetic and parasympathetic tone contribute to low frequency oscillations; the physiology underlying very low frequency and ultra-low frequency is not well understood (59).

The utility of low HRV in predicting SCD outcomes is not certain (65). In 900 patients without coronary heart disease (CHD), time domain measures of HRV were determined for all subjects with incident CHD and for all deaths that occurred (66). The study found that low HRV portended an elevated risk of CHD and death. In another study of 202 patients with moderate to severe HF (mean LVEF 24 ± 7% and HF class 2.3 ± 0.7), a diminished low frequency power obtained from an eight-minute EKG recording was associated with a threefold increase in the rate of SCD (67).

However, it may be that low HRV is a better predictor of nonarrhythmic mortality than SCD. In DINAMIT (as discussed above), low HRV was a selection criterion for trial entry (26). That the decrease in arrhythmic death was offset by the increase in nonarrhythmic death may be due to the inability of HRV to discriminate between the mode of death. HRV may have been a marker of advanced hemodynamic disease and pump failure, rather than a marker for arrhythmic death. In the ALIVE trial, a low HRV increased the risk of all-cause mortality (HR 1.46, 95% CI 1.1–1.94) but not arrhythmic mortality (68). Given these discrepant results, the role of HRV in prediction of SCD is unclear.

Baroreflex sensitivity (BRS) is a measure of the reflex bradycardia that follows an increase in systemic blood pressure. This reflex is mediated by arterial baroreceptors and may be measured after injection of phenylephrine or after spontaneous rises in blood pressure (64). Correlation between the two different tests is poor (69) and measures of baroreflex sensitivity are only moderately reproducible (70). Data on the ability of BRS to predict sudden death are conflicting. In the ATRAMI study in 1284 patients post-MI, HRV, and BRS were assessed at discharge (71). Depressed HRV and BRS carried a significant risk of cardiac mortality; when both parameters were depressed the risk increased further. Thus, ATRAMI demonstrated that since BRS adds to the prognostic value of HRV, the two measures are complimentary rather than redundant. However, in another study of 700 post-MI patients, HRV or BRS was not predictive of SCD (60). BRS also does not appear useful for risk stratification in patients with nonischemic cardiomyopathy (63).

HRT describes the change in sinus cycle length that follows a premature ventricular complex (PVC). After a PVC, there is an increase in blood pressure due to prolonged filling during the compensatory pause. Reflex parasympathetic activation occurs and the heart rate slows. HRT is measured by averaging approximately 15 to 20 beats after a PVC. Impaired HRT predicts both total mortality and SCD in post-MI patients (72,73). In an ATRAMI substudy, low HRT was associated with an approximately four-fold increase in relative risk of fatal and nonfatal cardiac arrest (73). HRT is an appealing measure as it can be performed from a small number of beats post-PVC on a 24-hour Holter monitor and does not require blood pressure monitoring like BRS.

In conclusion, it remains unclear what role HRV has in the prediction of SCD and it may be a more robust indicator of total mortality. BRS also predicts total mortality, and although the data are somewhat conflicting, there is evidence to support its ability to predict SCD in patients with CAD. HRT is a relatively new risk stratification tool which is associated with total mortality, but as with HRV and BRS its role in SCD prediction is less well-validated. For HRV, BRS, and HRT, more studies with longer follow-up and intervention trials are needed to define their role in risk stratification paradigms.

Nonsustained Ventricular Tachycardia

In the prereperfusion era, ventricular ectopy—ventricular couplets or NSVT—was associated with an increased risk of sudden death among patients with MI (74,75). In these observational studies the risk of SCD was mainly demonstrated in patients with a low LVEF, and whether NSVT was predictive of SCD independent of low LVEF is not clear. In the reperfusion era, a paucity of data exist. In the ATRAMI trial (76) NSVT, in addition to depressed BRS and HRV, was independently associated with increased mortality. The combination all three risk factors increased the risk of death 22-fold. In another trial of 700 post-MI patients, NSVT weakly predicted sudden death with a positive predictive accuracy of 12% (60). In MADIT and MUSTT, NSVT was a selection criterion for trial entry and the number needed to treat to save one life in MADIT and MUSTT was lower than that of subsequent trials that did require NSVT for trial entry (16,17,22). However, MADIT and MUSTT also used the EP study to risk-stratify patients, and similar risk reductions might have occurred if the EP study was used to risk-stratify patients who did not have NSVT as a qualifying arrhythmia. Thus one cannot infer a causal link between the presence of NSVT and the risk reductions seen in MADIT and MUSTT.

In patients with nonischemic cardiomyopathy, NSVT does not seem to be predictive of SCD. In DEFINITE (28), which used NSVT as part of the selection process, the absolute mortality reduction was 6.2%. In SCD-HeFT (29) where NSVT was not an inclusion criterion, there was a similar reduction in mortality of 7.2%, implying that NSVT does not provide additional risk stratification beyond LVEF and HF class. In the Marburg cardiomyopathy study (63) NSVT was associated with a higher risk of arrhythmia, but the trend was nonsignificant.

Therefore, in patients post-MI with ischemic cardiomyopathy, NSVT may predict SCD and total mortality; however, the incremental risk stratification in patients with LVEF ≤35% is unclear. The utility of obtaining routine Holter monitors for screening in this population is unclear and not currently recommended (77). NSVT may be more useful in patients post-MI with LVEF over the range of 35% to 40%; however, it is difficult to separate the predictive ability of NSVT versus EP study in this population. In patients with nonischemic cardiomyopathy, NSVT has not been demonstrated to reliably predict SCD.

QRS Duration

QRS duration refers to the duration of ventricular activation, and therefore, QRS prolongation reflects interventricular and/or intraventricular conduction delay or block. The prevalence of QRS prolongation in a community-based sample of HF patients was approximately 25% (78). In one study, for every 10 msec increase in QRS duration, the mortality rate increased by 10%. In a subgroup of patients with CAD and LVEF ≤30%, prolonged QRS duration remained an independent predictor of mortality (79). Furthermore, the morphology of the QRS complex appears to have relevance. In a MUSTT substudy, the presence of left bundle branch block and intraventricular conduction delay, but not right bundle branch block, was shown to increase the risk of SCD (80). While this suggests that a prolonged QRS, specifically left bundle branch block, may serve not only as a marker for advanced cardiac disease, it may play a causal role in increased mortality. As left bundle branch block results in ventricular dyssynchrony, it may also lead to depression of cardiac function (81). However, in patients who already have ICDs, QRS duration has not been shown to predict the delivery of appropriate shocks for VT/VF (82).

In patients with nonischemic cardiomyopathy, the DEFINITE trial did not show a relationship between QRS duration and all-cause mortality (28). In the Marburg Cardiomyopathy Study, neither left nor right bundle branch block predicted SCD (63). While SCD-HeFT reported a greater benefit of ICD therapy in mortality reduction in patients with a QRS >120 msec, the data include patients with both ischemic and nonischemic cardiomyopathies, and specific information in patients with just nonischemic cardiomyopathy is not available.

Thus, while QRS duration is an appealing measure for risk stratification due to its ease of use and availability, there are conflicting data that prolonged QRS duration identifies patients at higher risk for SCD with ischemic cardiomopathy, and a paucity of data to support its use in patients with nonischemic cardiomyopathy.

Genetics and Risk Stratification

Many disorders that predispose to SCD have been well characterized, such as the sodium channel gene SCN5A in the Brugada syndrome and long QT syndrome (LQT3), potassium channel mutations in the long QT syndrome, and calcium handling genes such as the ryandonine receptor (RYR2) in catecholaminergic polymorphic VT. The characterization of these disorders gives insight into the mechanisms of arrhythmias, and in some cases may be used to risk stratify patients for SCD. However, a paucity of information currently exists about the role of genetic disorders and risk of SCD in the general population. It is likely that SCD in the general population is a polygenic phenomenon. Identification of the genetic factors contributing to SCD may provide tools for risk stratification and targets for therapeutic measures.

That genetic factors contribute to SCD has been supported by population studies which show that SCD risk is often familial (83,84). In one study (83), a parental history of SCD before age 65 was associated with a 2.7-fold increased risk of SCD, after adjustment for familial aggregation of common risk factors. However, this study included SCD patients who were both ischemic and nonischemic at the time of cardiac arrest. In a complementary study, a parental history of SCD was associated with a 1.8-fold increased risk of SCD, while a parental history of MI was not associated with SCD (85). If both parents had a history of SCD, the risk of SCD in the offspring was increased nine-fold. In another study of patients with ST elevation MI, patients were grouped into those with VF arrest versus a control group with ST elevations in the absence of VF (84). A family history of SCD occurred significantly more frequently among patients with VF versus the controls without VF (43.1% versus 25.1%, respectively; OR 2.72, 95% CI 1.84–4.03).

The fact that family history of SCD may occur independently of myocardial ischemia suggests a genetic component may contribute to the ris
the risk from ischemia alone. The ris
as a greater number of relatives are
suggesting that multiple alleles for S
may play an additive or synergistic role.

Data are emerging that on the role of ion channel alleles in specific populations (86). In addition, as sympathetic activation likely influences the risk of ventricular arrhythmias, genes regulating the autonomic nervous system, coronary vasoconstriction, and the renin-angiotensin system may also play a role in SCD (87). Coagulation disorders may predispose to ventricular arrhythmias via coronary ischemia and thrombosis. Genes involved in platelet aggregation such as glycoprotein receptors have a putative role in SCD, but as of yet no definitive studies have demonstrated an association (87).

An understanding of the relationship between genotype and phenotype of the genes involved in SCD is essential. Monogenic disorders such as long QT syndrome have incomplete penetrance in family members who share the same mutation, suggesting allele-allele interactions or the influence of outside triggers (88). Neurohormonal triggers, environmental triggers, and medication interactions may all influence the severity of expression of a particular gene mutation. The eventual benefits of genetic studies of SCD include a genetic risk scoring tool to risk stratify patients, molecular therapeutic targets, and use of genetic profiling to avoid prescribing medications that may predispose to arrhythmias in a particular individual.

Magnetic Resonance Imaging (MRI) and Risk Stratification

Cardiac MRI may have a role in risk stratification for SCD due to its ability to detect myocardial scar. The use of gadolinium, which accumulates in infarcted tissue, has allowed delayed enhancement MRI to detect scar burden. Early experiments in dog models performed by coronary artery occlusion compared acute and chronic infarcts to pathologic specimens of the dog heart postmortem (89,90). Delayed enhancement MRI was remarkably accurate in imaging the infarcted tissue in comparison to the pathologic specimen. The spatial extent of hyperenhancement was the same as the spatial extent of myocyte necrosis at every stage post-MI. Reversible ischemia did not show delayed gadolinium uptake. Thus, delayed enhancement MRI can distinguish between reversible and irreversible injury, and

able and nonviable regions within the myocardium throughout infarct healing.

Whether the presence of scar and/or the amount of scar is predictive of SCD is yet to be determined. In a study of 48 patients with CAD who were referred for EP study, infarct size was compared with LVEF, with respect to their correlation with inducibility on EP study (91). They found that patients with sustained, monomorphic VT had larger infarcts than patients who did not have inducible arrhythmias, and patients with polymorphic VT or VF had intermediate infarct masses. Infarct mass and surface area were better predictors of inducibility of monomorphic VT than LVEF. The study was limited by its small sample size, but demonstrates that scar burden on MRI may correspond to inducibility on EP study. However, while inducibility on EP study is helpful in risk stratification of SCD, as discussed earlier even patients with a negative EP study have a high rate of future SCD. Thus, the true value of delayed enhancement MRI would be to demonstrate risk stratification beyond that of conventional methods.

In a study of 195 patients without known prior MI who underwent delayed enhancement MRI, investigators assessed the prognostic value of delayed enhancement compared to clinical variables (92). Delayed enhancement MRI demonstrated the strongest unadjusted associations with major adverse cardiac events and cardiac mortality (hazard ratios of 8.29 and 10.9, respectively; both *P* <0.0001). Interestingly, even patients with a small amount of scar (<2% of their myocardial mass), had more than a seven-fold increased risk for major adverse cardiac events. Further assessment of the prognostic value of infarct mass compared with LVEF in risk stratification will occur in the ongoing Defibrillators to Reduce Risk by Magnetic Resonance Imaging Evaluation (DETERMINE) study (93). In this multicenter study, patients with CAD, EF >35% (by any standard technique), and LV infarct mass >10% measured via contrast enhanced cardiac MRI will be randomized to optimal medical therapy plus an ICD versus optimal medical therapy alone.

Delayed enhancement MRI may prove to be a powerful noninvasive technique that based on quantification of scar burden can risk stratify patients for SCD and select patients who may need further therapy. Ongoing trials will clarify the role of MRI in risk stratification, and whether assessment of infarct mass will supplant LVEF as the best sole risk stratification tool.

Use of Risk Stratification Tools

The challenge underlying accurate assessment of an individual patient's risk of SCD lies in the fact that the electrical and anatomic milieu that predisposes to arrhythmias is a dynamic, not static state. For instance, a patient's risk of SCD may change as HF class or renal function changes, or if recurrent ischemic events occur. Thus, determination of a patient's long-term risk for SCD by testing at a fixed point in time may not lead to a proper assessment of true risk. The only current parameter longitudinally followed in clinical practice is the LVEF, but there may be a role for repeat testing of other parameters for risk stratification. In the MUSTT registry, the mortality curves between inducible patients and patients who were not treated with antiarrhythmic therapy start to diverge at one year (18), raising the possibility that the utility of an EP study would be enhanced if performed at more frequent intervals. Inducibility, rather than being thought of as a binary state, may be dynamic and change as a patient's underlying substrate changes. A similar rationale applies to other potential markers of SCD. The REFINE study evaluated 332 patients with EF ≤50% in the initial week post-MI (STEMI or NSTEMI) and then performed serial testing of LVEF, TWA, and HRT at 2 to 4 and 10 to 14 weeks post-MI (53). The median EF was 40% at one week and 47% at eight weeks post-MI. The authors found that no single test or combination of tests identified patients at increased risk at two weeks. However, testing at week 10 identified that patients with both an abnormal TWA and HRT along with LVEF <50%, had a relative risk of 5.2 times of SCD than that of patients without these markers. The trial suggests that immediate post-MI risk stratification by LVEF or other markers may not be helpful, as the post-MI state may subsequently improve or deteriorate, thus changing a patient's risk of SCD. In addition to demonstrating the time dependence or risk markers for SCD, the REFINE study also illustrates how the use of multiple tests for risk stratification increases the NPV. It may be that a single test will not have a sufficient negative predictive value to withhold ICD implantation, or a sufficient positive predictive value to recommend ICD implantation, but multiple tests may be predictive. Of course, the utility of a test or many tests depends on the underlying risk of the population being evaluated.

Post-MI patients with a LVEF ≤30% are high risk of SCD (9.5% at 20 months in MADIT II) and there is a need for tests with high NPV in this risk group. Patients with an LVEF of 30% to 50% are lower risk than patients with a LVEF less than 30%, but are a larger portion of the population. As such, there is a need for tests with high NPV in this population as well. Early post-MI risk stratification may be difficult given the changing arrhythmic milieu. Post-MI patients with a normal LVEF have a low overall risk of SCD EF and may not need further risk stratification.

Tests for risk stratification must be assessed for more than their ability to prognosticate SCD in observational studies (59). A particular test must demonstrate that it can be used to guide management of patients at risk for SCD. As such, the test needs to have specificity for arrhythmic death and not total mortality, given that our most powerful tool to "treat" SCD is an ICD. A test that does not distinguish between the two different modes of death may be a good overall prognosticator, but cannot guide who will benefit from SCD prophylaxis with an ICD. For instance, the EP study has been shown to guide ICD implantation in inducible patients and is predictive of arrhythmic death. This fundamental point should be taken into consideration when evaluating tests as risk stratification tools before they are adopted into clinical practice.

REFERENCES

1. American Heart Association. Heart Disease and Stroke Statistics—2008 Update. Dallas, TX: American Heart Association, 2008.
2. State specific mortality from sudden cardiac death—United States 1999. *MMWR CDC Surveill Summ* 2002; 51(6).123–6.
3. Albert CM, Chae CU, Grodstein F. Prospective study of sudden cardiac death among women in the United States. *Circulation* 2003; 107(16):2096–101.
4. Bayés de Luna A, Coumel P, Leclercq JF. Ambulatory sudden cardiac death: mechanisms of production of fatal arrhythmia on the basis of data from 157 cases. *Am Heart J* 1989; 117(1):151–9.
5. Huikuri HV, Castellanos A, Myerburg RJ. Sudden Death Due to Cardiac Arrhythmias. *N Engl J Med* 2001; 345(20):1473–82.
6. Myerburg RJ, Mitrani R, Interian A, Castellanos A. Interpretation of Outcomes of Antiarrhythmic Clinical Trials. Design Features and Population Impact. *Circulation* 1998; 97:1514–21.
7. Antiarrhythmics versus implantable defibrillators (AVID) investigators. A comparison of antiarrhythmic-drug therapy with implantable defibrillators in patients resuscitates from near-fatal ventricular arrhythmias. *N Engl J Med* 1997; 337(22):1576–83.
8. Domanski MJ, Sakseena S, Epstein AF, et al. Relative effectiveness of the implantable cardioverter-defibrillator and antiarrhythmic drugs in patients with varying degrees of left ventricular dysfunction who have survived malignant ventricular arrhythmias. AVID investigators. Antiarrhythmics Versus Implantable Defibrillators. *J Am Coll Cardiol* 1999; 34(4):1090–5.
9. Epstein AE, DiMarco JP, Ellenbogen KA, et al. ACC/AHA/HRS 2008 Guidelines for Device-Based Therapy of Cardiac Rhythm Abnormalities: a report of the American College of Cardiology/American Heart Association Task Force on Practice Guidelines (Writing Committee to Revise the ACC/AHA/NASPE 2002 Guideline Update for Implantation of Cardiac Pacemakers and Antiarrhythmia Devices) developed in collaboration with the American Association for Thoracic Surgery and Society of Thoracic Surgeons. *Circulation* 2008; 117(21):e350–408.
10. Kuck KH, Cappato R, Siebels J, Ruppel R. Randomized comparison of antiarrhythmic drug therapy with implantable defibrillators in patients resuscitated from cardiac arrest. The Cardiac Arrest Study Hamburg (CASH). *Circulation* 2000; 102(7):748–54.
11. Connolly SJ, Gent M, Roberts RS, et al. Canadian Implantable Defibrillator Study (CIDS). A randomized trail of the implantable cardioverter defibrillator against amiodarone. *Circulation* 2000; 101(11):1297–302.
12. Connolly SJ, Hallstrom AP, Cappato R, et al. Meta-analysis of the implantable cardioverter defibrillator secondary prevention trials: AVID, CIDS, CASH studies. *Eur Heart J* 2000; 21(24):2071–8.
13. Nichol G, Stiell IG, Laupacis A, Pham B, DeMaio V, Wells GA. A cumulative meta-analysis of the effectiveness of defibrillator-capable emergency medical services for victims of out-of-hospital cardiac arrest. *Ann Emerg Med* 1999; 34(4 Pt 1):517–25.
14. Tavazzi L, Volpi A. Remarks about postinfarction prognosis in light of the experience with the Gruppo Italiano per lo Studio della Sopravvivenza nell' Infarto Miocardico (GISSI) trials. *Circulation*. 1997; 95(5):1341–5.
15. Wilber DJ, Olshansky B, Moran JF, Scanlon PJ. Electrophysiological testing and nonsustained ventricular tachycardia. Use and limitations in patients with coronary artery disease and impaired ventricular function. *Circulation* 1990; 82(2).350–8.
16. Moss AJ, Hall WJ, Cannom DS, et al. Improved survival with an implanted defibrillator in patients with coronary artery disease at high risk for ventricular arrhythmia. Multicenter Automatic Defibrillator Implantation Trial (MADIT) Investigators. *N Engl J Med* 1996; 335(26):1933–40.
17. Buxton AE, Lee KL, Fisher JD, Josephson ME, Prystowsky EN, Hafley G. A randomized study of the prevention of sudden death in patients with coronary artery disease. Multicenter Unsustained Tachycardia Trial Investigators. *N Engl J Med* 1999; 341(25):1882–90.
18. Buxton AE, Kerry LL, Lorenzo D, et al. Electrophysiologic testing to identify patients with coronary artery disease who are at risk for sudden cardiac death. Multicenter Unsustained Tachycardia Trial Investigators. *N Engl J Med* 2000; 342(26):1937–45.
19. Buxton AE, Lee KL, Hafley GE, et al. Relation of ejection fraction and inducible ventricular tachycardia to mode of

death in patients with coronary artery disease: an analysis of patients enrolled in the multicenter unsustained tachycardia trial. *Circulation* 2002; 106(19):2466–72.

20. Tomaselli GF, Marbán E. Electrophysiological remodeling in hypertrophy and heart failure. *Cardiovasc Res* 1999; 42(2):270–83.
21. Nuss HB, Kääb S, Kass DA, Tomaselli GF, Marbán E. Cellular basis of ventricular arrhythmias and abnormal automaticity in heart failure. *Am J Physiol* 1999; 277(1 Pt 2):H80–91.
22. Moss AJ, Zareba W, Hall JW, et al. Prophylactic implantation of a defibrillator in patients with myocardial infarction and reduced ejection fraction. Multicenter Automatic Defibrillator Implantation Trial II Investigators. *N Engl J Med* 2002; 346(12):877–83.
23. Solomon SD, Zelenkofske S, McMurray JJV, et al. Sudden death in patients with myocardial infarction and left ventricular dysfunction, heart failure, or both. *N Engl J Med* 2005; 352(25):2581–8.
24. Pfeffer MA, McMurray JJV, Velazquez EJ, et al. Valsartan, Captopril, or Both in Myocardial Infarction Complicated by Heart Failure, Left Ventricular Dysfunction, or Both. Valsartan in Acute Myocardial Infarction Trial Investigators. *N Engl J Med* 2003; 349(20):1893–906.
25. Adabag AS, Therneau TM, Gersh BJ, Weston SA, Roger VL. Sudden death after myocardial infarction. *JAMA*. 2008; 300(17):2022–9.
26. Hohnloser SH, Kuck KH, Dorian P, et al. for the DINAMIT Investigators. Prophylactic use of an implantable cardioverter-defibrillator after acute myocardial infarction. *N Engl J Med* 2004; 351(24):2481–8.
27. Bigger JT Jr. Prophylactic use of implantable cardiac defibrillators in patients at high risk for ventricular arrhythmias after coronary-artery bypass graft surgery. Coronary Artery Bypass Graft (CABG)-Patch Trial Investigators. *N Engl J Med* 1997; 337(22):1569–75.
28. Kadish A, Dyer A, Daubert JP, et al. Prophylactic Defibrillator Implantation in Patients with Non-ischemic Dilated Cardiomyopathy. Defibrillators in Non-Ischemic Cardiomyopathy Treatment Evaluation (DEFINITE) Investigators. *N Engl J Med* 2004; 350(21):2151–8.
29. Bardy GH, Lee KL, Mark DB, et al. Amiodarone or an Implantable Cardioverter-Defibrillator for Congestive Heart Failure. Sudden Cardiac Death in Heart Failure Trial (SCD-HeFT) Investigators. *N Engl J Med* 2005; 352(3):225–37.
30. Volpi A, De Vita C, Franzosi MG, et al. Determinants of 6-month mortality in survivors of myocardial infarction after thrombolysis; results of the GISSI-2 database: the Ad hoc working froup of the Gruppo Italiano pers lo Studio della Sopravvivenza nell'Ifarcto Miocardico (GISSI)-2 Data base. *Circulation* 1993; 88(2):416–29.
31. Huikuri HV, Tapanainen JM, Lindgren K, et al. Prediction of sudden cardiac death after myocardial infarction in the beta-blocking area. *J Am Coll Cardiol* 2003; 42(4):652–8.
32. Bigger JT Jr., Fleiss JL, Kleiger R, Miller JP, Rolnitzky LM. The relationships among ventricular arrhythmias, left ventricular dysfunction, and mortality in the 2 years after myocardial infarction. *Circulation* 1984; 69(2):250–8.
33. Sanz G, Castaner A, Betriu A, et al. Determinants of prognosis in survivors of myocardial infarction: a prospective clinical angiographic study. *N Engl J Med* 1982:306(18):1065–70.
34. Daubert JP, Wojciech Z, Cannom DS, et al. Inappropriate implantable cardioverter defibrillator shocks in MADIT II. *J Am Coll Cardiol* 2008; 51(14):1357–65.
35. Singh SN, Poole J, Anderson J, et al. Role of amiodarone or implantable cardioverter/defibrillator in patients with atrial fibrillation and heart failure. *Am Heart J* 2006; 152(5):974.e7–11.
36. Kuchar DL, Thorburn CS, Sammel NL. Prediction of serious arrhythmic events after myocardial infarction: singla averaged electrocardiogram, Holter monitoring and radionuclide ventriculography. *J Am Coll Cardiol* 1987; 9(3):531–8.
37. Buxton AF, Lee KL, Hafley GE, et al. Limitations of ejection fraction for prediction of sudden death risk in patients with coronary artery disease: lessons from the MUSTT study. *J Am Coll Cardiol* 2007; 50(12):1150–7.
38. Goldenberg I, Vyas AK, Hall WJ, et al. Risk stratification for primary implantation of a cardioverter-defibrillator in patients with ischemic left ventricular dysfunction. *J Am Coll Cardiol* 2008; 51(3):288–96.
39. Narayan SM. T-wave alternans and the susceptibility to ventricular arrhythmias. *J Am Coll Cardiol* 2006; 47(2):269–81.
40. Pruvot EJ, Katra RP, Rosenbaum DS, Laurita KR. Role of calcium cycling versus restitution in the mechanism of repolarization alternans. *Circ Res* 2004; 94(8):1083–90.
41. Walker ML, Rosenbaum DS. Repolarization alternans: implications for the mechanism and prevention of sudden cardiac death. *Cardiovasc Res* 2003; 57(3):599–614.
42. Kaufman ES, Bloomfield DM, Steinman RC, et al. "Indeterminate" microvolt T-wave alternans tests predict high risk of death or sustained ventricular arrhythmias in patients with left ventricular dysfunction. *J Am Coll Cardiol* 2006; 48(7):1399–404.
43. Costantini O, Hohnloser SH, Kirk MM, et al. The ABCD (Alternans Before Cardioverter Defibrillator) Trial: Strategies Using T Wave Alternans to Improve Efficiency of Sudden Cardiac Death Prevention. *J Am Coll Cardiol* 2009; 53(6):471–9.
44. Cantillon DJ, Stein KM, Markowitz SM, et al. Predictive value of microvolt T-wave alternans in patients with left ventricular dysfunction. 2007; 50(2):166–73.
45. Bloomfield DM, Steinman RC, Nameros PB, et al. Microvolt T-wave alternans distinguishes between patients likely and patients not likely to benefit from implanted cardiac defibrillator therapy: a solution to the Multicenter Automatic Defibrillator Implantation Trial (MADIT) II conundrum. *Circulation* 2004; 110(14):1885–9.
46. Chow T, Kereiakes DJ, Onufer J, et al. Does microvolt T-wave alternans testing predict ventricular tachyarrhythmias in patients with ischemic cardiomyopathy and prophylactic defibrillators? *J Am Coll Cardiol* 2008; 52:1607–15.
47. Benditt DG, Chow T, Kereiakes DJ, et al. MASTER II - Microvolt T Wave Alternans Testing for Risk Stratification of Post MI Patients. Identifier: NCT00305214. http://clinicaltrials.gov/ct2/show/NCT00305214.
48. Brembilla-Perrot B, Donetti J, de la Chaise AT, Sadoul N, Aliot E, Juilliere Y. Diagnostic value of ventricular stimulation in patients with idiopathic dilated cardiomyopathy. *Am Heart J* 1991; 121(4 Pt 1):1124–31.
49. Teerlink JR, Jalaluddin M, Anderson S, et al. Ambulatory ventricular arrhythmias in patients with heart failure do not specifically predict an increased risk of sudden death. PROMISE

(Prospective Randomized Milrinone Survival Evaluation) Investigators. *Circulation* 2000; 101(1):40–6.

50. Salerno-Uriarte JA, De Ferrari GM, Klersy C, et al. Prognostic value of T-wave alternans in patients with heart failure due to nonischemic cardiomyopathy. ALPHA Study Group Investigators. *J Am Coll Cardiol* 2007; 50(19):1896–904.
51. Gold MR, Ip JH, Costantini O, Poole JE, et al. Role of microvolt T-wave alternans in assessment of arrhythmia vulnerability among patients with heart failure and systolic dysfunction: Primary results from the T-wave alternans Sudden Cardiac Death in Heart Failure Trial substudy. *Circulation* 2008; 118:2022–8.
52. Ikeda T, Yoshino H, Sugi K, et al. Predictive value of microvolt T-wave alternans for sudden cardiac death in patients with preserved cardiac function after acute myocardial infarction. *J Am Coll Cardiol*, 2006; 48(11):2268–74.
53. Exner DV, Kavanagh KM, Slaynych MP, et al. Noninvasive risk assessment early after a myocardial infarction: The REFINE study. *J Am Coll Cardiol* 2007; 50(24):2275–84.
54. De Bakker JM, van Capelle FJ, Janse MJ, et al. Reentry as a cause of ventricular tachycardia in patients with chronic ischemic heart disease: electrophysiologic and anatomic correlation. *Circulation* 1988; 77(3):589–606.
55. Simson MB, Untereker WJ, Spielman SR, et al. Relation between late potentials on the body surface and directly recorded fragmented electrograms in patients with ventricular tachycardia. *Am J Cardiol* 1983; 51(1):105–12.
56. Okin PM, Stein KM, Lippman N, Lerman BB, Kligfield P. Performance of the signal-averaged electrocardiogram: relationship to baseline QRS duration. *Am Heart J* 1995; 129(5):932–40.
57. Buckingham TA, Thessen CC, Stevens LL, Redd RM, Kennedy HL. Effect of conduction defects on the signal-averaged electrocardiographic determination of late potentials. *Am J Cardiol* 1988; 61(15):1265–71.
58. Gomes JA, Cain ME, Buxton AE, Josephson ME, Lee KL, Hafley GE. Prediction of long-term outcomes by signal-averaged electrocardiography in patients with unsustained ventricular tachycardia, coronary artery disease, and left ventricular dysfunction. *Circulation* 2001; 104(4):436–41.
59. Stein, KM. Noninvasive Risk Stratification for Sudden Death: Signal-Averaged Electrocardiography, Nosustained Ventricular Tachycardia, Heart Rate Variability, Baroreflex Sensitivity, and QRS Duration. *Prog Cardiovasc Dis* 2008, 51(2).106–17.
60. Huikuri HV, Tapanainen JM, Lindgren K, et al. Prediction of sudden cardiac death after myocardial infarction in the beta-blocking era. *J Am Coll Cardiol* 2003; 42(4):652–8.
61. Bauer A, Guznik P, Barthel P, et al. Reduced prognostic power of ventricular late potentials in post-infarction patients of the reperfusion era. *Eur Heart J* 2005; 26(8):747–8.
62. Ikeda T, Sakata T, Takami M, et al. Combined assessment of T-wave alternans and late potentials used to predict arrhythmic events after myocardial infarction. A prospective study. *J Am Coll Cardiol* 2000; 35(3):722–30.
63. Grimm W, Christ M, Bach J, Müller HH, Maisch B. Noninvasive arrhythmia risk stratification in idiopathic dilated cardiomyopathy: results of the Marburg Cardiomyopathy Study. *Circulation* 2003; 108(23):2883–91.
64. Goldberger JJ, Cain ME, Hohnloser SH, et al. American Heart Association/American College of Cardiology Foundation/Heart Rhythm Society scientific statement on noninvasive risk stratification techniques for identifying patients at risk for sudden cardiac death: a scientific statement from the American Heart Association Council on Clinical Cardiology Committee on Electrocardiography and Arrhythmias and Council on Epidemiology and Prevention. *Circulation* 2008; 118(14):1497–518.
65. Lahiri MK, Kannankeril PJ, Goldberger JJ. Assessment of autonomic function in cardiovascular disease. Physiological basis and prognostic implications. *J Am Coll Cardiol* 2008; 51(18):1725–33.
66. Dekker JM, Crow RS, Folsom AR, et al. Low heart rate variability in a 2-minute rhythm strip predicts risk of coronary heart disease and mortality from several causes: the ARIC study. Atherosclerosis Risk In Communities. *Circulation* 2000; 102(11):113–20.
67. La Rovere MT, Pinna GD, Maestri R. Short-term heart rate variability strongly predicts sudden cardiac death in chronic heart failure patients. *Circulation* 2003; 107(4):565–70.
68. Camm AJ, Pratt CM, Schwartz PJ, et al. Mortality in patients after a recent myocardial infarction: a randomized, placebo-controlled trial of azimilide using heart rate variability for risk stratification. AzimiLide post Infarct surVival Evaluation (ALIVE) Investigators. *Circulation* 2004; 109(8):990–6.
69. Maestri R, Pinna GD, Mortara A, La Rovere MT, Tavazzi L. Assessing baroreflex sensitivity in post-myocardial infarction patients: comparison of spectral and phenylephrine techniques. *J Am Coll Cardiol* 1998; 31(2):344–351.
70. Eckberg DL, Sleight P. *Human Baroreflexes in Health and Disease.* Oxford, UK: Clarendon Press, 1992.
71. La Rovere MT, Bigger JT Jr, Marcus FI, Mortara A, Schwartz PJ. Baroreflex sensitivity and heart-rate variability in prediction of total cardiac mortality after myocardial infarction. ATRAMI (Autonomic tone and reflexes after myocardial infarction) investigators. *Lancet* 1998; 351(9101):478–84.
72. Barthel P, Schneider R, Bauer A, et al. Risk stratification after acute myocardial infarction by heart rate turbulence. *Circulation* 2003; 108; (10):1221–6.
73. Ghuran A, Reid F, La Rovere MT, et al. Heart rate turbulence-based predictors of fatal and nonfatal cardiac arrest (the Autonomic Tone and Reflexes After Myocardial Infarction Substudy). *Am J Cardiol* 2002; 89(2):184–90.
74. Ruberman W, Weinblatt E, Goldberg JD, Frank CW, Chaudhary BS, Shapiro S. Ventricular premature complexes and sudden death after myocardial infarction. *Circulation* 1981; 64(2):297–305.
75. Taylor GJ, Humphries JO, Mellits EF, et al. Predictors of clinical course, coronary anatomy and left ventricular function after recovery from acute myocardial infarction. *Circulation* 1980; 62(5):960–70.
76. La Rovere MT, Pinna GD, Hohnloser SH. Baroreflex sensitivity and heart rate variability in the identification of patients at risk for life-threatening arrhythmias: implications for clinical trials. *Circulation* 2001; 103(16):2072–7.
77. Crawford MH, Bernstein SJ, Deedwania PC, et al. ACC/AHA Guidelines for Ambulatory Electrocardiography. A report of the American College of Cardiology/American Heart Association Task Force on Practice Guidelines (Committee to Revise the Guidelines for Ambulatory Electrocardiography). Developed in collaboration with the North American Society for Pacing and Electrophysiology. *J Am Coll Cardiol* 1999; 34(3):912–48.

78. Sandhu R, Bahler RC. Prevalence of QRS prolongation in a community hospital cohort of patients with heart failure and its relation to left ventricular systolic dysfunction. *Am J Cardiol* 2004; 93(2):244–6.

79. Kalahasti V, Nambi V, Martin DO, et al. QRS duration and prediction of mortality in patients undergoing risk stratification for ventricular arrhythmias. *Am J Cardiol* 2003; 92(7):798–803.

80. Zimetbaum PJ, Buxton AE, Batsford W, et al. Electrocardiographic predictors of arrhythmic death and total mortality in the multicenter unsustained tachycardia trial. *Circulation* 2004; 110(7):766–9.

81. Park RC, Little WC, O'Rourke RA. Effect of alternation of left ventricular activation sequence on the left ventricular end-systolic pressure-volume relation in closed-chest dogs. *Circ Res* 1985; 57(5):706–17.

82. Buxton AE, Sweeney MO, Wathen MS, et al. QRS duration does not predict occurrence of ventricular tachyarrhythmias in patients with implanted cardioverter-defibrillators. PainFREE Rx II Investigators. *J Am Coll Cardiol* 2005; 46(2):310–6.

83. Friedlander Y, Siscovick DS, Weinmann S, et al. Family history as a risk factor for primary cardiac arrest. *Circulation* 1998; (2):97:155–60.

84. Jouven X, Desnos M, Guerot C, Ducimetière P. Predicting sudden death in the population: the Paris Prospective Study I. *Circulation* 99(15):1978–83.

85. Dekker LR, Bezzina CR, Henriques JP, et al. Familial sudden death is an important risk factor for primary ventricular fibrillation: a case-control study in acute myocardial infarction patients. *Circulation* 2006; 114(11):1140–5.

86. Burke A, Creighton W, Mont E, et al. Role of SCN5A Y1102 polymorphism in sudden cardiac death in blacks. *Circulation* 2005; 112(6):798–802.

87. Prutkin JM, Sotoodehnia N. Genetics of Sudden Cardiac Arrest. *Prog Cardiovasc Dis* 2008; 50(6):390–403.

88. Priori SG, Napolitano C, Schwartz PJ. Low penetrance in the long-QT syndrome: clinical impact. *Circulation* 1999; 99(4):529–33.

89. Kim RJ, Fieno DS, Parrish TB, et al. Relationship of MRI delayed contrast enhancement to irreversible injury, infarct age, and contractile function. *Circulation* 1999; 100(19):1992–2002.

90. Fieno DS, Kim RJ, Chen EL, Lomasney JW, Klocke FJ, Judd RM. Contrast-enhanced magnetic resonance imaging of myocardium at risk: distinction between reversible and irreversible injury throughout infarct healing. *J Am Coll Cardiol* 2000; 36(6):1985–91.

91. Bello D, Fieno DS, Kim RJ, et al. Infarct morphology identifies patients with substrate for sustained ventricular tachycardia. *J Am Coll Cardiol* 2005; 45(7):1104–08.

92. Kwong RY, Chan AK, Brown KA, et al. Impact of unrecognized myocardial scar detected by cardiac magnetic resonance imaging on event-free survival in patients presenting with signs or symptoms of coronary artery disease. *Circulation* 2006; 113(23):2733–43.

93. Kadish, Alan. Defibrillators To Reduce Risk by Magnetic Resonance Imaging Evaluation (DETERMINE). Identifier: NCT00487279. http://clinicaltrials.gov/ct2/show/NCT00487279.

2 Management of Acute Coronary Syndromes

LUKE K. KIM
DMITRIY N. FELDMAN

OUTLINE

Acute coronary syndromes (ACS) encompass a wide spectrum of coronary artery disease from unstable angina (UA) to myocardial infarction (MI). According to the 2007 report from the American Heart Associations and Stroke Statistics Committee, about 700,000 Americans are expected to suffer from their first MI yearly, with almost 500,000 recurrent MIs occurring annually (1). Coronary heart disease (CHD) is responsible for about one out of every five deaths in the United States; ACS is the cause of over 1.5 million hospitalizations yearly and therefore plays a significant role in the cost of our health care.

Different mechanisms have been proposed for ACS including thrombus formation at a site of preexisting plaque rupture, dynamic obstruction, progressive mechanical obstruction, inflammation and increased myocardial oxygen demand (2). The diagnosis of ACS has been classified based on the underlying pathophysiology of the process, findings from the electrocardiogram (ECG) and cardiac biomarkers (Figure 2.1). Complete vessel occlusion from a plaque rupture and subsequent thrombus formation commonly results in a ST-elevation MI (STEMI) presentation. Other mechanisms can trigger a non-ST-elevation ACS presentation by causing cardiac ischemia without complete occlusion of the culprit artery. UA is distinguished from a non-ST-elevation MI (NSTEMI) by a lack of elevation in cardiac enzymes (CK, CK-MB, troponin I, or T) despite the presence of ischemic symptoms and/or ECG changes suggestive of ACS.

On the basis of clinical data early in the presentation, it is important to risk stratify patients into groups at high, intermediate, and low risk for complications (Table 2.1). The investigators from the Thrombolysis in Myocardial Infarction 11B (TIMI 11B) (3) and the Efficacy and Safety of Subcutaneous Enoxaparin in Non–Q-wave Coronary Events (ESSENCE) (4) trials suggested a scoring system with seven variables found to be independently predictive of short-term outcomes in patients with non-ST-elevation ACS. This scoring system (TIMI risk score) was developed to help with risk stratification in patients presenting with non-ST-elevation ACS. The variables include age ≥65 years, presence of at least three risk factors for CHD, prior coronary stenosis of ≥50%, presence of ST-segment deviation on admission ECG, at least two anginal episodes in the last 24 hours, elevated serum cardiac biomarkers, and the use of aspirin in the last seven

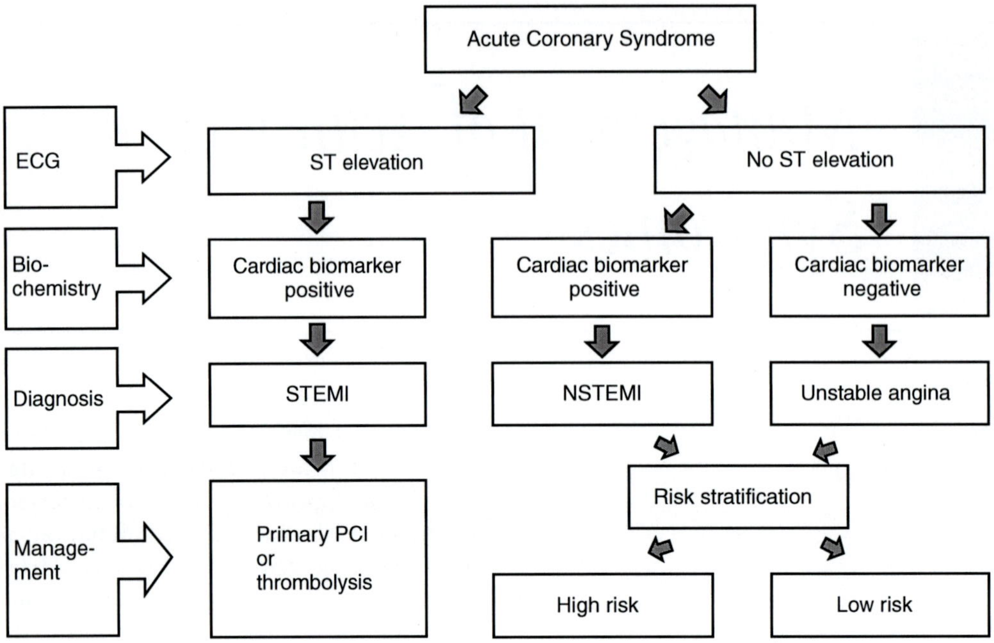

FIGURE 2.1 Algorithm for risk stratification and treatment of patients with acute coronary syndromes. (STEMI, ST-elevation myocardial infarction; NSTEMI, non-STEMI.)

days. The TIMI risk score has been found to be a useful tool for risk stratification and patient management in multiple trials. For instance, in the Treat Angina with Aggrastat and Determine Cost of Therapy with an Invasive or Conservative Strategy-Thrombolysis in Myocardial Infarction 18 (TACTICS-TIMI 18) trial, the high-risk patients with TIMI score ≥3 were identified and shown to benefit from an early invasive strategy in non-ST-elevation ACS as opposed to low-risk patients (5).

A slightly different scoring system (STEMI TIMI risk score) has been developed for patients presenting with STEMI (6). The TIMI risk score for STEMI patients is an arithmetic sum of eight variables with different number of points given for each variable. The variables include age, history of diabetes, hypertension or angina, systolic blood pressure <100 mm Hg, heart rate >100 bpm, Killip class II–IV, weight <76 kg, anterior ST elevation (or left bundle branch block), and time to reperfusion therapy >4 hours. A high TIMI risk score has been shown to be predictive of increased in-hospital mortality.

ACS carries a potentially grave prognosis if not treated promptly, particularly in patients with high-risk features mentioned above. Various medical and interventional therapies have been investigated in order to effectively treat the mechanisms underlying ACS. Treatment of STEMI patients requires an urgent reperfusion strategy with either thrombolysis or primary Percutaneous coronary intervention (PCI). Treatment of non-ST-elevation ACS patients may be less urgent, and the choice of invasive versus conservative strategy is made based on the risk stratification of ACS patients (Figures 2.2 and 2.3). There has been a significant progress in both medical and interventional treatments of ACS in the last few decades with marked improvement in both short- and long-term outcomes in patients presenting with ACS.

■ BETA-BLOCKERS

Beta-blockers inhibit beta-1 adrenergic receptors, primarily localized in the myocardial cells, causing a decrease in myocardial contractility. This, in turn, reduces oxygen demand by the myocardium and results in a decrease in myocardial ischemia. In addition, beta-blockers prolong diastole by slowing the heart rate and, consequently,

Table 2.1 American College of Cardiology/American Heart Association system for risk stratification of patients with non-ST-elevation acute coronary syndromes

	Risk		
Feature	**High Risk** *more than one of the features below*	**Intermediate Risk** *No high-risk features but must have one of the following*	**Low Risk** *No high- or intermediate-risk feature but may have any of the following*
History	Accelerating tempo of ischemic symptoms in preceeding 48 hours	Prior MI peripheral or cerebrovascular disease, or CABG, prior aspirin use	
Character of pain	Prolonged ongoing (>20 min) rest pain	Prolonged ongoing (>20 min) rest angina, now resolved with moderate/high likelihood of CAD Rest angina (>20 min) or relieved with rest or sublingual NTG Nocturnal angina New onset/progressive CCS class III/IV angina in the past 2 weeks without prolonged rest pain, but with moderate or high likelihood of CAD	Increased angina frequency, severity, duration Angina provoked at a lower threshold New onset angina with onset 2 weeks to 2 months prior to presentation
Clinical findings	Pulmonary edema, most likely due to ischemia New or worsening MR murmur S_3 or new/worsening rales Hypotension, bradycardia, tachycardia Age >75 years	Age >70 years	
Electrocardiogram	Angina at rest with transient ST-segment changes >0.5 mm Bundle-branch block, new or presumed new Sustained ventricular tachycardia	T-wave changes Pathological Q waves or resting ST-depression less than 1 mm in multiple lead groups	Normal or unchanged ECG
Cardiac biomarkers	Elevated cardiac TnT, Tnl, or CK-MB (e.g., TnT or Tnl, greater than 0.1 ng per ml)	Slightly elevated cardiac TnT, Tnl, or CK-MB (e.g., TnT greater than 0.01 but less than 0.1 ng per ml)	Normal

Source: From Ref. 18, with permission.
CABG, coronary artery bypass; MI, myocardial infarction; CAD, coronary artery disease; NTG, nitroglycerin; CCS, Canadian cardiovascular study; ECG, electrocardiogram.

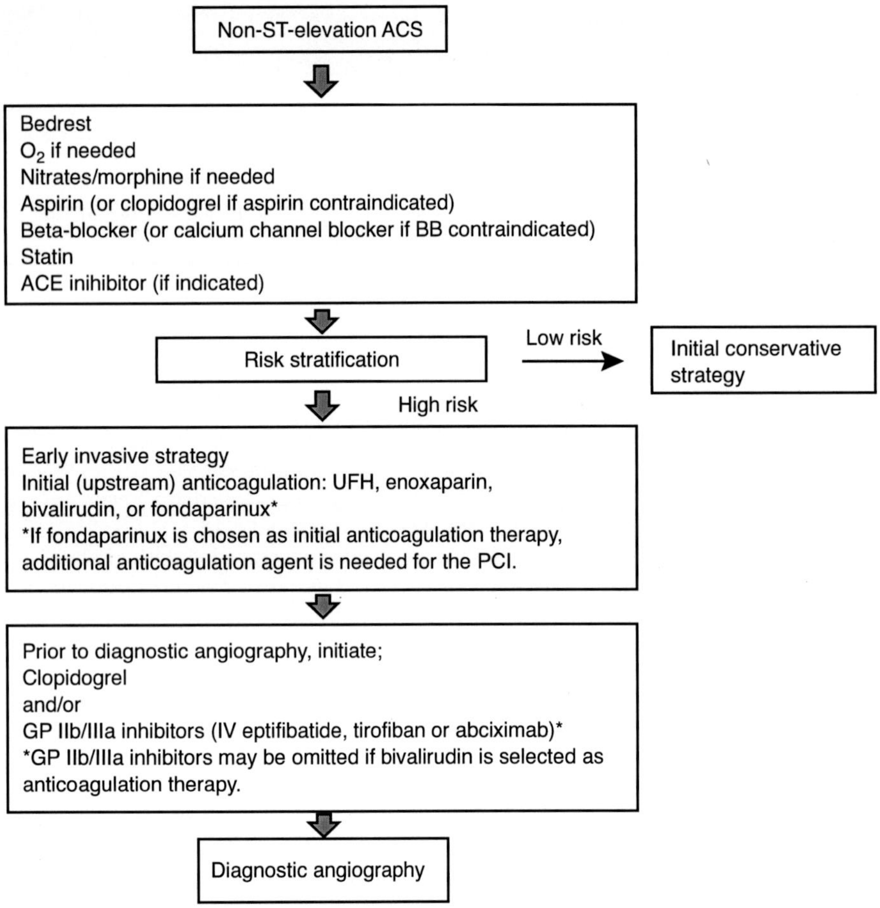

FIGURE 2.2 Algorithm for patients with non-ST-elevation acute coronary syndrome managed by an early invasive strategy. (ACS, acute coronary syndrome; UFH, unfractionated heparin; PCI, percutaneous coronary intervention.)

cause an increase in coronary blood flow. Several early trials have shown a benefit of beta-blockers in reducing ischemia and improving prognosis in ACS (7–9). A meta-analysis of patients with UA revealed a 13% reduction in the risk of MI after treatment with beta-blockers (8,9). Furthermore, in patients presenting with MI, a clear association between beta-blockers and a reduction in reinfarction and mortality was observed with timolol, propranolol and metoprolol (10–12). Since the earlier trials, more definitive data supporting the role of beta-blockers in a subset of patients with NSTEMI have been published (13–16). Most notably, the First International Study of Infarct Survival (ISIS-1), a landmark trial, which enrolled 16,027 patients with suspected MI, demonstrated a reduction in subsequent reinfarction and mortality with the use of intravenous beta-blockers followed by oral atenolol (13). The Clopidogrel and Metoprolol in Myocardial Infarction Trial (COMMIT) applied the same principle in 45,852 patients presenting with STEMI (17). This landmark trial revealed that the use of early beta-blocker therapy in STEMI reduces the risks of reinfarction and ventricular fibrillation. However, there was a small increase in frequency of cardiogenic shock in patients randomized to the beta-blocker group. Therefore, beta-blockers should be contraindicated in patients presenting with a cardiogenic shock or decompensated congestive heart failure (CHF). Other relative contraindications to beta-blockers include advanced heart block, bradyarrythmias, and active asthma. Unless these contraindications are present, the (ACC/AHA) guidelines list oral beta-blocker therapy within 24 hours as a class I indication in patients with ACS (18). In patients presenting with left ventricular dysfunction after MI as defined by an ejection fraction ≤40%, carvedilol has been shown to reduce reinfarction rate and mortality in the Carvedilol Post Infarction Survival Control in Left Ventricular Dysfunction (CAPRICORN) trial when compared with placebo (19).

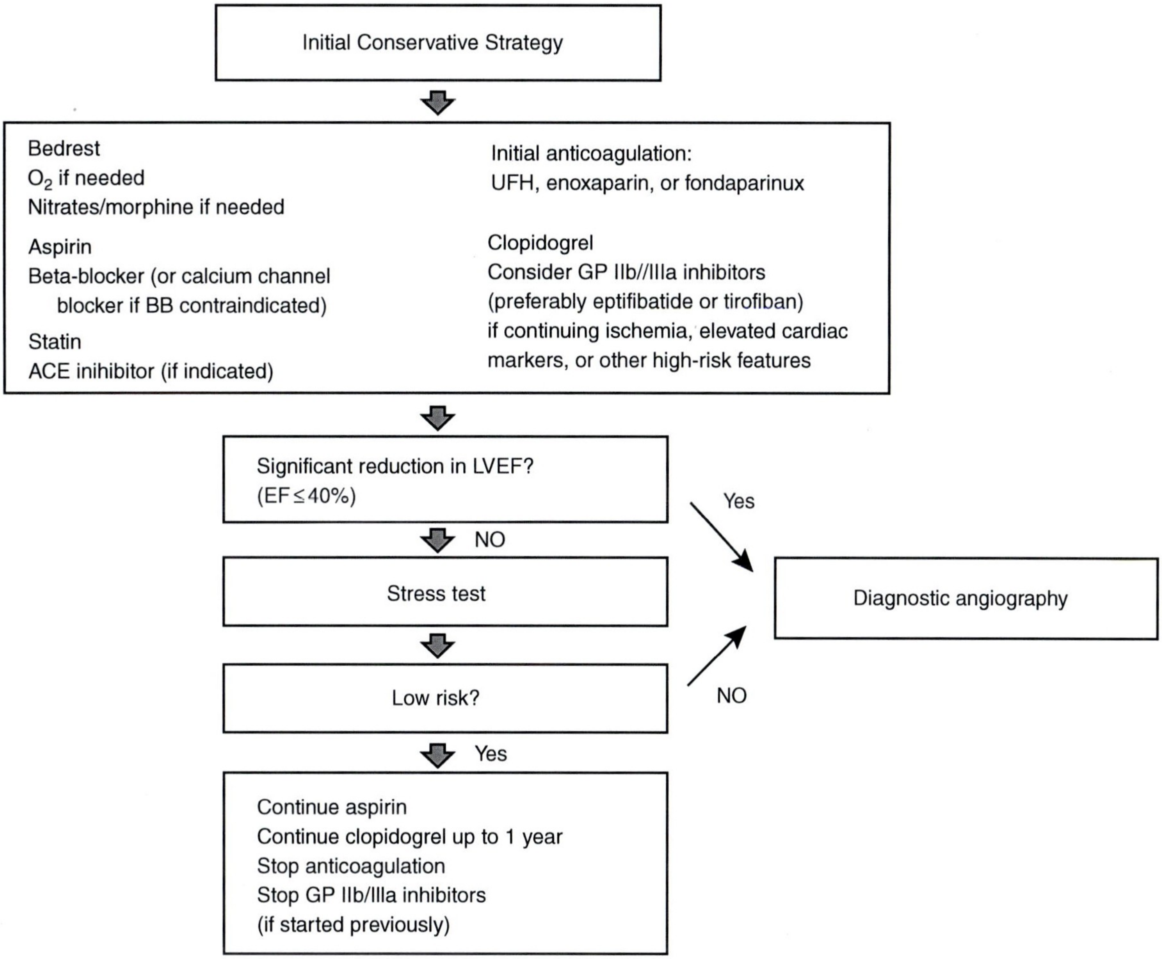

FIGURE 2.3 Algorithm for patients with non-ST-elevation acute coronary syndrome managed by an initial conservative strategy. (UFH, unfractionated heparin; LVEF, left ventricular ejection fraction.)

ANGIOTENSIN-CONVERTING ENZYME (ACE) INHIBITORS

ACE inhibitors attenuate ventricular remodeling and progression of regional myocardial dysfunction after MI. Several trials have attempted to confirm this benefit in a diverse spectrum of ACS patients. In the *Gruppo Italiano per lo Studio della Streptochi-nasi nell'Infarto Miocardico-3* (GISSI-3) trial, lisinopril started within 24 hours of acute MI resulted in a reduction in mortality (by 11%) and combined endpoint of mortality and left ventricular dysfunction (20). Similar benefit was observed in both the ISIS-4 and the Chinese Cardiac Study (CCS-1) (21,22). Importantly, patients with left ventricular dysfunction appeared to derive the greatest mortality benefit in these trials. In fact, the Cooperative New Scandinavian Enalapril Survival Study II (CONSENSUS II) demonstrated that early administration of intravenous enalapril did not result in an improved survival, but resulted in more hypotension when all patients were given an ACE inhibitor after MI (23). Therefore, later trials concentrated on identifying the group of patients that would benefit from ACE inhibitors. The Survival and Ventricular Enlargement (SAVE) trial randomized 2,231 patients presenting with MI with left ventricular ejection fraction ≤40% without overt CHF to captopril or placebo (24). All-cause mortality was reduced by 19% in addition to a significant reduction in CHF and recurrent MI. Even in patients with evidence of heart failure early after MI, ACE inhibitors reduced mortality by approximately 25%, along with a reduction of

esistant heart failure (25,26). In fact, f the SAVE trial, the Acute Infarction Study (AIRE) and the Trandolapril Evaluation study (TRACE) demonstrated both short- and long-term benefits in terms of reducing mortality, heart failure and reinfarctions. Therefore, the ACC/AHA guidelines categorize ACE inhibitors as a class I indication within the first 24 hours and recommend to be continued indefinitely for patients recovering from ACS with an ejection fraction ≤40% unless contraindicated (18). Due to the apparent benefits of ACE inhibitors in high-risk patients (27), the ACC/AHA guidelines also suggest ACE inhibitors as a class IIa indication even in the absence of left ventricular dysfunction in ACS.

■ ANGIOTENSIN II RECEPTOR BLOCKERS

Angiotensin II receptor blockers (ARBs) inhibit binding of angiotensin II to angiotensin 1 (AT1) receptor rather than preventing production of angiotensin II. This difference in mechanism from ACE inhibitors allows an inhibition of the renin-angiotensin system without affecting kinin metabolism. Therefore, ARBs have a minimally better side effect profile while still playing a significant role in attenuating myocardial remodeling. A few trials have demonstrated the benefit of ARBs in patients with left ventricular dysfunction after MI. In the Valsartan in Acute Myocardial Infarction (VALIANT) trial, 14,703 patients were enrolled and randomized to valsartan monotherapy, captopril monotherapy, or valsartan/captopril dual therapy (28). This trial demonstrated that in patients with MI complicated by CHF, left ventricular dysfunction or both, ARBs were not inferior to ACE inhibitors in terms of effects on mortality, heart failure and reinfarction. However, the combination therapy of ARB and ACE inhibitors resulted in more frequent adverse events without any improvement in cardiovascular outcomes. Currently, the ACC/AHA guidelines suggest ARBs as a class I indication in those with left ventricular dysfunction and CHF, but intolerant to ACE inhibitors (18). However, a combination therapy of ACE inhibitors and ARBs is classified as a class IIb recommendation due to the lack of clear additive benefit.

■ ALDOSTERONE ANTAGONISTS

Aldosterone antagonists act by binding mineralocorticoid receptors and function as potassium sparing diuretics. Aldosterone activates renin-angiotensin system in heart failure model along with promoting cardiac hypertrophy and fibrosis. Although the role of aldosterone antagonists in heart failure management has been well-established (29), clinical application in MI was not demonstrated until the Eplerenone Post-AMI Heart Failure Efficacy and Survival Study (EPHESUS) (30). In this trial, 6,632 patients with acute MI and left ventricular ejection fraction ≤40% were randomized to eplerenone, a selective aldosterone antagonist, versus placebo. Eplerenone use was associated with a reduction in all-cause mortality and the composite end point of death or hospitalization from cardiovascular causes. It is important to note that the majority of patients in this trial were already receiving optimal medical therapy in addition to eplerenone. According to the ACC/AHA guidelines, aldosterone receptor blockade should be prescribed for ACS patients without significant renal dysfunction or hyperkalemia who are already receiving therapeutic doses of a beta-blocker and ACE inhibitor, have an ejection fraction ≤40%, and have either symptomatic heart failure or diabetes mellitus (18).

■ STATINS

Statins are competitive inhibitors of Hydroxymethylglutaryl-COA (HMG-CoA)reductase enzyme responsible for cholesterol biosynthesis. In addition to their lipid lowering effect, statins have pleiotropic effects in CAD including plaque stabilization, reduction of inflammation, decreased thrombogenicity, and reversal of endothelial dysfunction among others. Several landmark trials have addressed the role of statins in secondary prevention of coronary events. The Scandinavian Simvastatin Survival Study (4S) enrolled 4,444 patients with angina or prior history of MI and average low density lipoprotein-cholesterol (LDL-C) of 188 mg/dL (31). By five years of follow-up, patients randomized to simvastatin had a 35% reduction in LDL-C along with a 30% relative reduction in overall mortality, a 39% reduction in nonfatal MIs, and a 34% reduction in revascularization procedures. Subsequent trials, the Cholesterol and Recurrent Events Trial (CARE) and the

Long-Term Intervention with Pravastatin in Ischaemic Disease Study (LIPID), confirmed a treatment benefit in post-MI patients with only moderately elevated LDL-C (32,33). With the role of the statins in secondary prevention well accepted, recent trials have sought to identify the benefit of statins in early stages of ACS. In the Myocardial Ischemia Reduction with Aggressive Cholesterol Lowering (MIRACL) trial, 3,086 patients were randomized to a high-dose atorvastatin or placebo in the early phase of ACS (34). Lipid-lowering therapy with 80 mg of atorvastatin reduced recurrent ischemic events in the first 16 weeks, with most benefit from a reduction in symptomatic ischemia requiring hospitalization. Since a high-dose atorvastatin was not compared to a low-dose of statin in this trial, the Pravastatin or Atorvastatin Evaluation and Infection Therapy trial (PROVE IT-TIMI 22) attempted to determine whether this was a truly dose-dependent effect by randomizing patients to a high-dose of atorvastatin versus a standard-dose of pravastatin (35). LDL cholesterol level was reduced from 106 mg/dL at baseline in each group to 95 mg/dL in the standard-dose pravastatin group and to 62 mg/dL in the high-dose atorvastatin group. Primary composite endpoint of all-cause mortality, MI, documented UA, revascularization, and stroke were reduced by 16% at two years. Based on these recent findings, National Cholesterol Education Program (NCEP) of the National Heart, Lung and Blood Institute proposed modifications to the ATP III guidelines suggesting an optional goal LDL-C <70 mg/dL for very high-risk patients, including all patients presenting with ACS (36). The 2007 ACC/AHA guidelines have adopted these modifications and recommended statins regardless of baseline LDL-C and diet modification for UA/NSTEMI patients (18). In addition, it is a class I indication for UA/NSTEMI patients to have a target LDL-C goal <100 mg/dL, with an optional goal <70 mg/dL for high-risk patients.

■ NITRATES

Nitrates reduce ischemia and improve coronary flow through vasodilation of the coronary arteries. In addition, myocardial oxygen demand is reduced by venodilation, which results in a decreased preload to the left ventricle. Although, nitrates are very effective at reducing angina and ischemic symptoms, large clinical trials have failed to demonstrate any improvement in survival (20,21). Certain contraindications to nitrates exist including right ventricular infarction, critical aortic stenosis, hypertrophic cardiomyopathy, and recent use of sildenafil. In the absence of such contraindications, the ACC/AHA guidelines suggest that patients with ACS with ongoing ischemic pain should receive sublingual nitroglycerin followed by intravenous nitroglycerin for treatment of persistent ischemia, heart failure, or hypertension. The use of nitroglycerin should not preclude therapy with other proven mortality-reducing interventions such as beta-blockers or ACE inhibitors.

■ CALCIUM CHANNEL BLOCKERS

Calcium channel blockers inhibit the influx of calcium into myocytes and vascular smooth muscle cells. Blockade of calcium flux leads to vasodilation, negative inotropy, and negative chronotropy. Dihydropyridines, such as nifedipine and amlodipine, have a greater selectivity for vascular smooth muscle cells compared with myocardium, and thereby produce a potent peripheral vasodilator effect. Early trials failed to demonstrate beneficial effects of nifedipine in patients with ACS (37,38). In fact, short-acting nifedipine was associated with an increased mortality in early phase of MI (39,40). Such increased mortality was thought to be secondary to episodes of hypotension and reflex sympathetic activation. Therefore, short-acting dihydropyridines are no longer recommended in ACS. On the other hand, nondihydropydines have been shown to have a potential role in patients with contraindications to beta-blockers (41). In the Diltiazem Reinfarction Study, patients receving diltiazem had a reduction in frequency of recurrent MI from 9.3% to 5.2% by 14 days after NSTEMI along with a 50% reduction in frequency of refractory angina (42). Furthermore, the Multicenter Diltiazem Postinfarction Trial (MDPIT) demonstrated a benefit of reducing recurrent cardiac events in patients receiving diltiazem after MI albeit not statistically significant (43). However, in patients with left ventricular ejection fraction ≤40%, diltiazem was associated with a higher frequency of CHF. The role of diltiazem was further investigated in the Incomplete Infarction Trial of European Research Collaborators Evaluating Prognosis post-Thrombolysis (INTERCEPT), which attempted to examine the use of diltiazem in patients with STEMI receiving thrombolysis (44). In contrast to previous studies, this trial did not demonstrate any significant reduction in the primary combined end point of cardiac death, nonfatal reinfarction, and refractory ischemia. The role of verapamil in ACS has been examined in several trials as well. In the Danish Verapamil Infarction Trial II (DAVIT II), patients treated with verapamil post-MI experienced a 17% lower incidence of death and reinfarction in the subset of patients without CHF (45). Given the above findings, the ACC/AHA guidelines recommend the use of nondihydropyridine calcium channel blockers only in ACS patients with continuing or recurring ischemia but who have preserved left ventricular function, in whom beta-blockers are contraindicated (18).

■ ANTIPLATELET AGENTS

Aspirin

Aspirin has been extensively studied in coronary artery disease. Aspirin causes an irreversible inactivation of the cyclooxygenase-1 enzyme required for the prostaglandin and thromboxane synthesis, which in turn diminishes platelet aggregation. It has been postulated that higher dose of aspirin can inhibit endothelial cell synthesis of prostacyclin responsible for vasodilation and inhibition of platelet aggregation. However, clinical relevance of this dose-dependent mechanism has never been demonstrated. One of the earlier trials, VA Cooperative Study, demonstrated that there was a 51% reduction in incidence of death or acute MI in patients who received aspirin for UA (46). Furthermore, the rate of nonfatal MI was reduced by approximately 50% in the aspirin group as well. The above findings were reproduced in later trials, and they clearly established the role of aspirin in UA (47,48). The Research on Instability in Coronary Artery Disease trial (RISC) tested the role of aspirin in NSTEMI/UA patients and demonstrated that aspirin was associated with a significant reduction in the combined endpoint of death and MI (49). This benefit persisted beyond one year, providing evidence for long-term benefit of aspirin in ACS. As the role of aspirin became essential in non-ST-elevation ACS, ISIS-2 was one of the landmark trials that attempted to expand the role of aspirin to STEMI (50). ISIS-2 randomized 17,187 patients presenting with acute STEMI to streptokinase, aspirin, both therapies, or neither, and demonstrated an additive effect of aspirin to thrombolytic therapy. Therefore, the ACC/AHA guidelines recommend addition of aspirin to all patients who present with ACS as soon as possible and for indefinite duration, except for those intolerant to aspirin, who should be receiving clopidogrel therapy.

Ticlopidine

Thienopyridines block the adenosine diphosphate (ADP) receptors on platelets, therefore decreasing platelet activation and aggregation. Ticlopidine was the first widely used thienopyridine that had an antiplatelet effect within 24 to 48 hours after its administration. The Studio della Ticlopidina nell'Angina Instabile Group trial (STAIG) was one of the first multicenter trials to evaluate the role of thienopyridines, particularly ticlopidine, in ACS (51). 652 patients with UA were randomized within 48 hours of presentation to conventional medical therapy alone versus ticlopidine in addition to conventional treatment. Ticlopidine was associated with a reduction in vascular mortality by 46.8% (4.8% versus 8.9%) and MI by 53.2% (5.1% versus 10.9%). However, ticlopidine was also reported to be associated with significant side effects, including thrombocytopenia, neutropenia and thrombocytopenic purpura-hemolytic uremic syndrome (52). Therefore, it is crucial that biweekly monitoring of blood counts be performed for four months after initiation of ticlopidine.

Clopidogrel

Due to unfavorable side effect profile of ticlopidine, clopidogrel became the thienopyridine of choice in ACS and PCI. In the Clopidogrel versus Aspirin in Patients at Risk of Ischemic Events (CAPRIE) trial, clopidogrel significantly reduced the combined endpoint of ischemic stroke, MI and vascular death in patients with atherosclerotic disease (53). Several landmark trials successfully expanded this role and the application of clopidogrel in ACS. The Clopidogrel in Unstable Angina to Prevent Recurrent Events (CURE) trial compared aspirin alone to aspirin plus clopidogrel in 12,562 patients who presented with non-ST-elevation ACS (54). Patients were randomized within 24 hours of symptom onset and the clopidogrel plus aspirin group received their treatment for a mean duration of nine months after an initial loading dose of 300 mg. The primary combined endpoint of cardiovascular death, MI, or stroke was reduced by 20% in the group receiving clopidogrel and aspirin (9.3% versus 11.4%). Although major bleeding complications were more common in the clopidogrel group, the absolute increase was only 1%, from 2.7% to 3.7%. When a subset of patients undergoing PCI was analyzed separately in the PCI-CURE substudy, pretreatment with clopidogrel plus aspirin prior to PCI led to both immediate and long-term benefits of reducing ischemic vascular events and death (55,56). However, there were several confounding factors in the PCI-CURE trial, which made routine clinical application of the trial data impractical. First, there was a significant delay (median of 10 days) to revascularization in this trial. Furthermore, GP IIb/IIIa inhibitors were used in only 21% of cases. Therefore, the Clopidogrel for Reduction of Events During Observation (CREDO) trial addressed these points and randomized 2,116 patients, more than half of whom were undergoing PCI for ACS, to receive a 300 mg clopidogrel loading dose or placebo in addition to aspirin 3 to 24 hours before urgent PCI, followed by a clopidogrel maintenance for one year compared with four weeks in the placebo group (57). This trial demonstrated that long-term clopidogrel therapy was associated with a 26.9% reduction in the combined risk of death, MI, or stroke (8.5% versus 11.5%) at one year. In addition, clopidogrel pretreatment at least six hours prior to PCI reduced the combined risk of death, MI, or urgent target vessel revascularization by 38.6% at 28 days.

With the role of clopidogrel being clearly defined in non-ST-elevation ACS, several trials also extensively studied its role in STEMI. The Clopidogrel as Adjunctive Reperfusion Therapy-Thrombolysis in Myocardial Infarction 28 (CLARITY-TIMI 28) trial randomized 3,491 patients with STEMI to either clopidogrel or placebo. These patients received fibrinolytics and aspirin, as well as heparin when appropriate, with angiogram being performed 48 hours after the event (58). This trial revealed that clopidogrel therapy reduced the composite endpoint of cardiovascular mortality, recurrent MI, and recurrent ischemia by 20% in STEMI patients postthrombolytic therapy. Furthermore, there was an improved patency rate of infarct-related artery in the group assigned to clopidogrel without any significant increase in major bleeding. The Clopidogrel and Metoprolol in Myocardial Infarction Trial/Chinese Cardiac Study-2 (COMMIT/CCS-2) was another landmark trial that provided further evidence for benefit of clopidogrel in STEMI patients (59). The trial enlisted 45,852 patients within 24 hours of suspected MI; 93% of patients had either ST elevation or left bundle branch block. Again, patients were randomized to clopidogrel plus aspirin versus aspirin alone in addition to standard medical therapy. After 4 weeks of treatment, addition of clopidogrel reduced the combined rate of death, reinfarction, and stroke by 9% (9.3% versus 10.1%) without a significant increase in bleeding rates. Since a significant portion of STEMI patients were treated with PCI, the PCI-CLARITY substudy attempted to identify the appropriate timing of clopidogrel loading (60). Upon subgroup analysis of data from CLARITY-TIMI 28 trial, in which patients underwent PCI two to eight days after thrombolysis, it was evident that patients who received clopidogrel loading within 45 minutes of thrombolysis had a decrease in the combined endpoint of cardiovascular death, MI, or stroke by 30 days (7.5% versus 12.0%).

To evaluate the optimal clopidogrel loading dose prior to PCI, the Antiplatelet Therapy for Reduction of Myocardial Damage during Angioplasty Study (ARMYDA-2) compared 600 mg versus 300 mg of clopidogrel loading given six hours prior to PCI (61). By 30 days, the composite endpoint of death, MI, or target vessel revascularization occurred in 4% in the 600 mg group compared to 12% in the 300-mg group ($P < 0.05$). However, a higher dose (900 mg) of clopidogrel in the Intracoronary Stenting and Antithrombotic Regimen-Choose Between 3 High Oral Doses for Immediate Clopidogrel Effect trial (ISAR-CHOICE) was associated with an increase in bleeding rates without any additional anti-ischemic benefit (62).

Given these data, the ACC/AHA has updated the guidelines on STEMI and now lists clopidogrel therapy for at least 14 days in patients with STEMI as a class I recommendation, regardless of whether they undergo reperfusion with fibrinolytic therapy or not (63). Furthermore, a loading dose of clopidogrel 300 mg is a class IIa recommendation in patients <75 years of age with STEMI who receive fibrinolytic therapy or who do not receive reperfusion therapy. For patients with STEMI undergoing primary PCI, a loading dose of clopidogrel 600 mg before or at the time of PCI is a class I indication according to the 2007 update of the ACC/AHA guidelines. In patients undergoing PCI within 12 to 24 hours of receiving fibrinolytic therapy, a loading dose of 300 mg may be considered instead. In terms of non-ST-elevation ACS, antiplatelet therapy in addition to aspirin should be initiated before diagnostic angiography with either clopidogrel or an intravenous GP IIb/IIIa inhibitor (Figure 2.2). Clopidogrel should be continued for at least 1 month and ideally for at least one year in patients presenting with ACS regardless of need for PCI (18). It is still recommended that clopidogrel be withheld for at least between five and seven days in patients for whom coronary artery bypass graft (CABG) surgery is planned, unless the urgency of revascularization outweighs the risks of bleeding.

Prasugrel

Recent findings have demonstrated that decreased response to clopidogrel leads to a higher risk of cardiovascular events including stent thrombosis. Prasugrel is a third-generation thienopyridine, which has been shown to generate active metabolite more efficiently leading to higher levels of platelet inhibition. The Prasugrel in Comparison to Clopidogrel for Inhibition of Platelet Activation and Aggregation-Thrombolysis in Myocardial Infarction 44 (PRINCIPLE-TIMI 44) trial compared prasugrel (60 mg loading dose followed by 10 mg maintenance dose) to a higher dose of clopidogrel (600 mg loading dose followed by 150 mg maintenance dose) in patients undergoing elective PCI (64). This trial demonstrated that prasugrel achieved superior platelet inhibition compared with a high dose of clopidogrel. In the Trial to Assess Improvement in Therapeutic Outcomes by Optimizing Platelet Inhibition with Prasugrel-Thrombolysis in Myocardial Infarction (TRITON-TIMI 38) trial, 13,608 patients with moderate- and high-risk ACS undergoing PCI were randomized to prasugrel (60 mg loading dose followed by 10 mg maintenance dose) or clopidogrel (300 mg loading dose followed by 75 mg maintenance dose) (65). This study demonstrated that prasugrel reduced the composite endpoint of death, nonfatal MI and nonfatal stroke by 20% in comparison to clopidogrel (9.9% versus 12.1%). In addition, the rate of stent thrombosis was significantly less with prasugrel (1.1% versus 2.4%). However, the rate of major hemorrhage was increased by 32% in the prasugrel group compared to the clopidogrel group. Subgroup analyses have identified those patients who were at high risk of bleeding with prasugrel. These risk factors included age ≥75 years, history of stroke or TIA, and body weight less than 60 kg. Therefore, prasugrel is an alternative antiplatelet agent, particularly for those patients who are resistant to clopidogrel or have high platelet reactivity while taking clopidogrel. Importantly, individual patient evaluation of bleeding risk should take place prior to starting prasugrel post-PCI in patients with ACS.

■ ANTITHROMBOTIC AGENTS

Unfractionated Heparin

Unfractionated heparin (UFH) inhibits platelet aggregation and fibrin formation by accelerating the action of antithrombin, which in turn inactivates factors IIa, IXa, and Xa. The benefit of heparin in UA has been well defined in early trials (48,49). In the RISC trial, a combination of aspirin and heparin reduced the incidence of MI and death during the first five days by 75% when compared with placebo. This result was successfully replicated in several small trials examining the role of heparin in UA. A meta-analysis of these trials revealed a 33% reduction in the combined risk of death or MI in patients treated with aspirin plus heparin compared with those treated with aspirin alone (66). With benefit of heparin clearly established in UA patients, later trials attempted to expand the role of heparin in NSTEMI.

In the Antithrombotic Therapy in Acute Coronary Syndromes trial (ATACS), there was a significant reduction in the combined endpoint of recurrent angina, MI, and death in the UFH plus aspirin group compared with aspirin alone (10.5% versus 27%) persisting until 12 weeks (67). A meta-analysis of 12 trials examining the role of UFH in non-ST-elevation ACS revealed that addition of UFH decreases the risk of MI/death by ~50% (68). However, there was no clinical benefit in long-term use of UFH beyond the first seven days. The ACC/AHA guidelines recommend UFH therapy as a class I indication in ACS regardless of the need for catheterization (18). If an invasive strategy is chosen, UFH should be stopped after a successful intervention. In conservatively managed patients, UFH should be continued for at least 48 hours, but the anticoagulation therapy should not be continued beyond eight days without another indication.

The recommended weight-adjusted regimen for UFH is an initial bolus of 60 U/kg (maximum 4,000 U) and an initial infusion of 12 U/kg/hour (maximum 1,000 U/hour). Due to a marked variability in the anticoagulant response in different individuals, the activated partial thromboplastin (aPTT) time needs to be monitored with a goal of 1.5 to 2 times the control value. Two consecutive therapeutic aPTT values need to be obtained in order to achieve a stable maintenance dose with subsequent daily aPTT to confirm the dose. UFH has been associated with a slight increase in major bleeding in most trials and serial blood counts should be obtained to monitor hemoglobin levels. In addition,

UFH can cause autoimmune heparin-induced thrombocytopenia. This rare but potentially lethal complication is associated with thrombosis and is treated by prompt withdrawal of UFH and initiation of alternative anticoagulation therapy.

Low-Molecular-Weight Heparin

Low-molecular-weight heparin (LMWH), like UFH, prevents clot propagation, but there are several advantages over UFH due to different mechanisms of action. The ratio of anti-Xa/anti-IIa activity is significantly higher in LMWH compared to UFH, thereby inhibiting thrombin generation more effectively with potentially less bleeding. Suppression of the release of von Willebrand factor also augments LMWH's anticoagulant effect. Furthermore, high bioavailability leads to a longer duration of systemic anticoagulation, and less binding to plasma proteins causing a more consistent anticoagulant effect. Therefore, LMWH is easier to administer than UFH since there is no need to follow anticoagulant levels. Several trials have compared LMWH to UFH in ACS patients.

Dalteparin was studied in the Fragmin during Instability in Coronary Artery Disease study (FRISC), which assigned 1,506 patients presenting with non-ST-elevation ACS to dalteparin versus a placebo (69). The rate of death and new MI was lower in the dalteparin group versus the placebo group (1.8% versus 4.8%) in the first six days, although no significant long-term benefit was observed. However, the Fragmin in Unstable Coronary Artery Disease Study (FRIC) also examined dalteparin versus UFH in non-ST-elevation ACS and concluded that there were no significant differences in mortality, MI, and recurrent angina (70). The Fraxiparine in Ischaemic Syndrome trial (FRAXIS) compared a different LMWH agent, nadroparin, to UFH in patients presenting with non-ST-elevation ACS (71). The trial did not reveal any benefit of nadroparin over UFH, but instead nadroparin was associated with a significant excess in bleeding complications with prolonged treatment.

Although the above agents have not demonstrated a clear benefit over UFH, several trials have defined a clear role of enoxaparin in ACS. The ESSENCE trial studied the effect of enoxaparin for two to eight days upon presentation with non-ST-elevation ACS, and showed a significant reduction in the combined endpoint of death, MI, or recurrent angina when compared with UFH at 14 days (16.6% versus 19.8%) (4). This benefit was still evident by one year of follow-up without a significant increase in bleeding. The TIMI 11B trial confirmed this finding and revealed a significant reduction in death, MI, or urgent revascularization in enoxaparin arm when compared with UFH (3). Of note, the greatest benefit was seen in high-risk patients with high TIMI scores. However, prolonged use of enoxaparin resulted in an increase in bleeding complication. A meta-analysis of these two trials showed a nearly 20% reduction in death and serious cardiac ischemic events within the first few days of treatment, and this benefit was sustained through 43 days (72). Furthermore, enoxaparin use was not associated with any increase in major hemorrhage, although the rate of minor hemorrhage was significantly higher in the enoxaparin group. A more recent meta-analysis examined the use of enoxaparin in the entire spectrum of ACS patients from UA to STEMI and revealed a significant reduction in the incidence of death or nonfatal MI (9.8% versus 11.4%) in the enoxaparin group when compared with UFH at 30 days (73).

With the introduction of different medical therapies for ACS, additional trials have sought to confirm superiority of enoxaparin to UFH with concurrent GP IIb/IIIa inhibitor therapy. In the Integrilin and Enoxaparin Randomized Assessment of Acute Coronary Syndrome Treatment trial (INTERACT), patients receiving enoxaparin in addition to aspirin and eptifibatide experienced a reduction in the rate of death, MI, or recurrent ischemia at 30 days (5% versus 9%) (74). The Aggrastat to Zocor trial (A to Z) confirmed the above findings in a large randomized trial involving 3,987 patients with non-ST-elevation ACS by demonstrating a nonsignificantly lower composite rate of death, MI, and refractory ischemia for enoxaparin versus UFH (8.4% versus 9.4%) at seven days (75).

The Superior Yield of the New Strategy of Enoxaparin, Revascularization, and Glycoprotein IIb/IIIa Inhibitors (SYNERGY) trial examined the role of enoxaparin in patients treated with an early invasive strategy (76). In this trial, 10,027 patients with non-ST-elevation ACS were randomized to enoxaparin versus UFH with GP IIb/IIIa inhibitors being added at physicians' discretion. Although enoxaparin was shown to be noninferior to UFH, enoxaparin use was associated with a significantly higher rate of major bleeding (9.1% versus 7.6%), suggesting that enoxaparin should be used cautiously in patients undergoing an early invasive strategy.

In terms of STEMI patients receiving thrombolytic therapy, the Assessment of the Safety and Efficacy of a New Thrombolytic Regimen-3 (ASSENT-3) trial compared enoxaparin versus UFH in patients receiving tenecteplase (77). This trial demonstrated a reduction in the combined endpoint of 30-day mortality, in-hospital reinfarction, and in-hospital refractory ischemia in the enoxaparin group (11.4% versus 15.4%). Similarly, the safety endpoint of intracranial hemorrhage and major bleeding was significantly lower in the enoxaparin group as well. Given the proven superiority of enoxaparin over UFH as an adjunctive therapy to thrombolytics, several trials have attempted to compare different antithrombotic agents to enoxaparin. In the Enoxaparin Versus Tinzaparin in Non-ST-segment Elevation Acute Coronary Syndromes trial (EVET), tinzaparin was found to be inferior to enoxaparin in non-ST-elevation ACS patients in terms of reduction of rates of recurrent angina, MI, and the rate of revascularization (78).

Fondaparinux

Fondaparinux, a selective inhibitor of activated factor X, was shown to have a similar efficacy to enoxaparin in reducing the risk of ischemic events at nine days (79). In fact, fondaparinux was associated with a reduced mortality at 30 days and 180 days with a substantial reduction in major bleeding. However, its use was associated with a higher rate of catheter-associated thrombus formation during PCI. Therefore, the ACC/AHA guidelines suggest regimens that use either enoxaparin or UFH or fondaparinux for patients with ACS being conservatively managed (Figure 2.3) (18). Furthermore, in patients with an increased risk of bleeding who are being managed conservatively, fondaparinux is recommended as a class I indication. In patients undergoing PCI, if fondaparinux was used initially, an additional anticoagulant with an anti-IIa activity, such as UFH, should be used during PCI to prevent thrombus formation.

Direct Thrombin Inhibitors

Direct thrombin inhibitors are able to inactivate thrombin in blood by directly binding to the catalytic site of thrombin rather than by acting through antithrombin molecule. Hirudin, a naturally occurring anticoagulant, was one of the first direct thrombin inhibitors to be tested for its utility in ACS. The Global Use of Strategies to Open Occluded Coronary Arteries trial IIb (GUSTO IIb) enrolled 12,141 ACS patients, including those with STEMI, and randomly assigned them to UFH or recombinant hirudin (80). Hirudin was associated with an early reduction of death or MI, but its beneficial effect decreased over time resulting in no mortality benefit, with only a modest reduction in reinfarction by 30 days. There was also an increase in the rate of moderate bleeding in the hirudin group compared with UFH. The role of recombinant hirudin in non-ST-elevation ACS was again examined in the Organisation to Assess Strategies for Ischemic Syndromes trial (OASIS-2) (81), where 10,141 patients with UA/NSTEMI were randomized to UFH or recombinant hirudin. By seven days, recombinant hirudin was associated with a significant reduction in cardiac death and new MI (3.6% versus 4.2%) along with a lower frequency of revascularization (6% versus 7%) in comparison to UFH. This benefit was observed at seven days and persisted until 35 days. However, as in GUSTO IIb, recombinant hirudin was associated with a significantly higher rate of major bleeding requiring more frequent transfusions (1.2% versus 0.7%). The role of recombinant hirudin in patients with non-ST-elevation ACS treated with PCI was investigated in the Hirudin in a European Trial versus Heparin in the Prevention of Restenosis after PTCA trial (HELVETICA) (82). In this trial, patients with UA undergoing PCI experienced fewer early cardiac events with hirudin compared with UFH (83). However, longer follow-up of patients in this trial showed no clinical benefit of hirudin.

For patients with STEMI treated with thrombolytic therapy, the TIMI 9B trial examined the role of hirudin (84). Heparin and hirudin demonstrated an equal effect as an adjunctive therapy to thrombolysis in patients with STEMI without a significant increase in major bleeding complications. The Hirulog Early Reperfusion/Occlusion trial (HERO) reproduced a similar finding with bivalirudin, a synthetic peptide that directly inhibits free and clot-bound thrombin (85). When given concurrently with streptokinase, bivalirudin was more effective than UFH in producing early infarct-related artery patency without increasing the risk of major bleeding. However, a larger randomized trial, HERO-2, revealed that bivalirudin had a similar mortality at 30 days compared with UFH when used in conjunction with streptokinase (86). There was a reduced rate of reinfarction in the bivalirudin group, but at the cost of increased mild and moderate bleeding.

Although the HERO-2 trial did not demonstrate a significant advantage of bivalirudin over UFH as an adjunctive therapy to thrombolytics, bivalrudin has been further investigated in a diverse spectrum of ACS patients due to its relatively safer profile compared with hirudin. In the TIMI 7 trial, 410 patients with UA who were treated with higher doses of bivalirudin experienced a reduced combined rate of death and MI (87). The role of bivalirudin was solidified by the Bivalirudin Angioplasty Study as the trial revealed that bivalirudin reduced the combined rate of death, MI, and repeat revascularization (6.2% versus 7.9%) compared to heparin in patients who underwent PCI secondary to UA (88). Subsequently, the Randomized Evaluation in PCI Linking Angiomax to Reduced Clinical Events (REPLACE-2) trial compared bivalirudin with provisional GP IIb/IIIa inihibitors to UFH plus routine GP IIb/IIIa inhibitors in 6,010 patients undergoing mostly elective PCI, with >20% of the patients undergoing PCI secondary to ACS (89). This trial successfully demonstrated noninferiority of bivalirudin in regard to the combined endpoint of death, MI, or revascularization in patients undergoing PCI.

As GP IIb/IIIa inhibitors became an integral part of ACS treatment, the Acute Catheterization and Urgent Intervention Triage Strategy trial (ACUITY) examined the role of bivalirudin in high-risk patients with ACS undergoing PCI (90). In this study, 13,819 patients presenting with non-ST-elevation ACS undergoing PCI were randomized to heparin plus a GP IIb/IIIa inhibitor, bivalirudin plus a GP IIb/IIIa inhibitor, or bivalirudin alone. By 30 days, it was evident that bivalirudin was noninferior to heparin in reducing composite end point of death, MI, and revascularization. In fact, bivalirudin alone was associated with a similar rate of composite ischemic end points with a significantly reduced rate of major bleeding compared with heparin plus a GP IIb/IIIa inhibitor group or bivalirudin plus a GP IIb/IIIa inhibitor group (3.0% versus 5.7% versus 5.3%). However, the rate of composite ischemic end points was higher with bivalirudin monotherapy than with heparin plus GP IIb/IIIa inhibitors (9.1% and 7.1%) among patients who did not receive a thienopyridine pretreatment. The Harmonizing Outcomes with Revascularization and Stents in Acute Myocardial Infarction trial (HORIZONS-AMI) examined whether similar benefits would be observed in STEMI patients (91); 3,602 patients with STEMI undergoing PCI were randomized to heparin plus GP IIb/IIIa inhibitor or bivalirudin alone. Treatment with bivalirudin resulted in a significantly lower mortality by 30 days (1.8% versus 2.9%) in comparison with heparin plus GP IIb/IIIa inhibitor group. In addition, there was a significantly lower rate of major bleeding events in the bivalirudin group (4.9% versus 8.3%). However, there was a small increase in acute stent thrombosis (within 24 hours) in the bivalirudin group, without any significant increase in stent thrombosis by 30 days. The ACC/AHA guidelines now recommend that a GP IIb/IIIa inhibitor may be omitted if bivalirudin is chosen as the agent of choice in ACS as long as clopidogrel pretreatment is administered.

Glycoprotein IIb/IIIa Inhibitor

Glycoprotein (GP) IIb/IIIa inhibitors prevent fibrinogen from cross-linking platelets and prevent platelet aggregation by occupying the receptor. Three GP IIb/IIIa inhibitors have been tested in numerous trials to identify their potential roles in ACS. Tirofiban is a nonpeptide molecule, which interferes with the GP IIb/IIIa inhibitor. The Platelet Receptor Inhibition in Ischemic Syndrome Management Study (PRISM) compared tirofiban to UFH in 3,232 patients with non-ST-elevation ACS (92). Tirofiban given for 48 hours prior to PCI in this patient population was shown to significantly reduce mortality (2.3% versus 3.6%) as compared with UFH only group. The Platelet Receptor Inhibition in Ischemic Syndrome Management in Patients Limited by Unstable Signs and Symptoms Study (PRISM-PLUS) attempted to further delineate this benefit by randomizing patients with non-ST-elevation ACS to UFH alone, tirofiban alone, or UFH plus tirofiban (93). This trial was terminated early in the group receiving tirofiban only due to excess mortality. However, by seven days after randomization, the frequency of death or MI was significantly reduced in the tirofiban plus UFH group and remained significant at six months (27.7% versus 32.1%) compared to UFH alone. The Randomized Efficacy Study of Tirofiban for Outcomes and Restenosis trial (RESTORE) examined the role of this medication in patients with ACS undergoing PCI (94). This trial demonstrated that primary composite end point of death, MI, angioplasty failure requiring CABG or unplanned stenting, and recurrent ischemia requiring repeat PCI was reduced by tirofiban (10.3% versus 12.2%). With the data from the above trials, tirofiban was approved by FDA for the treatment of ACS in conjunction with UFH.

Eptifibatide is another small molecule GP IIb/IIIa inhibitor, which has been studied extensively in ACS patients. It is a synthetic, nonimmunogenic heptapeptide, which mimics the Arg-Gly-Asp amino acid sequence by which fibrinogen binds to the GP IIb/IIIa receptor. In the Platelet Glycoprotein IIb/IIIa in Unstable Angina: Receptor Suppression Using Integrilin Therapy trial (PURSUIT), 10,948 patients were randomized to eptifibatide or placebo in conjunction with UFH and aspirin (95). By four days, the combined endpoint of death and nonfatal MI were reduced by 1.5% in the eptifibatide group (14.2% versus 15.7%). More remarkably, this benefit was apparent as early as 96 hours and persisted through 30 days with a greater benefit observed in patients undergoing early angioplasty. The Integrilin to Minimize Platelet Aggregation and Coronary Thrombosis-II trial (IMPACT-II) provided more answers regarding the role of eptifibatide in patients undergoing PCI (96). In the low-dose eptifibatide group, treatment with eptifibatide during PCI reduced the rates of early abrupt closure and ischemic events by 30 days (97). Several trials have also extensively studied the role of this agent as an adjunctive therapy to thrombolysis. In the IMPACT-AMI trial, the incidence and speed of reperfusion were enhanced when eptifibatide was combined with accelerated alteplase, aspirin, and heparin (98). However, GUSTO-V (99) and ASSENT-3 trials (100) showed conflicting data utilizing abciximab as a GP IIb/IIIa inhibitor. Due to insufficient data supporting the use of GP IIb/IIIa inhibitors with thrombolytics, currently GP IIb/IIIa inhibitors are not indicated as an adjunct therapy to thrombolysis. On the other hand, there is extensive literature that supports the use of GP IIb/IIIa inihibitors in PCI.

Abciximab, Fab fragment of a monoclonal antibody directed at the GP IIb/IIIa receptor, has been studied extensively in multiple ACS and PCI trials. The c7E3 Fab Antiplatelet Therapy in Unstable Refractory Angina trial (CAPTURE) enrolled patients with UA undergoing PCI and randomized them to abxicimab versus UFH (101). There was a significant reduction in the combined endpoint of death, MI, and revascularization at 30 days (11.3% versus 15.9%) with slightly more major bleeding events in patients receiving abciximab (3.8% versus 1.9%). Although this benefit dissipated by six months, other trials, such as the Evaluation of c7E3 for Prevention of Ischemic Complications trial (EPIC), have shown an improvement in long-term outcomes as long as three years after PCI (102). The EPIC trial randomized 2,099 high-risk patients to placebo versus abciximab, with a siginificant number of patients undergoing PCI secondary to severe UA or evolving MI. A bolus of abciximab followed by a 12-hour continuous infusion reduced the rate of death, MI, or revascularization by 35% at 30 days. This benefit was maintained at three years, and the greatest benefit was observed in patients with refractory UA or evolving MI. In this subgroup, abciximab was associated with a significant reduction in mortality at 3 years (5.1% versus 12.7%). The GUSTO IV-ACS trial attempted to extend the role of abxicimab to patients with ACS being managed conservatively without early invasive treatment (103). 7,800 patients with non-ST-elevation ACS were randomized to abciximab bolus plus 24-hour infusion, abxicimab plus 48-hour infusion or placebo along with concomitant aspirin and UFH. Unlike the previous PCI trials, there was no benefit associated with abciximab therapy at 30 days or one year regardless of the infusion duration.

Given the benefit of periprocedural clopidogrel, recent trials investigated the role of abciximab in conjunction with thienopyridines. In the Intracoronary Stenting and Antithrombotic Regimen: Rapid Early Action for Coronary Treatment 2 (ISAR-REACT 2) trial, 2,022 patients undergoing PCI secondary to non-ST-elevation ACS were randomized to abciximab versus placebo along with aspirin, heparin and pretreatment of 600mg of clopidogrel (104). By 30 days, there was a 25% reduction in ischemic events in the abciximab group (8.9% versus 11.9%). However, in a subgroup analysis, the benefit was only observed in patients with an elevated troponin I, suggesting a potential role of abxicimab in conjunction with clopidogrel in this subset of patients. The 2007 ACC/AHA guidelines suggest that for an initial invasive strategy, the antiplatelet therapy in addition to aspirin should be initiated before diagnostic angiography with either clopidogrel or an intravenous GP IIb/IIIa inhibitor (18). Furthermore, abciximab is indicated only if there is no appreciable delay to angiography, and PCI is likely to be performed. Otherwise, intravenous eptifibatide or tirofiban is the preferred choice of a GP IIb/IIIa inhibitor. For patients undergoing an initially invasive strategy, it is a class IIa recommendation to initiate the antiplatelet therapy with both clopidogrel and an intravenous GP IIb/IIIa inhibitor.

Thrombolytic Therapy

Thrombolytic therapy is an important therapy in STEMI that restores coronary flow and improves mortality. Several thrombolytic agents have been extensively studied to assess their efficacy in STEMI population. Streptokinase is a polypeptide derived from beta-hemolytic streptococcus. It activates plasmin through its binding to plasminogen and forms a complex which becomes an active enzyme. The GISSI-1 trial was a landmark trial enrolling 11,712 patients presenting with an acute STEMI (105). There was a remarkable reduction in the 21-day mortality in the streptokinase arm compared to placebo (10.7% versus 13%). This effect persisted through 12 months (17.2% versus 19%), demonstrating a clear role of thrombolytic therapy in STEMI. The benefit was most notable in the group where streptokinase was given <3 hours of presentation. This data were further supported in the ISIS-2 trial, which demonstrated an additive reduction in the risk of mortality when streptokinase was used in conjunction with aspirin (50). However, streptokinase is potentially antigenic and can cause an immunologic sensitization and allergic reaction, especially with repeated use exposure.

Alteplase (t-PA), on the other hand, is not antigenic and has no associated risk of allergic reaction. t-PA is fibrin-specific and has an increased affinity for plasminogen molecule. When bound to fibrin, t-PA attaches to thrombus and causes thrombolysis. Initial trials have demonstrated a significant reduction in the size of MI and an improvement of left ventricular EF in patients treated with recombinant t-PA versus placebo along with aspirin and UFH (106). The GUSTO-1 trial compared the efficacy of accelerated t-PA versus streptokinase in 41,021 patients that presented with an acute STEMI (107). This landmark trial demonstrated a 14% reduction in 30-day mortality favoring accelerated t-PA over streptokinase (6.3% versus 7.4%), and established accelerated t-PA plus intravenous UFH as the superior regimen. In a subgroup analysis, patients with age <75 years and anterior MI benefited the most from t-PA therapy, although the mortality reduction was observed across a wide variety of patients. Although the risk of major bleeding (including hemorrhagic stroke) was increased in the t-PA group compared with streptokinase group, the combined endpoint of death and stroke was significantly lower in the t-PA group. Once again, the GUSTO-1 trial demonstrated the emphasis of early intervention, as the patients with early thrombolysis had lower mortality rates (5.5% versus 9.0%).

Newer agents, such as reteplase, were recently investigated for further benefit in STEMI. Reteplase is a recombinant nonglycosylated form of human tissue plasminogen activator. In comparison to alteplase, reteplase has a longer half-life and binds fibrin with lower affinity, improving its ability to penetrate into clots. However, in the GUSTO-3 trial, reteplase did not provide any additional survival benefit compared with alteplase in the treatment of STEMI patients except for the benefit of easy administration (106). However, the International Joint Efficacy Comparison of Thrombolytics (INJECT) trial found reteplase to have at least an equivalent efficacy to streptokinase in terms of mortality, recurrent MI, stroke, and major bleeding (109). In fact, the use of reteplase was associated with a decreased risk of developing cardiogenic shock and CHF.

Tenecteplase is the newest thrombolytic agent, also extensively investigated recently. Tenecteplase is a recombinant fibrin-specific plasminogen activator derived from the native t-PA. It has a higher fibrin specificity and greater resistance to inactivation by its endogenous inhibitor in comparison to native t-PA. The TIMI-10B trial compared different doses of tenecteplase with a front-loaded alteplase in patients who presented with STEMI within 12 hours (110). Upon angiogram, the rate of TIMI 3 flow in the culprit vessel at 90 minutes was the same with the 40 mg dose of tenecteplase and alteplase. Further delineation of safety and efficacy of tenecteplase was performed in the ASSENT-2 trial, which randomized 16,950 patients to tenecteplase or t-PA (111). The 30-day mortality was similar in the tenecteplase group compared to the t-PA group (6.17% versus 6.15%), with no difference in the rates of intracranial hemorrhage. However, minor bleeding events were slightly reduced in the tenecteplase group.

Although the safety profile is improved with the recently studied thrombolytics, there are certain absolute contraindications to fibrinolytic therapy including history of any intracranial hemorrhage, history of ischemic stroke within the preceding three months, presence of a cerebral vascular malformation or a primary or metastatic intracranial malignancy, symptoms or signs suggestive of an aortic dissection, a bleeding diathesis or active bleeding with the exception of menses, and a significant closed-head trauma within the preceding three months (63). These contraindications preclude patients from receiving thrombolytic therapy and favor undergoing emergent PCI.

Invasive Versus Conservative Management Strategies for NSTEMI/UA

Although earlier trials failed to show the benefit of an invasive strategy over conservative therapy for NSTEMI, more contemporary studies have demonstrated potential benefits of an early invasive strategy in selected patients. In the Framingham and Fast Revascularization During Instability in Coronary Artery Disease trial (FRISC-II), 2,457 patients with non-ST-elevation ACS were randomized to either an invasive or a conservative strategy (112). The invasive strategy group underwent coronary angiogram within seven days and revascularization within ten days. Although there was a delay in revascularization, the invasive strategy was associated with a significantly lower incidence of death or MI at six months (9.4% versus 12.1%) (113). Furthermore, angina and hospital readmissions were significantly reduced as well. The follow-up at five years revealed persistent benefits with a reduction in all-cause mortality (9.7% versus 10.1%) and MI (12.9 % versus 17.7%) (114). The Randomized Intervention Trial of Unstable Angina 3 (RITA 3) sought to confirm the advantage of an invasive strategy in non-ST-elevation ACS patients (115). Although the rate of refractory angina was reduced as in the FRISC-II trial, there was no significant reduction of mortality or MI at four months and one year of follow-up. However, the study revealed a reduction in death and MI in the invasive strategy group by five years of follow-up (116). The benefits of an invasive strategy were observed mostly in patients at high-risk of death or MI, particularly in troponin-positive patients.

With the introduction of GP IIb/IIIa inhibitors in the spectrum of ACS therapy, the TACTICS-TIMI 18 trial randomized 2,220 patients with non-ST-elevation ACS to an invasive or conservative strategy in conjunction with tirofiban, heparin, and aspirin (5). At 6 months, the combined rate of death, nonfatal MI, and rehospitalization for ACS was reduced in the early invasive strategy group (15.9% versus 19.4%). More importantly, the rate of death or nonfatal MI was significantly reduced (7.3% versus 9.5%) as well, particularly in a high-risk group with a positive troponin marker. The Intracoronary Stenting with Antithrombotic Regimen Cooling-Off trial (ISAR-COOL) attempted to identify the appropriate timing of intervention in patients with ACS (117). Patients presenting with non-ST-elevation ACS were randomized to either an early invasive strategy group, who underwent angiography within six hours versus a delayed invasive strategy group, who underwent angiography after three to five days of pretreatment with GP IIb/IIIa inhibitors. The early invasive strategy was associated with a significant reduction in death or MI at 30 days (5.9% versus 11.6%).

With some of trials showing a beneficial effect of an early invasive strategy, several meta-analyses have evaluated these data (116,117). One meta-analysis revealed a significant reduction in MI, recurrent angina, and rehospitalizations in the early invasive group over a mean follow-up of 17 months (118). However, early invasive therapy was associated with a small increase in mortality and MI during the hospitalization, although there was a much greater reduction in all-cause mortality and MI upon long-term follow-up. With longer follow-up data available, a recent meta-analysis of these trials demonstrated an improved long-term survival (4.9% versus 6.5%) and a reduction in late MIs (7.6% versus 9.1%) and rehospitalizations (119). Therefore, the ACC/AHA guidelines classify the early invasive management strategy with PCI as a class I indication for patients with non-ST-elevation ACS without serious comorbidities, who have coronary lesions amenable to PCI and high-risk features or refractory angina despite maximal medical treatment (18). However, a recent clinical trial, the Invasive versus Conservative Treatment in Unstable Coronary Syndromes trial (ICTUS), showed that with the contemporary intensive medical therapy (aspirin, clopidogrel, high-dose statin, LMWH), an early invasive strategy was equivalent to a selectively invasive strategy in non-ST-elevation ACS (120). Therefore, the ACC/AHA guidelines give an option of initially conservative strategy for stable non-ST-elevation ACS patients as a class IIb indication. Importantly, noninvasive risk stratification of the medically treated patients with a stress test (Table 2.2) during or shortly after the hospitalization is an important part of management for these patients. The Duke treadmill score has been validated to assess prognosis in patients with suspected coronary artery disease (121). The score is calculated based on exercise time, ST deviation and treadmill angina index. In an analysis of 2,758 symptomatic patients, who underwent exercise stress testing, five-year mortality was 3%, 10%, and 35% for low-, moderate-, and high-risk patients, respectively (122). Therefore, it is a class I indication for patients with a high-risk finding

Table 2.2 American College of Cardiology/American Heart Association system for noninvasive risk stratification of patients with non-ST-elevation acute coronary syndromes, treated with a conservative strategy

	Risk Stratification		
	Low Risk	Intermediate Risk	High Risk
Feature			
Duke Treadmill Score	Greater than 5	–11 to 5	Less than –11
LVEF	Normal LV function	Mild/Moderate LV dysfunction	Severe LV dysfunction
Perfusion defects	Normal or small perfusion defect at rest or with stress	Moderate reversible perfusion defect	Large or multiple moderate reversible defects, LV dilation, or increased lung uptake
Stress echocardiographic findings	No stresss-induced wall motion abnormality	Stress-induced wall-motion abnormality involving ≤2 segments	Extensive stress-induced wall-motion abnormality

Source: From Ref. 18, with permission.

on noninvasive stress testing to be crossed over into the invasive strategy group. Other indications for an early invasive strategy include recurrent angina or ischemia with minimal activities despite intensive anti-ischemic therapy, a positive troponin marker, new ST-segment depressions on ECG, ischemia with CHF symptoms, depressed EF <40%, hemodynamic instability, sustained ventricular tachycardia, PCI within six months, or prior history of CABG.

Reperfusion Therapy in ST-Elevation MI

Although the efficacy of thrombolytic therapy has been well established, thrombolytics have been associated with significant bleeding complications, and their use has been limited to patients without contraindications to these agents. Earlier trials demonstrated a small benefit of emergent PCI over thrombolytic therapy in patients with STEMI. In the Primary Angioplasty in Myocardial Infarction trial (PAMI), the percutaneous angioplasty (PTCA) group experienced a significant decease in the in-hospital mortality along with a reduced rate of death or reinfarctions during hospitalization in comparison to the thrombolytic group (123). However, intracranial bleeding occurred more frequently among patients receiving thrombolytic therapy. By six months of follow-up, the overall rate of death or MI remained significantly reduced in the PTCA group (8.5 % and 16.8%).

With advances of adjunctive pharmacotherapy for PCI, multiple trials sought to confirm superiority of primary PCI to thrombolytic therapy in STEMI. In a review of 23 trials, primary PCI had better outcomes than thrombolytic therapy by reducing the combined endpoint of death, nonfatal reinfarction, and stroke (8% versus 14%), independent of the type of the thrombolytic agent used (124).

The Danish Trial in Acute Myocardial Infarction-2 (DANAMI-2) trial evaluated whether the strategy of reperfusion involving the transfer of patients to a PCI-center is superior to on-site fibrinolysis (125). The trial randomized 1,572 patients presenting with STEMI within 12 hours since the onset of symptoms to primary PCI versus t-PA. The trial showed that a combined 30-day rate of death, recurrent MI, or stroke was significantly lower in the PCI group (8.5% versus 14.2%), provided that the transfer took <2 hours. The Primary Angioplasty in AMI Patients from General Community Hospitals Transported to PCI Units versus Emergency Thrombolysis-2 trial (PRAGUE-2) also assessed the efficacy of transferring patients with STEMI to a tertiary center rather than treating them with thrombolytics on-site (126). The trial demonstrated that transferring STEMI patients for a PCI strategy markedly decreases mortality in patients presenting >3 hours since the onset of symptoms. However, for patients presenting <3 hours of symptom onset, thrombolytic therapy resulted in similar outcomes to PCI strategy. Thus, the timing of symptom onset and presentation to the hospital is important in making the decision whether to administer thrombolytic therapy to the STEMI patient on-site or transfer to a PCI facility.

Furthermore, the Should We Emergently Revascularize Occluded Coronaries for Cardiogenic Shock (SHOCK) trial asked whether PCI benefited patients presenting with cardiogenic shock secondary to STEMI. These patients were randomized to emergent revascularization or medical stabilization with a majority of the patients receiving an intra-aortic balloon pump therapy (127). The trial demonstrated that although there was no improvement in mortality by 30 days, a significant reduction in mortality was observed by six months of follow-up in the revascularization group (50.3% versus 63.1%). In both arms, mortality in patients presenting with cardiogenic shock was very high. Given these findings, the ACC/AHA guidelines have recommended that STEMI patients presenting to a hospital with a PCI capability should be treated with a primary PCI within 90 minutes of presentation (63). Furthermore, STEMI patients presenting to a hospital without PCI capability, and who cannot be transferred to a PCI center to undergo PCI within 90 minutes of presentation, should be treated with thrombolytic therapy within 30 min of presentation, unless fibrinolytic therapy is contraindicated. Rescue PCI is reasonable for patients in whom thrombolytic therapy has failed. Furthermore, with evidence from the SHOCK trial, early revascularization within 18 hours of shock onset is a class I indication for patients <75 years of age who develop cardiogenic shock within 36 hours of MI.

Although the benefit of primary PCI and rescue PCI have been clearly established, current data do not support the routine use of adjunctive PCI following successful thrombolysis. In the absence of recurrent ischemia, hemodynamic instability, life threatening ventricular arrhythmia and significant left ventricular dysfunction, studies have shown that routine use of PCI after successful thrombolysis does not improve left ventricular function or survival (128,129). Therefore, the ACC/AHA guidelines recommend routine PCI after successful thrombolysis without above complications as a class IIb indication. However, risk stratification of patients after successful thrombolysis with either noninvasive stress testing or diagnostic angiography should be strongly considered during or shortly after the hospitalization.

CONCLUSIONS

Recent advances in medical therapy have significantly altered the treatment of ACS and improved the short- and long-term outcomes of patients with ACS. In patients presenting with chest pain, careful history, physical examination, ECG and cardiac biomarkers can be used to diagnose and properly classify ACS (Table 2.1; Figure 2.1). For patients with STEMI, emergent revascularization needs to be considered along with immediate treatment with antithrombotic agents, antiplatelet agents, statins and beta-blockers. In non-ST-elevation ACS, similar medical treatment should be initially utilized (Figures 2.2 and 2.3). However, high-risk patients, particularly those with positive cardiac biomarkers, should be considered for more aggressive therapy including GP IIb/IIIa inhibition and early invasive management strategy.

REFERENCES

1. Rosamond W, Flegal K, Friday G, et al. Heart disease and stroke statistics—2007 update: a report from the American Heart Association Statistics Committee and Stroke Statistics Subcommittee. *Circulation* 2007; 115(5):e69 –171.
2. Zipes DP, Libby P, Bonow RO, et al. *Brauwald's Heart Disease: A Textbook of Cardiovascular Medicine*, 7th ed. Philadelphia: Saunders, 2005, pp. 1243–46.
3. Antman EM, McCabe CH, Enrique P, et al. Enoxaparin Prevents Death and Cardiac Ischemic Events in Unstable Angina/Non–Q-Wave Myocardial Infarction: Results of the Thrombolysis In Myocardial Infarction (TIMI) 11B Trial. *Circulation* 1999; 100(15):1593–601.
4. Cohen M, Demers C, Gurfinkel EP, et al. A comparison of low-molecular-weight heparin with unfractionated heparin for unstable coronary artery disease. Efficacy and Safety of Subcutaneous Enoxaparin in Non-Q-Wave Coronary Events Study Group. *N Engl J Med* 1997; 337(7):447–52.

5. Cannon CP, Weintraub WS, Demopoulos LA, et al. Comparison of early invasive versus early conservative strategies in patients with unstable angina and non-ST elevation myocardial infarction treated with early glycoprotein IIb/IIIa inhibition. *N Engl J Med* 2001; 344(25):1879–87.
6. Morrow DA, Antman EM, Charlesworth A, et al. TIMI risk score for ST-elevation myocardial infarction: A convenient, bedside, clinical score for risk assessment at presentation: An intravenous nPA for treatment of infarcting myocardium early II trial substudy. *Circulation* 2000; 102(17):2031–7.
7. Gottlieb SO, Weisfeldt ML, Ouyang P, et al. Effect of the addition of propranolol to therapy with nifedipine for unstable angina pectoris: A randomized, double-blind, placebo-controlled trial. *Circulation* 1986; 73(2):331–7.
8. Yusuf S, Wittes J, Friedman L, et al. Overview of results of randomized clinical trials in heart disease. II. Unstable angina, heart failure, primary prevention with aspirin, and risk factor modification. *JAMA* 1988; 260(15):2259–63.
9. Freemantle N, Cleland J, Young P, et al. beta Blockade after myocardial infarction:systematic review and meta regression analysis. *BJM* 1999; 318(7200):1730–7.
10. Timolol-induced reduction in mortality and reinfarction in patients surviving acute myocardial infarction. *N Engl J Med* 1981; 304(14):801–7.
11. Hjalmarson A, Elmfeldt D, Herlitz J, et al. Effect on mortality of metoprolol in acute myocardial infarction. A double-blind randomised trial. *Lancet* 1981; 2(8251):823–7.
12. Beta Blocker Heart Attack Trial Research Group. A randomized trial of propranolol in patients with acute myocardial infarction. Mortality results. *JAMA* 1982; 247(12):1707–14.
13. Randomised trial of intravenous atenolol among 16 027 cases of suspected acute myocardial infarction: ISIS–1. First International Study of Infarct Survival Collaborative Group. *Lancet* 1986; 2(8498):57–66.
14. Hjalmarson A, Herlitz J, Holmberg S, et al. The Goteborg metoprolol trial. Effects on mortality and morbidity in acute myocardial infarction. *Circulation* 1983; 67(6):I26–32.
15. Yusuf S, Sleight P, Rossi P, et al. Reduction in infarct size, arrhythmias and chest pain by early intravenous beta blockade in suspected acute myocardial infarction. *Circulation* 1983; 67(6):I32–41.
16. Shivkumar K, Schultz L, Goldstein S, et al. Effects of propanolol in patients entered in the Beta-Blocker Heart Attack Trial with their first myocardial infarction and persistent electrocardiographic ST-segment depression. *Am Heart J* 1998; 135(2):261–7.
17. Chen ZM, Pan HC, Chen YP, Early intravenous then oral metoprolol in 45852 patients with acute myocardial infarction: randomised placebo-controlled trial COMMIT (ClOpidogrel and Metoprolol in Myocardial Infarction Trial). *Lancet* 2005; 366(9497):1622–32.
18. Anderson JL, Adams CD, Antman EM, et al. ACC/AHA 2007 Guidelines for the Management of Patients With Unstable Angina/Non-ST-Elevation Myocardial Infarction. *JACC* 2007; 50(7):e1–157.
19. Dargie HJ. Effect of carvedilol on outcome after myocardial infarction in patients with left-ventricular dysfunction: the CAPRICORN randomised trial. *Lancet* 2001; 537(9266):1385–90.
20. GISSI-3: Effects of lisinopril and transdermal glyceryl trinitrate singly and together on 6-week mortality and ventricular function after acute myocardial infarction. Gruppo Italiano per lo Studio della Sopravvivenza nell'infarto Miocardico. *Lancet* 1994; 343(8906):1115–22.
21. ISIS-4: A randomised factorial trial assessing early oral captopril, oral mononitrate, and intravenous magnesium sulphate in 58,050 patients with suspected acute myocardial infarction. ISIS–4 (Fourth International Study of Infarct Survival) Collaborative Group. *Lancet* 1995; 345(8951):669–85.
22. Oral captopril versus placebo among 13,634 patients with suspected acute myocardial infarction: Interim report from the Chinese Cardiac Study (CCS–1). *Lancet* 1995; 345(8951):686–7.
23. Swedberg K, Held P, Kjekshus J, et al. Effects of the early administration of enalapril on mortality in patients with acute myocardial infarction. Results of the Cooperative New Scandinavian Enalapril Survival Study II (CONSENSUS II). *N Engl J Med* 1992; 327(10):678–84.
24. Pfeffer MA, Braunwald E, Moyé LA, et al. Effect of captopril on mortality and morbidity in patients with left ventricular dysfunction after myocardial infarction. Results of the survival and ventricular enlargement trial. The SAVE Investigators. *N Engl J Med* 1992; 327(10):669–77.
25. Effect of ramipril on mortality and morbidity of survivors of acute myocardial infarction with clinical evidence of heart failure. The Acute Infarction Ramipril Efficacy (AIRE) Study Investigators. *Lancet* 1993; 342(8875):821–8.
26. KØber L, Torp-Pedersen C, Carlsen JE, et al. A clinical trial of the Angiotensin-Converting-Enzyme Inhibitor trandolapril in patients with left ventricular dysfunction after myocardial infarction. The Trandolapril Cardiac Evaluation (TRACE) study group. *N Engl J Med* 1995; 333(25):1670–6.
27. Yusuf S, Sleight P, Pogue J, et al. The Heart Outcomes Prevention Evaluation Study Investigators. Effects of an Angiotensin-Converting-Enzyme Inhibitor, Ramipril, on Death From Cardiovascular Causes, Myocardial Infarction, and Stroke in High-Risk Patients. *N Engl J Med* 2000; 342(3):145–53.
28. Pfeffer MA, McMurray JJ, Velazquez EJ, et al. Valsartan, Captopril, or Both in Myocardial Infarction Complicated by Heart Failure, Left Ventricular Dysfunction, or Both. *N Engl J Med* 2003; 349(20):1893–906.
29. Pitt B, Zannad F, Remme WJ, et al. The effect of spironolactone on morbidity on morbidity and mortality in patients with severe heart failure Randomized Aldactone Evlautation Study Investigators. *N Engl J Med* 1999; 341(10):709–17.
30. Pitt B, Remme W, Zannad F, et al. Eplerenone, a selective aldosterone blocker, in patients with left ventricular dysfunction after myocardial infarction. *N Engl J Med* 2003; 348, 1309–21.
31. Randomised trial of cholesterol lowering in 4444 patients with coronary heart disease: The Scandinavian Simvastatin Survival Study (4S). *Lancet* 1994; 344(14):1383–9.
32. Sacks FM, Pfeffer MA, Moye LA, et al. The effect of pravastatin on coronary events after myocardial infarction in patients with average cholesterol levels. Cholesterol and Recurrent Events Trial investigators. *N Engl J Med* 1996; 335(14):1001–9.
33. Prevention of cardiovascular events and death with pravastatin in patients with coronary heart disease and a broad range of initial cholesterol levels. The Long-Term Intervention with Pravastatin in Ischaemic Disease (LIPID) Study Group. *N Engl J Med* 1998; 339(19):1349–57.

34. Schwartz GG, Olsson AG, Ezekowitz MD, et al. Effects of atorvastatin on early recurrent ischemic events in acute coronary syndromes: the MIRACL study: A randomized controlled trial. *JAMA* 2001; 285(13):1711–8.
35. Cannon CP, Braunwald E, McCabe CH, et al. Intensive versus moderate lipid lowering with statins after acute coronary syndromes. *N Engl J Med* 2004; 350(15):1495–504.
36. Executive Summary of The Third Report of The National Cholesterol Education Program (NCEP) Expert Panel on Detection, Evaluation, And Treatment of High Blood Cholesterol In Adults (Adult Treatment Panel III). *JAMA* 2001; 285(19):2486–97.
37. Wilcox RG, Hampton JR, Banks DC, et al. Trial of early nifedipine in acute myocardial infarction: the TRENT study. *Br Med J* 1986; 293(6556):1204–8.
38. Secondary prevention reinfarction Israeli nifedipine trial (SPRINT). A randomized intervention trial of nifedipine in patients with acute myocardial infarction. The Israeli Sprint Study Group. *Eur Heart J* 1988; 9(4):354–64.
39. Muller JE, Morrison J, Stone PH, et al. Nifedipine therapy for patients with threatened and acute myocardial infarction: a randomized, double-blind, placebo-controlled comparison. *Circulation* 1984; 69(4):740–7.
40. Goldbourt U, Behar S, Reicher-Reiss H, et al. Early administration of nifedipine in suspected acute myocardial infarction: the Secondary Prevention Reinfarction Israeli Nifedipine Trial 2 Study. *Arch Intern Med* 1993; 153(3):345–53.
41. Ryan TJ, Anderson JL, Antman EM, et al. ACC/AHA guidelines for the management of patients with acute myocardial infarction. A report of the American College of Cardiology/American Heart Association Task Force on Practice Guidelines (Committee on Management of Acute Myocardial Infarction). *JACC* 1996; 28(5):1328–428.
42. Gibson RS, Boden WE, Theroux P, et al. Diltiazem and reinfarction in patients with non-Q-wave myocardial infarction. Results of a double-blind, randomized, multicenter trial. *N Engl J Med* 1986; 315(7):423–9.
43. The effect of diltiazem on mortality and reinfarction after myocardial infarction. The Multicenter Diltiazem Postinfarction Trial Research Group. *N Engl J Med* 1988; 319(7):385–92.
44. Boden WE, van Gilst WH, Scheldewaert RG, et al. Diltiazem in acute myocardial infarction treated with thrombolytic agents: a randomised placebo-controlled trial. Incomplete Infarction Trial of European Research Collaborators Evaluating Prognosis post-Thrombolysis (INTERCEPT). *Lancet* 2000; 355(9217):1751–6.
45. Effect of verapamil on mortality and major events after acute myocardial infarction (the Danish Verapamil Infarction Trial II—DAVIT II). *Am J Cardiol* 1990; 66(10):779–85.
46. Lewis HD, Davis JW, Archibald DG, et al. Protective effects of aspirin against acute myocardial infarction and death in men with unstable angina. Results of a Veterans Administration Cooperative Study. *N Engl J Med* 1983; 309(7):396–403.
47. Cairns JA, Gent M, Singer J, et al. Aspirin, sulfinpyrazone, or both in unstable angina. Results of a Canadian multicenter trial. *N Engl J Med* 1985; 313(22):1369–75.
48. Theroux P, Ouimet H, McCans J, et al. Aspirin, heparin, or both to treat acute unstable angina. *N Engl J Med* 1988; 319(17):1105–11.
49. Risk of myocardial infarction and death during treatment with low dose aspirin and intravenous heparin in men with unstable coronary artery disease. The RISC Group. *Lancet* 1990; 336(8719):827–30.
50. Randomised trial of intravenous streptokinase, oral aspirin, both, or neither among 17,187 cases of suspected acute myocardial infarction: ISIS–2. ISIS–2 (Second International Study of Infarct Survival) Collaborative Group. *Lancet* 1988; 2(8607):349–60.
51. Balsano F, Rizzon P, Violi F, et al. Antiplatelet treatment with ticlopidine in unstable angina. A controlled multicenter clinical trial. The Studio della Ticlopidina nell'Angina Instabile Group. *Circulation* 1990; 82(1):17–26.
52. Steinhubl SR, Tan WA, Foody JM, et al. Incidence and clinical course of thrombotic thrombocytopenic purpura due to ticlopidine following coronary stenting. EPISTENT Investigators. Evaluation of Platelet IIb/IIIa Inhibitor for Stenting. *JAMA* 1999; 281(9):806–10.
53. CAPRIE Steering Committee. A randomised, blinded, trial of clopidogrel versus aspirin in patients at risk of ischaemic events (CAPRIE). *Lancet* 1996; 348(9038):1329–39.
54. Yusuf S, Zhao F, Mehta SR, et al. Clopidogrel in Unstable Angina to Prevent Recurrent Events Trial Investigators. Effects of clopidogrel in addition to aspirin in patients with acute coronary syndromes without ST-segment elevation. *N Engl J Med* 2001; 345(7):494–502.
55. Mehta SR, Yusuf S, Peters R, et al. Effects of pretreatment with clopidogrel and aspirin followed by long-term therapy in patients undergoing percutaneous coronary intervention: the PCI-CURE study. *Lancet* 2001; 358(9281):527–33.
56. Yusuf S, Mehta SR, Zhao F, et al. Early and late effects of clopidogrel in patients with acute coronary syndromes. *Circulation* 2003; 107(7):966–72.
57. Steinhubl SR, Berger PB, Mann JT 3rd, et al. Early and sustained dual oral antiplatelet therapy following percutaneous coronary intervention: a randomized controlled trial. *JAMA* 2002; 288(19):2411–20.
58. Sabatine MS, Cannon CP, Gibson CM, et al, for the CLARITY-TIMI 28 investigators. Addition of clopidogrel to aspirin and fibrinolytic therapy for myocardial infarction with ST-segment elevation. *N Engl J Med* 2005; 352(12):1179–89.
59. Chen ZM, Jiang LX, Chen YP, et al. COMMIT (ClOpidogrel and Metoprolol in Myocardial Infarction Trial) collaborative group. Addition of clopidogrel to aspirin in 45,852 patients with acute myocardial infarction: randomised placebo-controlled trial. *Lancet* 2005; 366(9497):1607–21.
60. Sabatine MS, Cannon CP, Gibson CM, et al. Effect of clopidogrel pretreatment before percutaneous coronary intervention in patients with ST-elevation myocardial infarction treated with fibrinolytics. The PCI-CLARITY study. *JAMA* 2005; 294(10):1224–32.
61. Patti G, Colonna G, Pasceri V, et al. Randomized trial of high loading dose of clopidogrel for reduction of periprocedural myocardial infarction in patients undergoing coronary intervention results from the ARMYDA-2 (Antiplatelet therapy for Reduction of MYocardial Damage during Angioplasty) Study. *Circulation* 2005; 111(16):2099–106.
62. Von Beckerath N, Taubert D, Pogatsa-Murray G, et al. Absorption, Metabolization, and Antiplatelet Effects of 300-, 600-, and 900-mg Loading Doses of Clopidogrel. Results of the ISAR-CHOICE (Intracoronary Stenting and Antithrombotic Regimen: Choose Between 3 High Oral Doses for Immediate Clopidogrel Effect) Trial. *Circulation* 2005; 112(19):2946–50.

63. Antman EM, Hand M, Armstrong PW, et al. 2007 Focused Update of the ACC/AHA 2004 guidelines for the Management of Patients with ST-Elevation Myocardial Infacrtion. *Circulation* 2008; 117(2):296–329.
64 Wiviott SD, Trenk D, Frelinger AL, et al. Prasugrel compared with high loading- and maintenance-dose clopidogrel in patients with planned percutaneous coronary intervention: the Prasugrel in comparison to clopidogrel for inhibition of platelet activation and aggregation-thrombolysis in myocardial infarction 44 trial. *Circulation* 2007: 116(25):2923-32.
65 Wiviott SD, Braunwald E, McCabe CH, et al. Prasugrel versus clopidogrel in patients with acute coronary syndromes. *N Engl J Med* 2007; 357(20):2001-15.
66. Oler A, Whooley MA, Oler J, et al. Adding heparin to aspirin reduces the incidence of myocardial infarction and death in patients with unstable angina. A meta-analysis. *JAMA* 1996; 276(10):811–15.
67. Cohen M, Adams PC, Parry G, et al. Combination antithrombotic therapy in unstable rest angina and non-Q-wave infarction in nonprior aspirin users. Primary end points analysis from the ATACS trial. Antithrombotic Therapy in Acute Coronary Syndromes Research Group. *Circulation* 1994; 89(1):81–8.
68. Eikelboom JW, Anand SS, Malmberg K, et al. Unfractionated heparin and low-molecular-weight heparin in acute coronary syndrome without ST elevation: a meta-analysis. *Lancet* 2000; 355(9219):1936–42.
69. Low-molecular-weight heparin during instability in coronary artery disease, Fragmin during Instability in Coronary Artery Disease (FRISC) study group. *Lancet* 1996; 347(9001):561–8.
70. Klein W, Buchwald A, Hillis SE, et al. Comparison of low-molecular-weight heparin with unfractionated heparin acutely and with placebo for 6 weeks in the management of unstable coronary artery disease. Fragmin in unstable coronary artery disease study (FRIC). *Circulation* 1997; 96(1):61–8.
71. Comparison of two treatment durations (6 days and 14 days) of a low molecular weight heparin with a 6-day treatment of unfractionated heparin in the initial management of unstable angina or non-Q wave myocardial infarction: FRAX.I.S. (FRAxiparine in Ischaemic Syndrome). *Eur Heart J* 1999; 20(21):1553–62.
72. Antman EM, Cohen M, Radley D, et al. Assessment of the treatment effect of enoxaparin for unstable angina/non-Q-wave myocardial infarction. TIMI 11B-ESSENCE meta-analysis. *Circulation* 1999; 100(15):1602–8.
73. Murphy SA, Gibson CM, Morrow DA, et al. Efficacy and safety of the low-molecular weight heparin enoxaparin compared with unfractionated heparin across the acute coronary syndrome spectrum: a meta-analysis. *Eur Heart J* 2007; 28(17):2077–86.
74. Goodman SG, Fitchett D, Armstrong PW, et al. Randomized evaluation of the safety and efficacy of enoxaparin versus unfractionated heparin in high-risk patients with non-ST-segment elevation acute coronary syndromes receiving the glycoprotein IIb/IIIa inhibitor eptifibatide. *Circulation* 2003; 107(2):238–44.
75. Blazing MA, de Lemos JA, White HD, et al. Safety and efficacy of enoxaparin vs unfractionated heparin in patients with non-ST-segment elevation acute coronary syndromes who receive tirofiban and aspirin: a randomized controlled trial. *JAMA* 2004; 292(1):55–64.
76. Ferguson JJ, Califf RM, Antman EM, et al. Enoxaparin vs unfractionated heparin in high-risk patients with non-ST-segment elevation acute coronary syndromes managed with an intended early invasive strategy: primary results of the SYNERGY randomized trial. *JAMA* 2004; 292(1):45–54.
77. Assessment of the Safety and Efficacy of a New Thrombolytic Regimen (ASSENT)-3 Investigators. Efficacy and safety of tenecteplase in combination with enoxaparin, abciximab, or unfractionated heparin: the ASSENT-3 randomised trial in acute myocardial infarction. *Lancet* 2001; 358(9282):605–13.
78. Michalis LK, Katsouras CS, Papamichael N, et al. Enoxaparin versus tinzaparin in non-ST-segment elevation acute coronary syndromes: the EVET trial. *Am Heart J* 2003; 146(2):304–10.
79. Yusuf S, Mehta SR, Chrolavicius S, et al. Comparison of Fondaparinux and Enoxaparin in Acute Coronary Syndromes. *N Engl J Med* 2006; 354(14):1464–76.
80. A comparison of recombinant hirudin with heparin for the treatment of acute coronary syndromes. The Global Use of Strategies to Open Occluded Coronary Arteries (GUSTO) IIb investigators. *N Engl J Med* 1996; 335(11):775–82.
81. Effects of recombinant hirudin (lepirudin) compared with heparin on death, myocardial infarction, refractory angina, and revascularisation procedures in patients with acute myocardial ischaemia without ST elevation: A randomised trial. Organisation to Assess Strategies for Ischemic Syndromes (OASIS-2) Investigators. *Lancet* 1999; 353(9151):429–38.
82. Serruys PW, Herrman JP, Simon R, et al. A comparison of hirudin with heparin in the prevention of restenosis after coronary angioplasty. Helvetica Investigators. *N Engl J Med* 1995; 333(12):757–63.
83. Mehta SR, Eikelboom JW, Rupprecht HJ, et al. Efficacy of hirudin in reducing cardiovascular events in patients with acute coronary syndrome undergoing early percutaneous coronary intervention. *Eur Heart J* 2002; 23(2):117–23.
84. Antman EM. Hirudin in Acute Myocardial Infarction. Thrombolysis and Thrombin Inhibition in Myocardial Infarction (TIMI) 9B Trial. *Circulation* 1996; 94(5):911–21.
85. White HD, Aylward PE, Frey MJ, et al. Randomized, Double-blind Comparison of Hirulog Versus Heparin in Patients Receiving Streptokinase and Aspirin for Acute Myocardial Infarction (HERO). *Circulation* 1997; 96(7):2155–61.
86. White H. Thrombin-specific anticoagulation with bivalirudin versus heparin in patients receiving fibrinolytic therapy for acute myocardial infarction: the HERO-2 randomised trial. *Lancet* 2001; 358(9296):1855–63.
87. Fuchs J and Cannon CP. Hirulog in the treatment of unstable angina. Results of the Thrombin Inhibition in Myocardial Ischemia (TIMI) 7 trial. *Circulation* 1995; 92(4):727–33.
88. Bittl JA, Chaitman BR, Feit F, et al. Bivalirudin versus heparin during coronary angioplasty for unstable or postinfarction angina: Final report reanalysis of the Bivalirudin Angioplasty Study. *Am Heart J* 2001; 142(6):952–9.
89. Lincoff AM, Bittl JA, Harrington RA, et al. Bivalirudin and provisional glycoprotein IIb/IIIa blockade compared with heparin and planned glycoprotein IIb/IIIa blockade during percutaneous coronary intervention: REPLACE-2 randomized trial. *JAMA* 2003; 289(7):853–63.
90. Stone GW, McLaurin BT, Cox DA, et al. Bivalirudin for patients with acute coronary syndromes. *N Engl J Med* 2006; 355(21):2203–16.

91. Stone GW, Witzenbichler B, Guagliumi G, et al. Bivalirudin during Primary PCI in Acute Myocardial Infarction. *N Engl J Med* 2008; 358(21):2218–30.
92. A comparison of aspirin plus tirofiban with aspirin plus heparin for unstable angina. Platelet Receptor Inhibition in Ischemic Syndrome Management (PRISM) Study Investigators. *N Engl J Med* 1998; 338(21):1498–1505.
93. Inhibition of the platelet glycoprotein IIb/IIIa receptor with tirofiban in unstable angina and non-Q-wave myocardial infarction. Platelet Receptor Inhibition in Ischemic Syndrome Management in Patients Limited by Unstable Signs and Symptoms (PRISM-PLUS) Study Investigators. *N Engl J Med* 1998; 338(21):1488–97.
94. Effects of Platelet Glycoprotein IIb/IIIa Blockade With Tirofiban on Adverse Cardiac Events in Patients With Unstable Angina or Acute Myocardial Infarction Undergoing Coronary Angioplasty. The RESTORE Investigators. *Circulation* 1997; 96(5):1445–53.
95. Inhibition of platelet glycoprotein IIb/IIIa with eptifibatide in patients with acute coronary syndromes. The PURSUIT Trial Investigators. Platelet Glycoprotein IIb/IIIa in Unstable Angina: Receptor Suppression Using Integrilin Therapy. *N Engl J Med* 1998; 339(7):436–43.
96. Randomized placebo-controlled trial of effect of eptifibatide on complications of percutaneous coronary intervention: IMPACT-II. Integrilin to minimize platelet aggregation and coronary thrombosis-II. *Lancet* 1997; 349(9063):1422–8.
97. Novel dosing regimen of eptifibatide in planned coronary stent implantation (ESPRIT): a randomized, placebo-controlled trial. *Lancet* 2000; 356(9247):2037–44.
98. Ohman EM, Kleiman NS, Gacioch G, et al. Combined accelerated tissue-plasminogen activator and platelet glycoprotein IIb/IIIa integrin receptor blockade with Integrilin in acute myocardial infarction. Results of a randomized, placebo-controlled, dose-ranging trial. IMPACT-AMI Investigators. *Circulation* 1997; 95(4):846–54.
99. Topol EJ. Reperfusion therapy for acute myocardial infarction with fibrinolytic therapy or combination reduced fibrinolytic therapy and platelet glycoprotein IIb/IIIa inhibition: the GUSTO V randomised trial. *Lancet* 2001; 357(9272):1905–14.
100. Efficacy and safety of tenecteplase in combination with enoxaparin, abciximab, or unfractionated heparin: the ASSENT-3 randomised trial in acute myocardial infarction. *Lancet* 2001; 358(9282):605–13.
101 The CAPTURE study. Randomised placebo-controlled trial of abciximab before and during coronary intervention in refractory unstable angina: the CAPTURE study. *Lancet* 1997; 349(9063):1429–35.
102. Use of a monoclonal antibody directed against the platelet glycoprotein IIb/IIIa receptor in high risk coronary angioplasty. The EPIC Investigation. *N Engl J Med* 1994; 330(14):956–61.
103. Simoons ML. Effect of glycoprotein IIb/IIIa receptor blocker abciximab on outcome in patients with acute coronary syndromes without early coronary revascularisation: The GUSTO IV-ACS randomised trial. *Lancet* 2001; 357(9272):1915–24.
104. Kastrati A, Mehilli J, Neumann FJ, et al. Abciximab in Patients With Acute Coronary Syndromes Undergoing Percutaneous Coronary Intervention After Clopidogrel Pretreatment. *JAMA* 2006; 295(13):1531–8.
105. Effectiveness of intravenous thrombolytic treatment in acute myocardial infarction. Gruppo Italiano per lo Studio della Streptochinasi nell'Infarto Miocardico (GISSI). *Lancet* 1986; 1(8478):397–402.
106. Van de Werf F and Arnold AE. Intravenous tissue plasminogenactivator and size of infarct, left ventricular function, and survival in acute myocardial infarction. *Br Med J* 1988; 297(6660):1374–9.
107. The GUSTO Investigators. An international randomized trial comparing four thrombolytic strategies for acute myocardial infarction. *N Engl J Med* 1993; 329(10):673–82.
108. A comparison of reteplase with alteplase for acute myocardial infarction. The Global Use of Strategies to Open Occluded Coronary Arteries (GUSTO III) Investigators. *N Engl J Med* 1997; 337(16):1118–23.
109. Randomised, double-blind comparison of reteplase double-bolus administration with streptokinase in acute myocardial infarction (INJECT): trial to investigate equivalence. International Joint Efficacy Comparison of Throm, bolytics. *Lancet* 1995; 346(8971):329–36.
110. Cannon CP, Gibson CM, McCabe CH, et al. TNK-tissue plasminogen activator compared with front-loaded alteplase in acute myocardial infarction:results of the TIMI 10B trial. Thrombolysis in Myocardial Infarction (TIMI) 10B Investigators. *Circulation* 1998; 98(25):2805–14.
111. Van De Werf F, Adgey J, Ardissino D, et al. Single-bolus tenecteplase compared with front-loaded alteplase in acute myocardial infarction: the ASSENT-2 double-blind randomised trial. Assessment of the Safety and Efficacy of a New Thrombolytic Investigators. *Lancet* 1999; 354(9180):716–22.
112. Invasive compared with non-invasive treatment in unstable coronary-artery disease: FRISC II prospective randomised multicentre study. FRagmin and Fast Revascularisation during InStability in Coronary artery disease Investigators. *Lancet*, 1999; 354(9180):708–15.
113. Wallentin B, Lagerqvist B, Husted S, et al. Outcome at 1 year after an invasive compared with a non-invasive strategy in unstable coronary-artery disease: the FRISC II invasive randomised trial. *Lancet* 2000; 356(9223):9–16.
114. Lagerqvist B, Husted S, Kontny F, et al. 5-year outcomes in the FRISC-II randomized trial of an invasive versus a non-invasive strategy in non-ST-elevation acute coronary syndrome: a follow-up study. *Lancet* 2006; 368(9540):998–1004.
115. Fox KA, Poole-Wilson PA, Henderson RA, et al, for the Randomized Intervention Trial of unstable Angina (RITA) investigators. Interventional Versus Conservative Treatment for Patients With Unstable Angina or Non-ST-Elevation Myocardial Infarction: the British Heart Foundation RITA 3 Randomised Trial. Randomized Intervention Trial of unstable Angina. *Lancet* 2002; 360(9335):743–51.
116. Fox KA, Poole-Wilson P, Clayton TC, et al. 5-year outcome of an interventional strategy in non-ST-elevation acute coronary syndrome: the British Heart Foundation RITA 3 randomised trial. *Lancet* 2005; 366(9489):914–20.
117. Neumann FJ, Kastrati A, Pogatsa-Murray G, et al. Evaluation of Prolonged Antithrombotic Pretreatment ("Cooling-Off" Strategy) Before Intervention in Patients With Unstable Coronary Syndromes. *JAMA* 2003; 290(12):1593–9.
118. Mehta SR, Cannon CP, Fox KA, et al. Routine vs selective invasive strategies in patients with acute coronary syndromes: a collaborative meta-analysis of randomized trials. *JAMA* 2005; 293(23):2908–17.

119. Bavry AA, Kumbhani DJ, Rassi AN, et al. Benefit of early invasive therapy in acute coronary syndromes: a meta-analysis of contemporary randomized clinical trials. *JACC* 2006; 48(7):1319–25.
120. de Winter RJ, Windhausen F, Cornel JH, et al. Early Invasive versus Selectively Invasive Management for Acute Coronary Syndromes. *N Engl J Med* 2005; 353(11):1095–104.
121. Mark DB, Hlatky MA, Harrell FE Jr, et al.Exercise treadmill score for predicting prognosis in coronary artery disease. *Ann Intern Med* 1987:106(6):793–800.
122. Shaw LJ, Peterson ED, Shaw LK, et al. Use of a prognostic treadmill score in identifying diagnostic coronary disease subgroups. *Circulation* 1998:98(16):1622–30.
123. Grines CL, Browne KF, Marco J, et al. A comparison of immediate angioplasty with thrombolytic therapy for acute myocardial infarction. *N Engl J Med* 1993; 328(10):673–9.
124. Keeley EC, Boura JA, Grines CL, et al. Primary angioplasty versus intravenous thrombolytic therapy for acute myocardial infarction: a quantitative review of 23 randomised trials. *Lancet* 2003; 361(9351):13–20.
125. Andersen HR, Nielsen TT, Rasmussen K, et al., for the DANAMI-2 Investigators. A comparison of coronary angioplasty with fibrinolytic therapy in acute myocardial infarction. *N Engl J Med* 2003; 349(8):733–42.
126. Widimsky P, Budesínský T, Vorác D, et al., for the PRAGUE Study Group Investigators. Long distance transport for primary angioplasty vs. immediate thrombolysis in acute myocardial infarction. Final results of the randomized national multicentre trial PRAGUE-2. *Eur Heart J* 2003; 24(1):94–104.
127. Hochman JS, Sleeper LA, Webb JG, et al. Early revascularization in acute myocardial infarction complicated by cardiogenic shock. *N Engl J Med* 1999; 341(9):625–34.
128. The TIMI Study Group. Comparison of invasive and conservative strategies after treatment with intravenous tissue plasminogen activator in acute myocardial infarction: results of the thrombolysis in myocardial infarction (TIMI) phase II trial. *N Engl J Med* 1989; 320(10):618–27.
129. Terrin ML, Williams DO, Kleiman NS, et al. Two- and three-year results of the Thrombolysis in Myocardial Infarction (TIMI) Phase II clinical trial. *J Am Coll Cardiol* 1993; 22(7):1763–72.

3 Percutaneous Coronary Intervention in the Modern Era

HASAN A. AHMAD
ROBERT M. MINUTELLO

OUTLINE

More than one million percutaneous coronary interventions (PCI) are performed annually in the United States. This number illustrates the remarkable adoption of this procedure in modern cardiology practice and its evolution since it was first performed in 1977 by Andreas Gruentzig. While angioplasty was initially a treatment option for isolated proximal coronary artery lesions, the development of stents, improvement in operator techniques, and advances in adjunctive pharmacotherapy expanded its application to more complex lesions. Moreover, drug-eluting stents (DES) heralded in a new era of PCI with a broad adoption of PCI across the clinical spectrum of coronary artery disease (CAD). Currently, several issues confront the practice of PCI and promising innovations offer the potential for further improvement. Given significant improvements in medical therapy for CAD over the last decade, the appropriate role of PCI in stable coronary disease is unclear. Modern PCI techniques have allowed treatment of multivessel and complex CAD previously amenable only to coronary artery bypass surgery. The goal of this chapter is to provide an overview of the key challenges facing PCI and the potential of new innovations to further improve the clinical application of this procedure.

■ PCI AND STABLE CORONARY ARTERY DISEASE

Over 13 million people have CAD in the United States with at least half having some degree of angina pectoris. For chronic stable CAD, current ACC/AHA guidelines recommend PCI for symptom relief after failure of medical therapy as well as for select patients with a large ischemic burden associated with single or two-vessel CAD. These recommendations are based on studies designed prior to advances in modern medical therapy. The majority of these studies have demonstrated that PCI in stable CAD predominantly relieves angina,

definite, demonstrable benefit on cardiac). Moreover, a recent meta-analysis comparing PCI (including angioplasty and bare metal stents) to medical therapy similarly concluded that in patients with chronic stable CAD, PCI does not offer any benefit in terms of death and myocardial infarction (2).

Few of these trials, however, used modern interventional techniques or adjunctive pharmacotherapy. Given the limitations of these data, a modern trial comparing optimal medical therapy versus optimal medical therapy and contemporary PCI was formulated. The Clinical Outcomes Utilizing Revascularization and Aggressive Drug Evaluation (COURAGE) trial analyzed 2287 patients with stable angina who received state of the art medical therapy and were randomized to either PCI or an initial noninterventional strategy. After a median follow-up of 4.6 years, there was no benefit with PCI with respect to death or myocardial infarction (19.0% in the PCI group and 18.5% in the medical-therapy group, P = NS), but rates of freedom from angina favored PCI throughout the study (3). COURAGE, however, excluded patients with severe angina (CCS IV) or a markedly positive stress test and although a majority of patients had multivessel disease, most received only one stent suggesting incomplete revascularization. Moreover, patients were randomized after screening coronary angiography, which may have introduced inherent selection bias for angiographically less severe disease. In contrast to COURAGE, a recent meta-analysis from the Duke registry with 18,481 patients demonstrated that PCI as initial therapy was superior to medical therapy in low-severity CAD, conferring a survival benefit (4).

There are several plausible explanations for the findings seen in COURAGE. Advances in medical therapy, especially the use of statins, have had a dramatic effect on risk factor modification. The reduction in cardiac events by 16% by statins alone may reduce the additive benefits from PCI and alter the natural progression of CAD. Next, the degree of ischemia in COURAGE patients may have determined the degree of benefit from PCI, as there is a trend for improved hard outcomes in symptomatic patients with demonstrable ischemia on imaging studies such as exercise scintigraphy. In the COURAGE nuclear substudy, PCI treated patients had significant ischemia reduction and lower risk for death or MI, particularly if baseline ischemia was moderate to severe (5). This finding echoes the SWISSI II trial, where treatment with PCI in patients with proven silent ischemia demonstrated a reduction of cardiac and total mortality (6). Recently, the FAME study investigators showed that reduced fractional flow reserve may be another tool to help guide ischemia-driven revascularization with PCI. The use of this device during PCI to determine lesion hemodynamic significance may result in an overall reduction in hard clinical end points (7). All of these findings clearly suggest the need to demonstrate significant ischemia in order to fully benefit from PCI. Lastly, the vast minority of patients in COURAGE did not receive DES, which have repeatedly shown to reduce cardiac events across clinical trials and registries.

In summary, the failure of medical therapy, a history of recent MI (<3 months), demonstration of significant inducible ischemia, detection of unequivocally reduced fractional flow reserve, or the presence of specific angiographic features of coronary stenoses should guide utilization of PCI in patients with stable coronary lesions (8).

■ PCI FOR ACUTE CORONARY SYNDROMES

Acute coronary syndromes (ACS) encompass the clinical scenarios of unstable angina (USA), non-ST-elevation myocardial infarction (NSTEMI) and ST-elevation infarction (STEMI), and together account for approximately 2.5 million hospital discharges annually. For USA/NSTEMI, multiple risk assessment scores, such as GRACE and TIMI, attempt to quantify risk according to patients' clinical characteristics (9,10). Numerous trials and meta analyses have shown that patients with high risk scores (i.e., GRACE ≥89, TIMI ≥4) benefit most from an early invasive strategy, in particular those with positive cardiac biomarkers and/or ST-segment changes (11–13).

For STEMI, primary PCI is superior to fibrinolysis based on multiple trials (14) and the benefits of reperfusion therapy are time dependent (15,16) and greatest in those at high risk (17). Contemporary PCI guidelines emphasize primary PCI within 90 minutes of first medical contact (18) and successful primary PCI depends on operator and hospital expertise (19). Routine facilitated PCI for STEMI has been shown to be of no benefit (20) and may potentially be harmful; however, a pharmaco-invasive strategy using rescue PCI after failed fibrinolysis or within 3 to 24 hours of successful fibrinolysis has been shown to reduce recurrent MI and mortality (21,22). Hospital quality performance measures (23) have emphasized early reperfusion therapy in STEMI in an attempt to reduce overall door-to-balloon/door-to-reperfusion times.

In summary, patients with ACS comprising USA and NSTEMI should be risk stratified with TIMI or GRACE scores and moderate to high-risk patients should be treated with an early invasive strategy (24). For STEMI patients at a facility with appropriate expertise and resources, reperfusion with primary PCI should be performed within 90 minutes. Moreover, patients treated with fibrinolytics have been shown to benefit from a routine invasive strategy after thrombolytic therapy and should be transferred early to a PCI equipped hospital.

■ DRUG-ELUTING STENTS AND BARE METAL STENTS

Coronary bare metal stents (BMS) were introduced in 1993 and significantly reduced the procedural complication rates of percutaneous transluminal balloon angioplasty (PTCA) such as acute and subacute vessel closure, intimal dissection, elastic recoil of the vessel wall and reduced angioplasty-related restenosis rates. The Stent Restenosis Study (STRESS) and the Belgium Netherlands Stent (BENESTENT) trials were landmark BMS studies and enrolled patients with discrete stenoses in large-caliber vessels (25,26). Angiographic restenosis rates were 31.6% and 22%, respectively, and rates of in-stent restenosis as defined by the need for repeat revascularization of the target vessel were 10.2% and 13.5%, which compared favorably to restenosis rates of 30% to 60% after balloon angioplasty.

DES introduced in 2003 were celebrated as a major breakthrough given a significant reduction of in-stent restenosis observed with this technology. Restenosis after stenting is due to a neointimal proliferative response that begins shortly after the mechanical trauma of stent deployment and endothelial injury. In approximately 20% of cases this normal healing response is pronounced, resulting in lumen compromise and restenosis, defined in binary fashion as greater than 50% renarrowing. The response typically occurs within six to nine months after stent deployment. DES prevents in-stent restenosis mainly by inhibiting smooth muscle cell activation and proliferation. A DES consists of a metal stent platform, a pharmacological agent, and a biocompatible polymer designed to control release of this drug over time. The ideal agent must safely exert sufficient antirestenotic effects while maintaining a wide enough therapeutic index at the site of implantation to allow for eventual stent endothelialization and adequate vessel healing. The two antiproliferative agents studied most extensively in human clinical trials are sirolimus and paclitaxel, the former acts via inhibition of cell growth and proliferation by arresting the cell cycle and the latter by stabilizing microtubules which arrests mitosis and cell proliferation. The original sirolimus-eluting Cypher and the paclitaxel-eluting Taxus stents have been joined by newer compounds and stents such as the zotarolimus-eluting Endeavor and the everolimus-eluting Xience/Promus stents, both of whose pharmacologic agents work mechanistically similar to sirolimus.

Pivotal trials of DES such as SIRIUS, TAXUS, ENDEAVOR, and SPIRIT found rates of revascularization in target lesions of 3% to 6%, which reflects a 75% relative reduction in restenosis compared with BMS (27–30). Long-term analysis from the Cypher and Taxus studies have shown a fairly consistent overall reduction of clinical events related to restenosis and at the same time have potentially identified a small risk of late stent thrombosis for both products. (Table 3.1 lists technical factors related to stenting which may contribute to thrombosis in DES.) This is particularly true in patients who do not continue dual antiplatelet therapy. Stent thrombosis is defined as an abrupt onset of an ACS accompanied by biochemical and or electrocardiographic evidence of myocardial injury and confirmed with angiographic evidence of a flow-limiting thrombus near a previously placed stent. Angiography may not be always possible and a clinical impression of stent thrombosis is a reasonable surrogate (Table 3.2). Several large scale studies have shown that acute (within 24 hours) and subacute (within 2–30 days) stent thrombosis for DES is similar to BMS ranging from 0.6% to 1.4% as long as dual antiplatelet therapy is continued uninterrupted (31,32). Early stent thrombosis is a multi-factorial but is likely primarily related to technical aspects of stent implantation (33). Late thrombotic events are very rare with BMS. Stent thrombosis, when it occurs, is serious, often manifested by acute myocardial infarction or death.

Initial anecdotal reports of subacute stent thrombosis first surfaced after introduction of the Cypher stent in 2003 when 360 cases (out of a total 575,000 stents implanted) were reported. However, a significant risk of late stent thrombosis (30 days to one year) (LST) and very late stent thrombosis (after one year) (VLST) became evident. Late BMS thrombosis is uncommon (<1%), occurs at a mean of 2.4 to 3.6 months and is rare beyond 6 months. LST was first described with the use of intracoronary radiation therapy (34–36). In DES, LST is frequently related to interruption or premature termination of dual antiplatelet therapy. A meta-analysis of 14 clinical trials (37) with longer follow-up noted that the incidence of very late thrombosis (VLST) of DES (occurring after one year, after the index procedure) was 0.5% compared with 0.28% in those who received BMS ($P = 0.22$). Although the event rate was not statistically significant, the median time for thrombosis in the DES group was 18 months compared with 3.5 months for the BMS group. LST after 6 months was four times higher in the DES group compared with BMS (0.44% versus 0.06%, $P = 0.014$) and at 12 months or beyond was 0.5% for the DES group compared with no events in the BMS group. Newer data, however, including a large recent meta analysis have suggested that there is no appreciable difference in rates of stent thrombosis with a significant improvement in overall outcomes of DES versus BMS (38,39).

The exact mechanism of late stent thrombosis in DES is multi-factorial and includes factors related to inflammation, endothelial injury and incomplete healing. One million DES have been deployed worldwide

Table 3.1 Factors related to stent thrombosis

Stent design
• Polymer coating
• Strut design and composition
• Pharmacologic agent
Procedural characteristics
• Stent underexpansion / malapposition
• Poor epicardial blood flow
• Vessel dissection / thrombosis
Clinical considerations
• Acute coronary syndrome
• Plaque morphology
• Vessel size / lesion length

Table 3.2 Stent thrombosis definition

Academic Research Consortium Definitions	
• Define ST	Acute coronary syndrome with angiographic or autoposy evidence of thrombus or occle
• Probable ST	Unexcepted death within 30 days following PCI or acute MI involving the target vessel territory without angiographic confirmation
• Possible ST	All unexplained deaths occurring at least 30 days following PCI
Temporal classification	
• Acute ST	During PCI or within 24 hours
• Subacute ST	Between 1 and 30 days following PCI
• Late ST	Between 1 month and 1 year following PCI
• Very late ST	More than 1 year following PCI

Abbreviations: PCI, percutaneous coronary intervention; ST, stent thrombosis.

and are used in the majority of PCIs where stents are deployed in a patient population quiet different from those enrolled in DES trials. Factors such as risk of restenosis, risk of bleeding, and the potential need for discontinuing clopidogrel should be considered prior to DES implantation. Patients in whom a BMS should be considered include:

1. Those with a very low risk of restenosis—restenosis requiring revascularization within 9 months is unlikely (4–10%) if a BMS is implanted in a *de novo* lesion in a native vessel, the lesion is not ostial or at a bifurcation, the artery has a reference diameter of at least 3.5 mm, the lesion length is less than 10 mm, and the patient does not have diabetes.
2. Patients with a bleeding condition who cannot take antiplatelet therapy long term.
3. Patients who undergo percutaneous coronary revascularization before undergoing a surgical procedure and who will need to interrupt their antiplatelet drugs before surgery.

Utilization of DESs may yield better results in the following scenarios:

4. Lesion characteristics such as diffuse disease, medium to small vessel diameter (<3.0 mm), ostial lesions, in-stent restenosis, and saphenous vein grafts.
5. Patients with diabetes.

In cases where DES are preferred, IVUS guidance to optimize stent deployment should be strongly considered, especially in anatomically critical or complex lesions.

Patient selection is crucial in reducing rates of stent thrombosis. The SCAAR registry initially showed increased rates of stent thrombosis with DES; however, as practice patterns changed, this increase disappeared and there was no difference in stent thrombosis between DES and BMS (38). Nevertheless, given these findings, the duration of dual antiplatelet therapy with clopidogrel and aspirin is recommended for at least 12 months.

PCI FOR MULTIVESSEL DISEASE AND COMPLEX LESIONS

Given advances in endovascular therapeutic technologies, PCI is now performed across nearly the full spectrum of clinical and angiographic scenarios. In terms of angiographic variables, multivessel disease remains an important topic and its relevance is paramount in studies comparing PCI to CABG. Since the 1980s, 11 randomized trials involving patients with multivessel CAD have been performed. RITA, GABI, CABRI, EAST and BARI assessed the results of balloon angioplasty versus CABG while ERACI II, ARTS, SOS, MASS-II, and AWESOME compared PCI with bare metal stenting and CABG. Pooled analysis among these trials shows no difference in the frequency of death or myocardial infarction (MI) between the two treatment modalities, but higher rates of repeat revascularization in patients receiving PCI (40). Several issues impact the performance of PCI in these trials, including the fact that utilization of antiplatelet and lipid lowering therapy was suboptimal. Moreover, stroke was routinely not included as an endpoint (which would have favored PCI) and follow up was too short to assess the impact of late graft occlusion. The ARTS II and ERACI III trials utilized DES, and both showed comparable result between DES and CABG (41,42). The most recent and influential trial utilizing DES and comparing CABG to PCI in multivessel disease is the SYNTAX trial (43). The SYNTAX trial is the first to quantify the degree of anatomic complexity using a number, the "SYNTAX SCORE," and utilize this variable as a predictor for outcomes (44). One year results showed that there were comparable overall safety outcomes (Death, CVA, MI,) in CABG and PCI patients at 12 months (7.7% versus 7.6 %). Symptomatic graft occlusion and stent thrombosis were similar but there was a significantly higher rate of revascularization in the PCI group (13.5% versus 5.9 %), and a significantly higher rate of CVA in the CABG group (2.2% versus 0.6%). Based on the available data, PCI appears to be an acceptable option for patients with multivessel disease, especially in patients with lower SYNTAX scores. This angiographic score, along with clinical variables, should guide physicians to the more appropriate, patient-specific revascularization strategy.

PCI FOR LEFT MAIN DISEASE

A significant left main stenosis (LMS), defined as a lesion with >50% stenosis, is present in 4% to 6% of all patients undergoing coronary angiography and in 30% of CABG patients. Given its proximal location and large diameter, it presents itself as an attractive target for PCI. However, LMS occurs as an isolated lesion only 6% to 9% of the time, contains significant calcification 50% of the time and is accompanied by multivessel disease 70% to 80% of the time. The majority of lesions occur in the distal segment of the artery (Figure 3.1), resulting in bifurcated or trifurcated lesions which are technically challenging and also have a relatively higher rate of restenosis. CABG for LMS has long been the standard of care and the current ACC/AHA guidelines state that PCI for left main stem stenosis is a class III indication. However, the use of PCI in LMS has increased with the advent of DES, and a recent survey indicated that LMS was treated with PCI in 29% of European and 18% of U.S. patients (45). Much of the rationale behind CABG as the standard of care for LMS is based on surgical data from the past three decades, much of which involves patients who received suboptimal medical therapy and/or received angioplasty without stenting

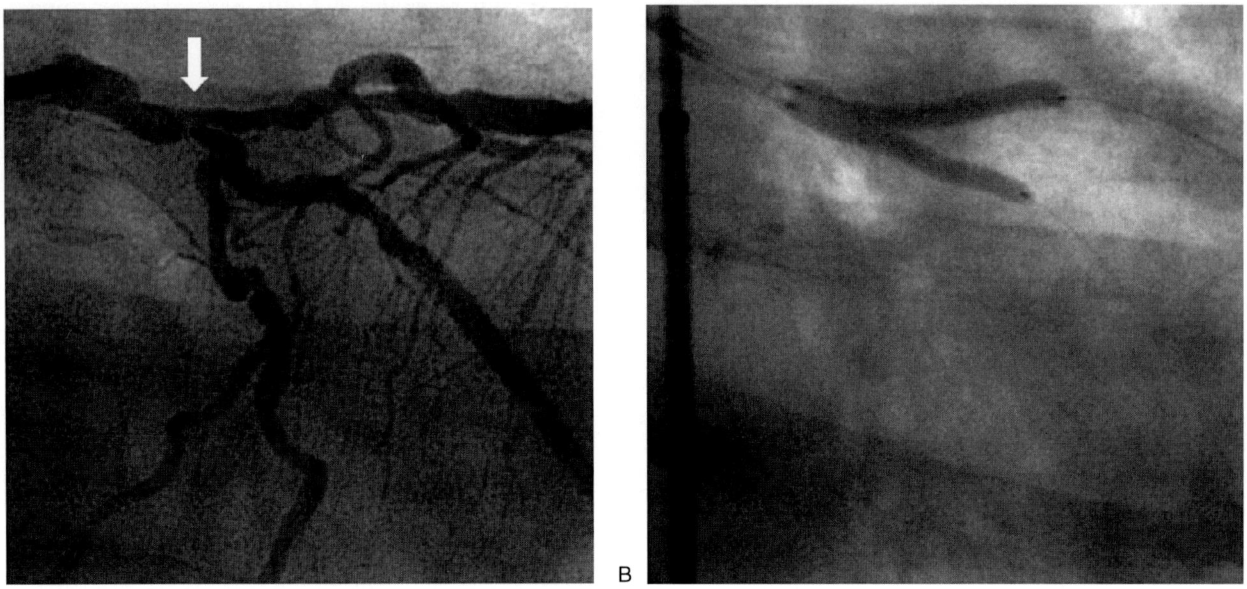

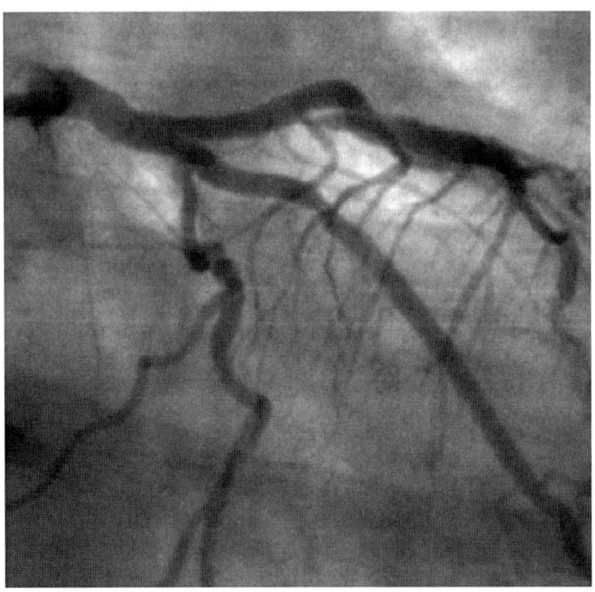

FIGURE 3.1 Serial angiograms of a patient with a non-STEMI and high-grade left main disease at the bifurcation (A, arrow) who was deemed clinically not to be a surgical candidate and whose SYNTAX score was high at 38. Two stents are simultaneously and rapidly inflated and deflated in the left main extending into the left anterior descending and the circumflex, respectively (B). The final angiogram (C) and subsequent intravascular ultrasound reveal good lumen expansion and result.

(46). Eight studies of BMS for LMS with over 1100 patients between 1999 and 2003 showed an in hospital mortality of 6%, 1 to 2 year mortality of 17% and repeat revascularization rate of 29% (47). Two registries of patients with LMS undergoing CABG or PCI showed similar mortality rates at one year but revascularization rates of 20 to 26% with PCI versus 3 to 4% with CABG (48,49). DES has lowered revascularization rates and improved outcomes, with recent studies showing an in-hospital mortality of 2.4% and repeat revascularization of 13%. (47). These studies were limited by small numbers, incomplete angiographic restenosis follow-up, short duration of follow up and lack of control groups in four studies. In addition, the presence of significant distal or bifurcation LMS in 42% to 94% of patients probably affected the outcome given the known adverse outcomes with distal LMS (50). Treatment of nonbifurcation, proximal LMS with DES appears to be a much safer and effective treatment option (51).

The SYNTAX trial, designed to compare PCI with CABG in the current era, included 705 patients with LMS. As reported above, this trial used a coronary lesion complexity score to provide guidance on an optimal revascularization strategy. In this subgroup, there was no difference in major adverse cardiac and cerebrovascular events (MACCE) (death, MI, CVA, revascularization) between the CABG and PCI arms (13.7% versus 15.8%) with a higher rate of revascularization in the PCI group (11.8% versus 6.5%) being offset by a higher rate of CVA in the CABG group (2.7% versus 0.3%). However, patients with higher SYNTAX scores appeared to benefit from CABG, in particular patient with concomitant multivessel disease. In conclusion, left main stenting can be considered a viable option in patients in the correct angiographic and clinically setting, with the SYNTAX score being the most contemporary tool to help determine eligibility.

■ BIFURCATION STENTING

Bifurcation lesions are difficult to approach percutaneously, and account for 15% to 18% of all PCIs. Turbulent flow dynamics and high shear stress likely predispose coronary bifurcations to the development of atherosclerosis. When compared with nonbifurcation interventions, bifurcation interventions demonstrate lower procedural success rates, higher procedural costs, longer hospitalizations, and higher clinical and angiographic restenosis rates. There are six different classification schemes for bifurcation lesions (33). A variety of approaches have been described in the treatment of these lesions, and each involve an algorithm of how and when to stent the side branch of the bifurcation. Multiple two-stent bifurcation strategies exist, including T-stenting (Figure 3.2), simultaneous-kissing stents, the crush, and the culotte. Each strategy has its advantages and disadvantages with limited direct comparisons among the techniques. Stenting with DES with a single stent in the main branch remains the default approach and most widely used approach (52,53). An algorithm for bifurcation stenting is shown in Figure 3.3. Importantly, dedicated bifurcation stents, such as the Petal™ (Boston Scientific, Natick, MA), are being developed and studied. These have the potential to markedly change the way in which bifurcation lesions are intervened upon in the future.

■ PCI FOR CHRONIC TOTAL OCCLUSIONS

A chronic total occlusion (CTO) is defined as a >3-month-old obstruction of a native coronary artery with TIMI 0 flow and, and is prevalent in over 20% of patients with angiographically documented CAD. Histologically, a CTO is composed of atherosclerotic plaque and thrombus with multiple layers of clot at multiple sites of plaque fissure. Clinically and physiologically a CTO with well-developed collaterals mimics a 90% lesion. Patients with CTOs may well have angina during periods of increased oxygen demand but lack the risk of abrupt vessel closure due to plaque rupture with the resulting degree of myocardial necrosis seen in ACS. PCI for a CTO remains a major challenge despite recent technological advances, and is the most common reason for failure of a PCI. The rationale behind performing PCI for CTOs revolves around the potential for improvement of clinical symptoms, normalization of a positive stress test, elimination of the need for subsequent CABG, and improvement in myocardial function. A few large registries provide current knowledge on the long-term impact of a CTO PCI. One

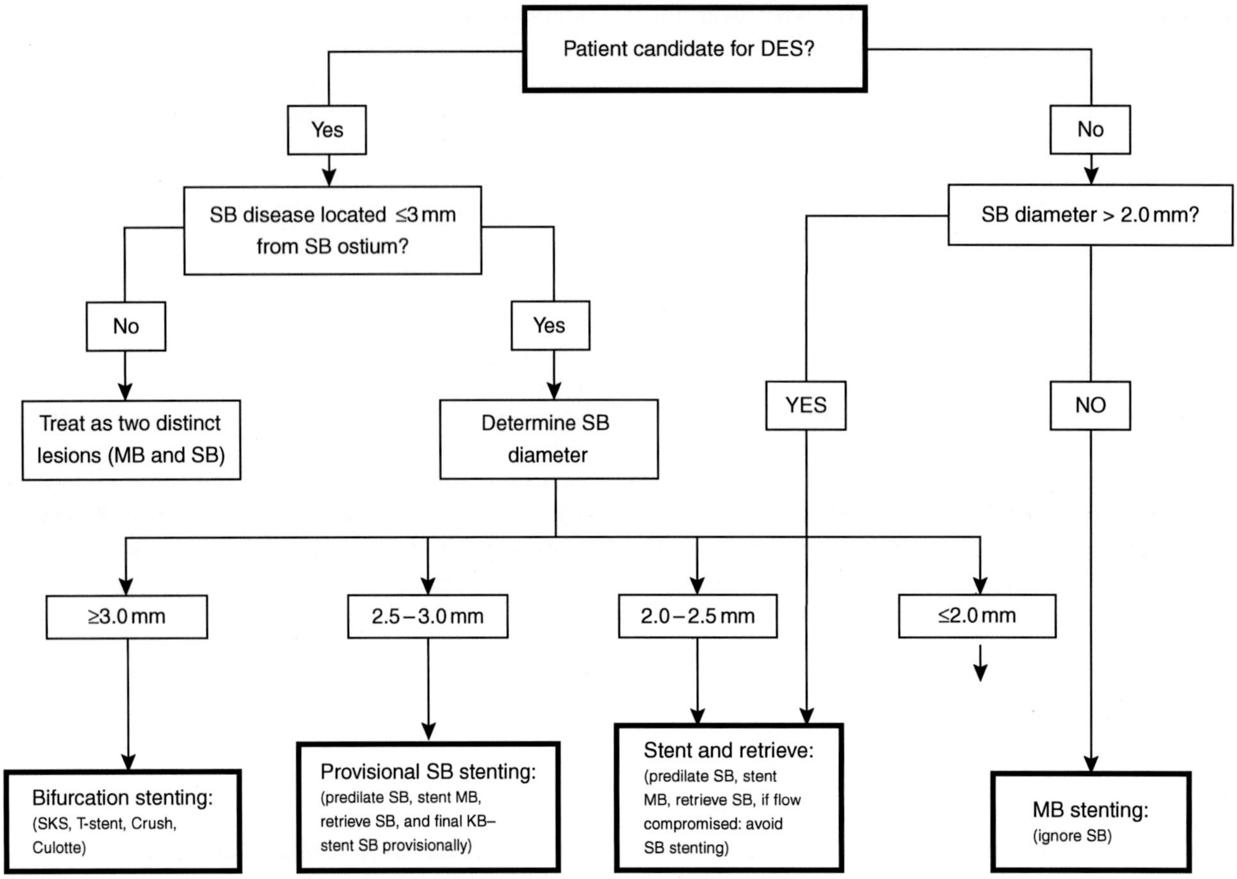

FIGURE 3.2 Bifurcation lesion algorithm for coronary intervention. (DES, drug-eluting stent; SB, side branch; MB, main branch; SKS, simultaneous kissing stents; KB, kissing balloons.)

large registry followed 2,007 patients over a 20-year period from 1980 to 1999 (54). Follow up over 10 years showed similar survival in those with successful CTO PCI compared with those with successful PCI of a non-occlusive lesion and significantly higher survival when compared to those with CTO revascularization failure. Recently presented data from the Milan-New York registry followed 1362 patients from 2000 to 2007 (55). The procedural success was 66.8%, DES were used in 61% of cases and BMS in 30% of cases. After three years of follow-up, mortality and need for cardiac surgery was lower in patients with successful CTO PCI compared with those with failed CTO PCI, with the largest benefit observed the subgroup receiving successful PCI of the left anterior descending artery. The Florence PCI registry followed 486 patients with successful PCI and at least one CTO between 2003 and 2006 (56). At two years, the group with successful PCI had a higher cardiac survival and lower cardiac surgery rate. Other registries have demonstrated improvement in LV function in patients with a successful CTO PCI. The indications for recanalization attempt by PCI are based on duration and length of occlusion balanced against benefits in terms of improvements in symptoms and exercise capacity. If a patient is being considered for CABG to alleviate symptoms related to a CTO, an attempt with PCI is a reasonable first approach (Figure 3.3). Multivessel disease poses additional challenges and careful consideration should be given to revascularization of a vessel providing collaterals to an occluded vessel. Major factors influencing the technical success of CTO recanalization include age less than 3 months, length <15 mm, absence of TIMI 0 flow, presence of a stump, and presence of bridging collaterals. Although there is a small, theoretically higher risk of coronary perforation with CTO PCIs, complications

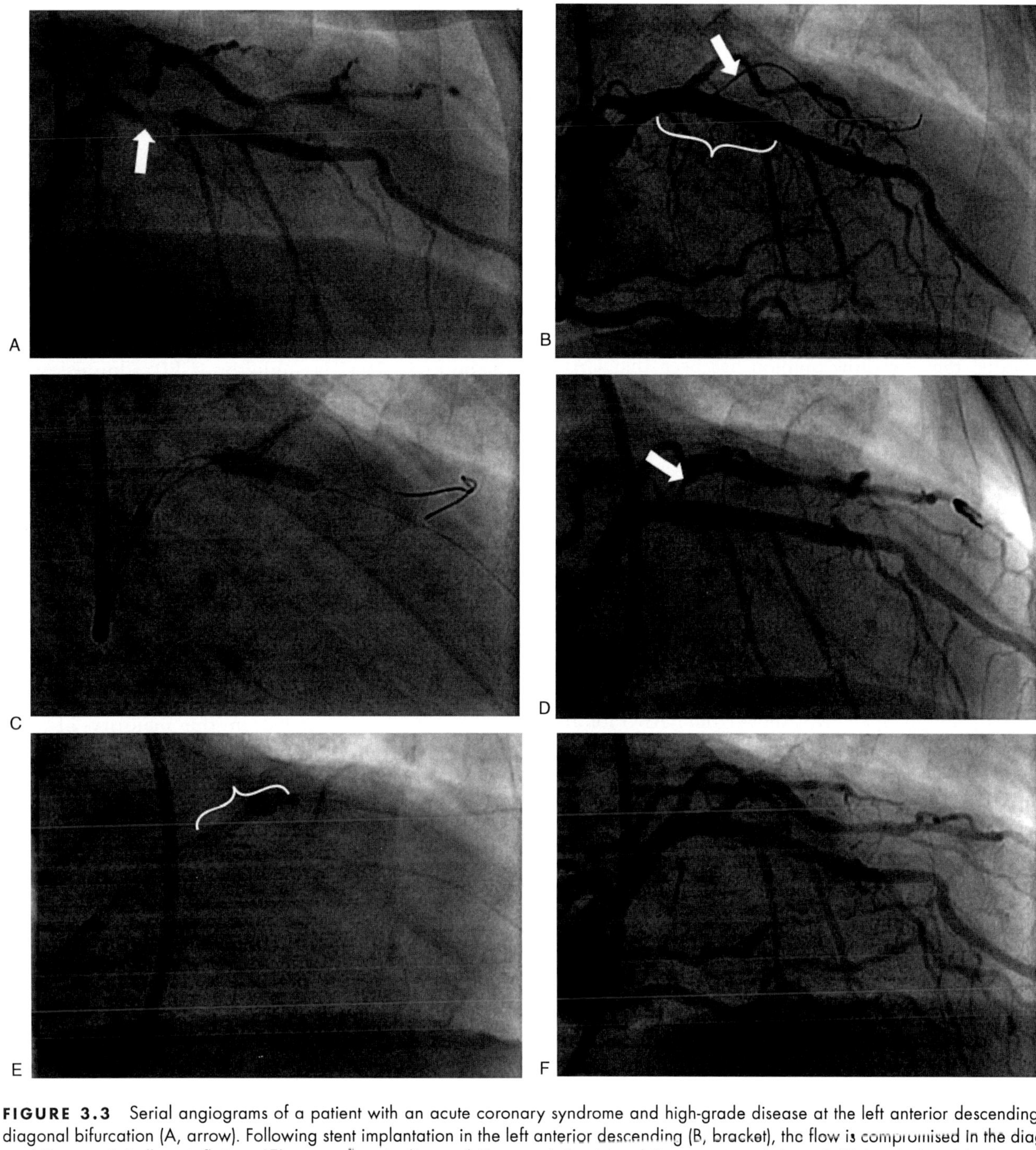

FIGURE 3.3 Serial angiograms of a patient with an acute coronary syndrome and high-grade disease at the left anterior descending/diagonal bifurcation (A, arrow). Following stent implantation in the left anterior descending (B, bracket), the flow is compromised in the diagonal (B, arrow). Balloon inflations (C) restore flow in diagonal (D, arrow). Provisional T stenting in side branch (E, bracket) and final angiographic result (F).

are by in large similar in type and frequency that those seen in general PCI.

In summary, CTOs are a frequent occurrence in patients needing revascularization, but they pose a low risk when treated conservatively. Future cardiac events in patients with CTOs are frequently caused by progression of disease in the other vessels rather than the occluded vessel itself, and the modest benefit obtained from recanalization must be balanced against the complexity of the PCI and relatively lower success rate.

■ PCI AND CABG: COMPLEMENTARY RATHER THAN COMPETITIVE STRATEGIES

Both PCI and CABG are available revascularization strategies for multivessel CAD. Based on several studies comparing CABG with angioplasty alone or with stenting, the prevailing opinion has been that CABG results in less repeat revascularization, and better anginal relief compared with PCI, without a demonstrable survival benefit except perhaps in diabetic patients. Registry data from New York State showed a 4.9% rate of revascularization with CABG compared with 35% with PCI (57). As PCI has advanced, however, the rates of repeat revascularization have declined substantially from 50% in the BARI trial to 28% in ERACI II trial at five years and 11.8% in the ARTS II study at five years. Registry data favoring CABG may be due in part to selection bias owing to the fact that PCI is typically the revascularization method utilized for clinically higher risk patients (ACS, STEMI, shock) and CABG for anatomically complex patients (LMS, multivessel, CTO). The SYNTAX trial, attempting to correct for both this clinical and anatomic heterogeneity/bias, had one year data indicating no difference in mortality between CABG and PCI, but higher rates of repeat revascularization with PCI were seen in patients with higher lesion complexity. These data suggest that patients with complex coronary anatomy are likely to benefit from CABG and those with less complex anatomy are likely to benefit from PCI. Therefore PCI and CABG may be complementary rather than competing revascularization strategies.

■ ANTIPLATELET AND ANTITHROMBOTIC THERAPIES IN PCI

Adjunctive pharmacotherapy is an essential aspect of percutaneous coronary intervention. Optimization of both antithrombotic and antiplatelet therapies remains integral to improved procedural success (58,59). Intra-venous unfractionated heparin has been the most utilized antithrombotic agent, and serves to prevent catheter and device-mediated thrombosis intra-procedurally during PCI. Heparin, however, is limited by an unpredictable dose response, inhibition by plasma proteins, as well as theoretical platelet activation (60). Bivalirudin, a direct thrombin inhibitor, is being increasingly used during PCI, both in the elective and ACS setting. Several studies have shown similar efficacy with respect to cardiac events and ischemic endpoints, with a concomitant reduction in bleeding when comparing bivalirudin to heparin and glycoprotein IIb/IIIa inhibitor (GPI) administration (61–64).

Since platelets are pivotal to thrombus formation both in ACS as well as in stent thrombosis, therapies designed to inhibit platelet activation and aggregation are crucial to successful outcomes (58,59,65). Parenteral GPI agents, namely eptifibatide and abciximab, have been studied extensively in patient undergoing PCI in the setting of an ACS, with numerous trials showing benefit of these agents in reducing cardiac events (66,67). While the preponderance of the data show benefit of GPI, in the current era of bivalirudin and clopidogrel preloading, it remains unclear whether GPI are needed in the majority of ACS patients (68). Recent data from HORIZONS-AMI and ACUITY trials show similar outcomes in high-risk PCI groups, namely UA/NSTEMI and STEMI patients, when comparing bivalirudin compared to heparin and a GPI (62–64). Subgroup analyses show that this is particularly the case when clopidogrel is administered early and prior to index PCI (69). Some studies have shown that the antiplatelet activity of upstream clopidogrel obviates the need for a GPI, particularly in elective PCI (70,71). While the practice is not universal, the current ACC/AHA recommendations have upstream clopidogrel therapy as a class 1a indication in the setting of ACS (72). Nevertheless, it is general consensus of opinion that GPIs do have a role in PCI, particularly in high-risk patients with angiographic and clinical features suggesting a greater procedural risk (73).

Dual antiplatelet (DAP) therapy with clopidogrel and aspirin remains the cornerstone of post-PCI pharmacologic management (58,59). The current recommended duration of clopidogrel post-stent placement is for at least one month following BMS placement and 12 months following DES placement (72). These data for extended clopidogrel treatment arise from registries suggesting a small but significant increase in late stent thrombosis likely due to delayed endothelialization and/or a persistent inflammatory response in the setting of DES implantation (74). Following widespread adaptation of prolonged DAP therapy in DES use, recent data show no significant difference in late thrombotic events as compared to BMS (75). Nonetheless, in patients at higher bleeding risk and in who DAP therapy cannot be definitively continued for 12 months, BMS should be considered in lieu of DES given BMS's more reliable and faster endothelial formation (76).

While clopidogrel, along with aspirin, is effective at reducing cardiac and thrombotic events post-PCI, it remains relatively unpredictable in its platelet-inhibitory response (77). Studies have shown that over 20% of patients receiving clopidogrel have inadequate platelet-inhibition following PCI (78). Moreover, its onset of action is long, making it less than ideal to administer in the cath lab immediately before the procedure (79). A number of PCI centers are beginning to utilize platelet activity assays to directly measure the efficacy of anti-platelet agents, allowing for a more tailored strategy to post-PCI platelet inhibition. An ongoing trial is investigating whether this patient-specific approach can lead to an improvement of outcomes post-PCI (82). Prasugrel is a newer agent, which affords greater predictability and reliability of platelet inhibition, as well as a more rapid onset of action (80). Clinical studies have shown a reduction of cardiac events post-PCI in prasugrel when compared to clopidogrel, at the expense of increased bleeding (81).

In summary, for routine elective PCI either unfractionated heparin or bivalirudin may be utilized, with GPIs used in high-risk cases. Dual antiplatelet therapy with aspirin and clopidogrel should be routinely used prior to and post-PCI. Preloading with clopidogrel is preferred at least 6 hours before and preferably one day prior to elective cases. For high risk or emergent PCI the antithrombotic agents are the same but since clopidogrel preloading may not always be possible, GPIs may be used at the operator's discretion and continued postprocedure for up to 18 hours. Dual antiplatelet therapy with clopidogrel and aspirin should be continued for one month for BMS, 12 months for DES, and single antiplatelet therapy should be continued indefinitely.

■ ROLE OF NEWER IMAGING STRATEGIES AND PCI

Asymptomatic nonobstructive CAD can remain dormant for decades before there is a transition to symptomatic, occlusive atherothrombotic disease related to plaque rupture or plaque erosion. Plaques at high risk for rupture have specific features which may be identified by newer imaging techniques. Virmani and colleagues (83) have subdivided vulnerable plaques into distinctive pathologic categories seen at autopsy: (a) plaque ruptures, also termed thin fibrous cap atheromas (TCFAs), which account for 55% to 60% of acute cardiac deaths and are associated with a thin fibrous cap, large necrotic core, and inflammation in the shoulder of the plaque; (b) superficial erosions, which are present in 30% to 35% of cardiac deaths, are characterized by an absence of endothelium, lipids pool, or necrotic core, and are rich in proteoglycans and smooth muscle cells; and (c) calcified nodules, which account for 2% to 7% of cardiac deaths, with thrombus and fibrin interspersed between nodules of calcium. The annual incidence of high-risk plaques turning into clinical events ranges from 4% in single vessel disease to 13% in triple-vessel disease.

Proper evaluation and treatment of high-risk plaques has the potential for preventing the majority of myocardial infarctions. Angiography is an excellent tool for lesions that narrow the arterial lumen, but positively remodeled lesions may maintain lumen area despite substantial plaque. Another imaging modality being utilized with increasing frequency is multi-detector coronary CT angiography which is able to visualize the presence of calcified, fibrotic, and soft lesions, but current spatial resolution limitations makes plaque vulnerability determinations difficult and unreliable. Seven novel intracoronary techniques to detect vulnerable plaques have potential clinical applications: intravascular ultrasound (IVUS), virtual histology (VH), palpography, optical coherence tomography (OCT), intravascular magnetic resonance imaging (ivMRI), angioscopy, and spectroscopy. IVUS is a commonly used tool and is excellent for visualizing the arterial wall and extent of atherosclerosis, especially positive remodeling. However given inadequate axial resolution, it is a poor modality for detecting TCFAs, necrotic core areas, and plaque inflammation. VH is an IVUS based modality which may allow assessment of four major plaque components: fibrotic tissue, fibro-fatty tissue, calcific necrotic core, and calcium. The ongoing Providing Regional Observations to Study Predictors of Events in the Coronary Tree (PROSPECT) trial is the first prospective natural history study designed to evaluate the prognostic value of IVUS-VH derived plaque composition in nonobstructive segments. OCT is a catheter based optical imaging modality and measures back reflected infrared light with the highest resolutions of all of all invasive modalities. Excellent histopathologic correlations have been obtained both for human coronary tissue and animal models with greater than 90% sensitivity and specificity for differentiating among lipid rich, fibro-calcific, and fibrous plaque compositions. OCT is especially useful for measuring TCFA, plaque inflammation, plaque neovascularization and intraplaque hemorrhage but it has limited value in quantifying positive remodeling (33). Future validation of these techniques may allow their application to high-risk patients to foster "lesion directed therapy" in addition to long-term systemic therapy in order to reduce coronary events and improve survival. Examples of lesion directed therapy include photodynamic therapy (PDT) which has been shown to reduce macrophages from atherosclerotic plaques in animal models (33,84). New strategies might create opportunities for "prophylactic angioplasty" that could stabilize plaques identified as unstable.

Advances in Coronary CT angiography (CTA) have had significant impact on the use of PCI with regard to patient selection, noninvasive detection of significant lesions and restenosis, and procedure planning as it relates to stent sizing and PCI equipment. A paradigm for CTA guided interventions is shown in Figure 3.4 (85). An area of great interest is the utilization of 3DCTA in the catheterization lab, whereby the CTA images can be imported and linked to the C-arm and angiographic imaging can begin with the best angle preselected from CTA map. The C-arm rotation is accompanied by automatic rotation of the CTA map to an angle with the least foreshortening and overlap. This approach would permit more accurate stent sizing, facilitated stent placement, and decreased number of coronary angiogram images. This technique would be especially useful in CTO lesions, where CTA can guide PCI by providing visualization of the path of an otherwise angiographically-invisible occluded artery.

■ FUTURE DIRECTIONS IN STENT ENGINEERING: BIOABSORBABLE STENTS

The advent of metallic stents followed by DES were major advances in the field of interventional cardiology. By providing scaffolding, stents prevent abrupt vessel closure and reduce restenosis compared with angioplasty. DES addressed pitfalls related to restenosis and neointimal hyperplasia, but delayed endothelial healing and stent thrombosis requiring extended antiplatelet therapy remain major concerns. A new technology which may address these issues is the use of bioabsorbable materials in stents that erode over time, leaving no residual implant. Such biodegradable stents would have to function at the level of a current generation DES and provide the same long-term safety profile before they can be adopted. The most tested biodegradable polymers include PGA (polyglycolic acid), PDLLA (poly-D, L-lactide) and PLLA (poly-L-lactid acid). These polymers are ideally suited for coronary implantation given their tensile strength, elongation time, low inflammatory response and rapid degradation rate. Lactide and glycolide based polymers undergo degradation by hydrolysis which leads to the formation of water soluble, low molecular weight components which are metabolized into carbon dioxide and water. Absorbable metals such as magnesium and iron, being they are essential elements and appear to be biocompatible, serve as alternatives to to bioabsorbable polymers.

The first PLLA based stents were developed in the 1980s and successfully used in animal models. They were followed by the more thrombogenic PGA based stent at Kyoto University and the Cleveland clinic/ Mayo/Thoraxcenter stent consisting of five biodegradable polymers which suffered from marked inflammation and neointimal proliferation in porcine models (86). The Igaki-Tamai PLLA based heat and balloon expandable stent has been more promising, showing a relatively low angiographic restenosis rates of 5.3% and a good safety profile (87). The newer Bioabsorbable Vascular Solutions (BVS) Everolimus-eluting stent is undergoing feasibility testing in the ABSORB trial. Initial results in humans show neointimal growth rates similar to current DES (88). The first absorbable

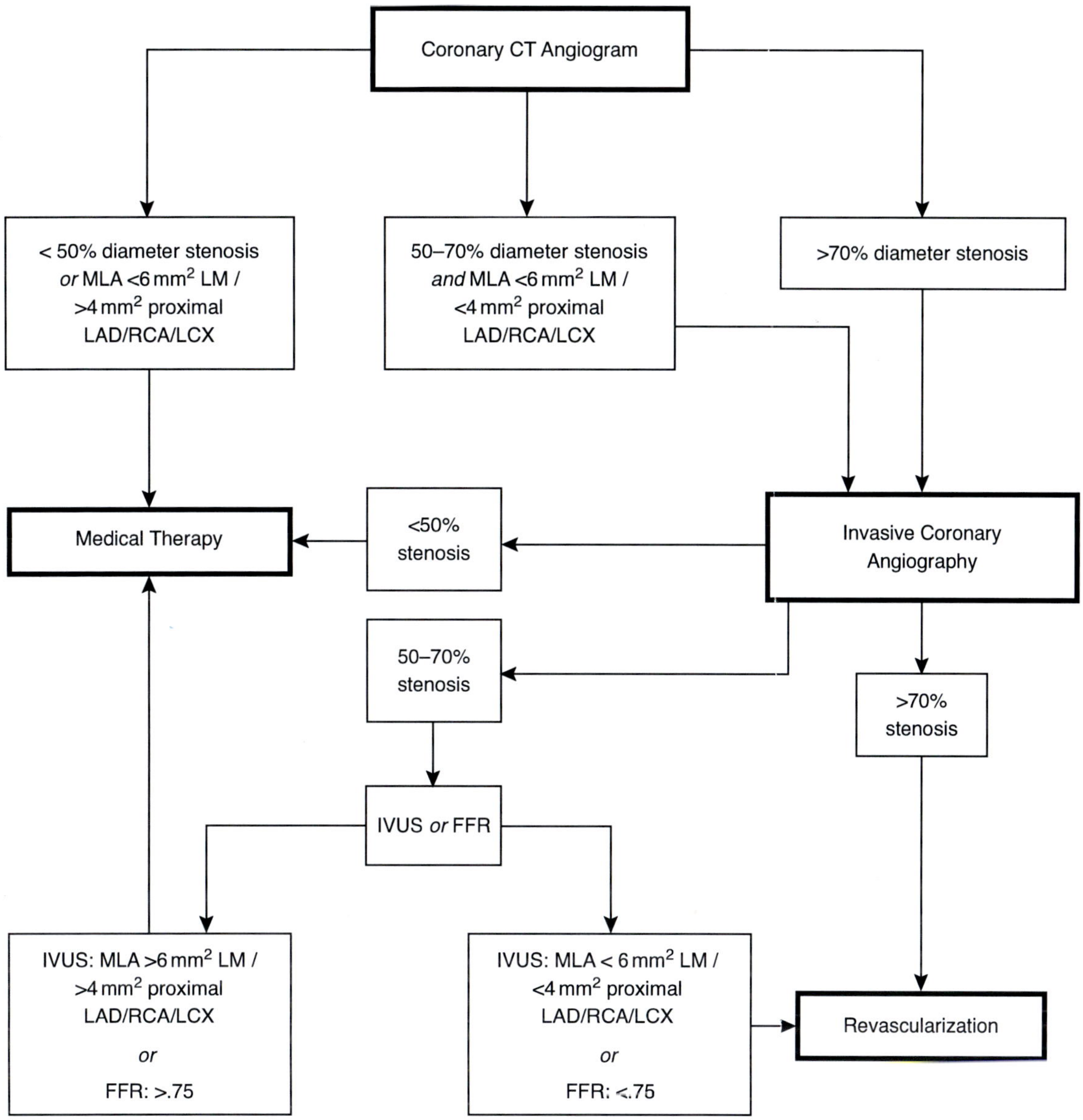

FIGURE 3.4 Use of coronary CT angiogram to determine revascularization for coronary artery disease. (FFR, fractional flow reserve; IVUS, intravascular ultrasound; LM, left main; MLA, minimum lumen area; LAD, left anterior descending artery; RCA, right coronary artery; LCX, left circumflex artery.)

magnesium stent was studied in the PROGRESS-AMS trial which showed adequate safety, but restenosis rates similar to BMS (89). Addition of an antiproliferative agent agent in combination with a magnesium based stent may reduce these revascularization rates. With further refinements and addition of a drug delivery system, bioabsorbable stents have the potential to greatly advance the practice of PCI and other endovascular interventions.

■ REFERENCES

1. Katritsis DG, Ioannidis JPA. Percutaneous coronary intervention versus conservative therapy in nonacute coronary artery disease: a meta-analysis. *Circulation* 2005; 111(22):2906–12.
2. Bucher HC, Hengstler P, Schindler C, Guyatt GH. Percutaneous transluminal coronary angioplasty versus medical treatment for non-acute coronary heart disease: meta-analysis of randomised controlled trials. *BMJ* 2000 Jul 8; 321(7253):73–7.
3. Boden WE, O'Rourke RA, Teo KK, et al. Optimal medical therapy with or without PCI for stable coronary disease.

COURAGE Trial Research Group. *N Engl J Med* 2007; 356(15):1503–16.

4. Smith PK, Califf RM, Tuttle RH, et al. Selection of surgical or percutaneous coronary intervention provides differential longevity benefit. *Ann Thorac Surg* 2006 Oct; 82(4):1420–9.
5. Shaw LJ, Berman DS, Maron DJ, et al. Optimal medical therapy with or without percutaneous coronary intervention to reduce ischemic burden: results from the Clinical Outcomes Utilizing Revascularization and Aggressive Drug Evaluation (COURAGE) trial nuclear substudy. *Circulation* 2008 Mar 11; 117(10):1283–91.
6. Erne P, Schoenenberger AW, Burckhardt D, et al. Effects of percutaneous coronary interventions in silent ischemia after myocardial infarction: the SWISSI II randomized controlled trial. *JAMA* 2007; 297(18):1985–91.
7. Tonino PA, De Bruyne B, Pijls NH, et al. Fractional flow reserve versus angiography for guiding percutaneous coronary intervention. FAME Study Investigators. *N Engl J Med* 2009 Jan 15; 360(3):213–24.
8. Katritsis D, Meier B. Percutaneous Coronary Intervention for Stable Coronary Artery Disease. J Am Coll Cardiol 2008; 52(11):889–93.
9. Antman EM, Cohen M, Bernink PJ, et al. The TIMI risk score for unstable angina/non-ST elevation MI: A method for prognostication and therapeutic decision making. *JAMA* 2000; 284(7):835–42.
10. Mehta SR, Granger CB, Boden WE, et al. Early versus delayed invasive intervention in acute coronary syndromes. *N Engl J Med* 2009; 360(21):2165–75.
11. Cannon CP, Weintraub WS, Demopoulos LA, et al. Comparison of early invasive and conservative strategies in patients with unstable coronary syndromes treated with the glycoprotein IIb/IIIa inhibitor tirofiban. *N Engl J Med* 2001; 344(25):1879–87.
12. Fox KA, Poole-Wilson P, Clayton TC, et al. 5-year outcome of an interventional strategy in non-ST-elevation acute coronary syndrome: the British Heart Foundation RITA 3 randomised trial. *Lancet* 2005; 366(9489):914–20.
13. Mehta SR, Cannon CP, Fox KA, et al. Routine vs selective invasive strategies in patients with acute coronary syndromes: a collaborative meta-analysis of randomized trials. *JAMA* 2005; 293(23):2908–17.
14. Keeley EC, Boura JA, Grines CL. Primary angioplasty versus intravenous thrombolytic therapy for acute myocardial infarction: a quantitative review of 23 randomised trials. *Lancet* 2003; 361(9351):13–20.
15. Nallamothu BK, Bates ER. Percutaneous coronary intervention versus fibrinolytic therapy in acute myocardial infarction: is timing (almost) everything? *Am J Cardiol* 2003; 92(7):824–6.
16. Gersh BJ, Stone GW, White HD, Holmes DR Jr. Pharmacological facilitation of primary percutaneous coronary intervention for acute myocardial infarction: is the slope of the curve the shape of the future?. *JAMA* 2005; 293(8):979–86.
17. Thune JJ, Hoefsten DE, Lindholm MG, et al. Simple risk stratification at admission to identify patients with reduced mortality from primary angioplasty. *Circulation* 2005; 112(13):2017–21.
18. Masoudi FA, Bonow RO, Brindis RG, et al. ACC/AHA 2008 statement on Performance Measurement and Reperfusion Therapy: a report of the ACC/AHA Task Force on Performance Measures (Work Group to address the challenges of Performance Measurement and Reperfusion Therapy). *J Am Coll Cardiol* 2008; 52(24):2100–12.
19. Srinivas VS, Hailpern SM, Koss E, Monrad ES, Alderman MH. Effect of Physician Volume on the Relationship Between Hospital Volume and Mortality During Primary Angioplasty. *J Am Coll Cardiol* 2009; 53(7):574–9.
20. Van de Verf F. Primary versus tenecteplase-facilitated percutaneous coronary intervention in patients with ST-segment elevation acute myocardial infarction (ASSENT-4 PCI): randomised trial. Assessment of the Safety and Efficacy of a New Treatment Strategy with Percutaneous Coronary Intervention (ASSENT-4 PCI) investigators Lancet. 2006 Feb 18;367(9510):569–78.
21. Cantor WJ, Fitchett D, Borgundvaag B, Ducas J, Heffernan M, Cohen EA, Morrison LJ, Langer A, Dzavik V, Mehta SR, Lazzam C, Schwartz B, Casanova A, Goodman SG; TRANSFER-AMI Trial Investigators. Routine early angioplasty after fibrinolysis for acute myocardial infarction N Engl J Med. 2009 Jun 25;360(26):2705–18.
22. Wijeysundera HC, Vijayaraghavan R, Nallamothu BK, Foody JM, Krumholz HM, Phillips CO, Kashani A, You JJ, Tu JV, Ko DT. Rescue angioplasty or repeat fibrinolysis after failed fibrinolytic therapy for ST-segment myocardial infarction: a meta-analysis of randomized trials. J Am Coll Cardiol. 2007 Jan 30;49(4):422–30.
23. Krumholz HM, Anderson JL, Bachelder BL, et al. ACC/AHA 2008 performance measures for adults with ST-elevation and non-ST-elevation myocardial infarction. A report of the American College of Cardiology/American Heart Association Task Force on Performance Measures. *J Am Coll Cardiol* 2008; 52(24):2046–99.
24. Anderson JL, Adams CD, Antman EM, et al. ACC/AHA 2007 guidelines for the management of patients with unstable angina/non-ST-Elevation myocardial infarction: a report of the American College of Cardiology/American Heart Association Task Force on Practice Guidelines (Writing Committee to Revise the 2002 Guidelines for the Management of Patients With Unstable Angina/Non-ST-Elevation Myocardial Infarction) developed in collaboration with the American College of Emergency Physicians, the Society for Cardiovascular Angiography and Interventions, and the Society of Thoracic Surgeons endorsed by the American Association of Cardiovascular and Pulmonary Rehabilitation and the Society for Academic Emergency Medicine. *J Am Coll Cardiol* 2007; 50(7):e1–157.
25. Fischman DL, Leon MB, Baim DS, et al. A randomized comparison of coronary-stent placement and balloon angioplasty in the treatment of coronary artery disease. *N Engl J Med* 1994; 331:496–501.
26. Serruys PW, de Jaegere P, Kiemeneij F, et al. A comparison of balloon-expandable-stent implantation with balloon angioplasty in patients with coronary artery disease. *N Engl J Med* 1994; 331:489–95.
27. Moses JW, Leon MB, Popma JJ, et al. Sirolimus-eluting stents versus standard stents in patients with stenosis in a native coronary artery. *N Engl J Med* 2003; 349:1315–23.
28. Stone GW, Ellis SG, Cox DA, et al. A polymer-based, paclitaxel-eluting stent in patients with coronary artery disease. *N Engl J Med* 2004; 350(3):221–31.

29. Fajadet J, Wijns W, Laarman GJ, et al. Randomized, double-blind, multicenter study of the Endeavor zotarolimus-eluting phosphorylcholine-encapsulated stent for treatment of native coronary artery lesions: clinical and angiographic results of the ENDEAVOR II trial. *Circulation* 2006; 114(8):798–806.
30. Stone GW, Midei M, Newman W, et al. Comparison of an everolimus-eluting stent and a paclitaxel-eluting stent in patients with coronary artery disease: a randomized trial. *JAMA* 2008; 299:1903–13.
31. Mauri L, Hsieh WH, Massaro JM, Ho KK, D'Agostino R, Cutlip DE. Stent thrombosis in randomized clinical trials of drug-eluting stents. *N Engl J Med* 2007; 356:1020–9.
32. Stone GW, Moses JW, Ellis SG, et al. Safety and efficacy of sirolimus- and paclitaxel-eluting coronary stents. *N Engl J Med* 2007; 356:998–1008.
33. Topol EJ. *Textbook of Interventional Cardiology*, 5th ed. Philadelphia: WB Saunders, 2008.
34. Waksman R, Bhargava B, Mintz GS, et al. Late total occlusion after intracoronary brachytherapy for patients with in-stent restenosis. *J Am Coll Cardiol* 2000; 36(1):65–8.
35. Waksman R, Ajani AE, White RL, et al. Prolonged anti-platelet therapy to prevent late thrombosis after intracoronary gamma-radiation in patients with in-stent restenosis: Washington Radiation for In-Stent Restenosis Trial plus 6 months of clopidogrel (WRIST PLUS). *Circulation* 2001; 103(19):2332–5.
36. Waksman R, Ajani AE, Pinnow E, et al. Twelve versus six months of clopidogrel to reduce major cardiac events in patients undergoing gamma-radiation therapy for in-stent restenosis: Washington Radiation for In-Stent restenosis Trial (WRIST) 12 versus WRIST PLUS. *Circulation* 2002; 106(7):776–8.
37. Bavry AA, Kumbhani DJ, Helton TJ, Borek PP, Mood GR, Bhatt DL. Late thrombosis of drug-eluting stents: a meta-analysis of randomized clinical trials. *Am J Med* 2006; 119(12):1056–61.
38. Lagerqvist B, James SK, Stenestrand U, Lindbäck J, Nilsson T, Wallentin L. Long-term outcomes with drug-eluting stents versus bare-metal stents in Sweden. *N Engl J Med* 2007; 356(10):1009–19.
39. Douglas PS, Brennan JM, Anstrom KJ, et al. Clinical Effectiveness of Coronary Stents in Elderly Persons: Results From 262,700 Medicare Patients in the American College of Cardiology-National Cardiovascular Data Registry. *J Am Coll Cardiol* 2009; 53:1629–41.
40. Mercado N, Wijns W, Serruys PW, et al. One-year outcomes of coronary artery bypass graft surgery versus percutaneous coronary intervention with multiple stenting for multisystem disease: a meta-analysis of individual patient data from randomized clinical trials. *J Thorac Cardiovasc Surg* 2005; 130(2):512–19.
41. Serruys P, Daemen J, Morice MC, et al. Three-year follow-up of the ARTS-II: sirolimus-eluting stents for the treatment of patients with multivessel coronary artery disease. *EuroIntervention* 2008; 3(4):450–9.
42. Rodriguez A, Maree A, Grinfeld L, et al. Revascularization strategies of coronary multiple vessel disease in the Drug Eluting Stent Era: one year follow-up results of the ERACI III Trial. *EuroIntervention* 2006; 2:53–60.
43. Serruys PW, Morice MC, Kappetein AP, et al. Percutaneous coronary intervention versus coronary-artery bypass grafting for severe coronary artery disease. *N Engl J Med* 2009 Mar 5; 360(10):961–72.
44. Sianos G, Morel MA, Kappetein AP, et al. The SYNTAX score: an angiographic tool grading the complexity of coronary artery disease. *EuroIntervention* 2005; 1(2):219–27.
45. Kappetein AP, Dawkins KD, Mohr FW, et al. Current percutaneous coronary intervention and coronary artery bypass grafting practices for three-vessel and left main coronary artery disease. Insights from the SYNTAX run-in phase. *Eur J Cardiothorac Surg* 2006; 29:486–91.
46. Yusuf S, Zucker D, Peduzzi P, et al. Effect of coronary artery bypass graft surgery on survival: overview of 10-year results from randomized trials by the Coronary Artery Bypass Graft Surgery Trialists Collaboration. *Lancet* 1994; 344:563–70.
47. Taggart S, Kaul W, Boden WE, et al. Revascularization for unprotected left main stem coronary artery stenosis stenting or surgery. *J Am Coll Cardiol* 2008; 51(9):885–92.
48. Chieffo A, Morici N, Maisano F, et al. Percutaneous treatment with drug-eluting stent implantation versus bypass surgery for unprotected left main stenosis: a single-center experience. *Circulation* 2006; 113:2542–7.
49. Palmerini T, Marzocchi A, Marrozzini C, et al. Comparison between coronary angioplasty and coronary bypass surgery for the treatment of unprotected left main coronary artery stenosis (the Bologna registry). *Am J Cardiol* 2006; 98:54–9.
50. Valgimigli M, Malagutti P, Rodriguez-Granillo GA, et al. Distal left main coronary disease is a major predictor of outcome in patients undergoing percutaneous intervention in the drug-eluting stent era: an integrated clinical and angiographic analysis based on the RESEARCH and T-SEARCH registries. *J Am Coll Cardiol* 2006; 47:1530–7.
51. Chieffo A, Park SJ, Valgimigli M, et al. Favorable long-term outcome after drug-eluting stent implantation in nonbifurcation lesions that involve unprotected left main coronary artery. A multicenter registry. *Circulation* 2007; 116:158–62.
52. Colombo A, Moses JW, Morice MC, et al. Randomized study to evaluate sirolimus-eluting stents implanted at coronary bifurcation lesions. *Circulation* 2004; 109(10):1244–9.
53. Pan M, de Lezo JS, Medina A, et al. Rapamycin-eluting stents for the treatment of bifurcated coronary lesions: a randomized comparison of a simple versus complex strategy. *Am Heart J* 2004; 148(5):857–64.
54. Suero JA, Marso SP, Jones PG, et al. Procedural outcomes and long-term survival among patients undergoing percutaneous coronary intervention of a chronic total occlusion in native coronary arteries: a 20-year experience. *J Am Coll Cardiol* 2001; 38(2):409–14.
55. Obunai K. The Milan-New York CTO registry. Presented at: Transcatheter Therapeutics Annual Scientific Symposium. Washington, DC: October 13, 2008.
56. Valenti R, Migliorini A, Signorini U, et al. Impact of complete revascularization with percutaneous coronary intervention on survival in patients with at least one chronic total occlusion. *Eur Heart J* 2008; 29(19):2336–42.
57. Hannan EL, Racz MJ, Walford G, et al. Long-term outcomes of coronary-artery bypass grafting versus stent implantation. *N Engl J Med* 2005; 352:2174–83.

58. Schomig A, Neumann FJ, Kastrati A, et al. A randomized comparison of antiplatelet and anticoagulant therapy after the placement of coronary-artery stents. *N Engl J Med* 1996; 334:1084–9.
59. Leon MB, Baim DS, Popma JJ, et al. A clinical trial comparing three antithrombotic-drug regimens after coronary-artery stenting. *N Engl J Med* 1998; 339:1665–71.
60. Xiao Z, Théroux P. Platelet activation with unfractionated heparin at therapeutic concentrations and comparisons with a low-molecular-weight heparin and with a direct thrombin inhibitor. *Circulation* 1998; 97:251–6.
61. Lincoff AM, Bittl JA, Harrington RA, et al. Bivalirudin and provisional glycoprotein IIb/IIIa blockade compared with heparin and planned glycoprotein IIb/IIIa blockade during percutaneous coronary intervention: REPLACE-2 randomized trial. *JAMA* 2003; 289:853–63.
62. Stone GW, McLaurin BT, Cox DA, et al. Bivalirudin for patients with acute coronary syndromes. *N Engl J Med* 2006; 355:2203–16.
63. Stone GW, White HD, Ohman EM, et al. Bivalirudin in patients with acute coronary syndromes undergoing percutaneous coronary intervention: a subgroup analysis from the Acute Catheterization and Urgent Intervention Triage strategy (ACUITY) trial. *Lancet* 2007; 369:907–19.
64. Stone GW, Witzenbichler B, Guagliumi G, et al. Bivalirudin during primary PCI in acute myocardial infarction. *N Engl J Med* 2008; 358:2218–30.
65. Hamdalla H, Steinhubl SR. Oral antiplatelet therapy for percutaneous coronary revascularization. *Catheter Cardiovasc Interv* 2007; 69:637–42.
66. Topol EJ, Moliterno DJ, Herrmann HC, et al. Comparison of two platelet glycoprotein IIb/IIIa inhibitors, tirofiban and abciximab, for the prevention of ischemic events with percutaneous coronary revascularization. *N Engl J Med* 2001; 344:1888–94.
67. Labinaz M, Ho C, Banerjee S, et al. Meta-analysis of clinical efficacy and bleeding risk with intravenous glycoprotein IIb/IIIa antagonists for percutaneous coronary intervention. *Can J Cardiol* 2007; 12:963–70.
68. Cohen M, Hoekstra J, Giugliano R, et al. Treatment strategies in non-ST-elevation acute coronary syndromes in patients undergoing percutaneous coronary intervention: an evidence-based review of clinical trial results and treatment guidelines: report on a roundtable discussion. *J Interv Cardiol* 2008; 21:283–99.
69. Lincoff AM, Steinhubl SR, Manoukian SV, et al. Influence of timing of clopidogrel treatment on the efficacy and safety of bivalirudin in patients with non-ST-elevation acute coronary syndromes undergoing percutaneous coronary intervention. An analysis of the ACUITY Trial. *JACC Cardiovasc Interv* 2008; 1(6):639–48.
70. Kastrati A, Mehilli J, Schühlen H, et al. The ISAR REACT trial. A clinical trial of abciximab in elective PCI after pretreatment with clopidogrel. *N Engl J Med* 2004; 350:232–8.
71. Pannu R, Andraws R. Effects of glycoprotein IIb/IIIa inhibitors in patients undergoing percutaneous coronary intervention after pretreatment with clopidogrel: a meta-analysis of randomized trials. *Crit Pathw Cardiol* 2008; 7:5–10.
72. King SB III, Smith SC Jr, Hirshfeld JW Jr, Jacobs AK, Morrison DA, Williams DO. 2007 focused update of the ACC/AHA/SCAI 2005 guideline update for percutaneous coronary intervention. *J Am Coll Cardiol* 2008; 51:172–209.
73. Feldman DN, Wong SC, Bergman G, Minutello RM. Provisional glycoprotein IIb/IIIa blockade in patients receiving bivalirudin during percutaneous coronary intervention. *J Invasive Cardiol* 2009; 21(6):258–63.
74. Jaffe R, Strauss BH. Late and very late thrombosis of drug-eluting stents: evolving concepts and perspectives. *J Am Coll Cardiol* 2007; 50:119–27.
75. Stone GW, Moses JW, Ellis SG, et al. Safety and efficacy of sirolimus- and paclitaxel-eluting coronary stents. *N Engl J Med* 2007; 356:998–1008.
76. Bavry AA, Bhatt DL. Appropriate use of drug-eluting stents: balancing the reduction in restenosis with the concern of late thrombosis. *Lancet* 2008; 371:2134–43.
77. Gurbel PA, Bliden KP, Hiatt BL, O'Connor CM. Clopidogrel for coronary stenting: response variability, drug resistance, and the effect of pretreatment platelet reactivity. *Circulation* 2003; 107:2908–13.
78. Gurbel PA, Bliden KP, Etherington A, Tantry US. Assessment of clopidogrel responsiveness: measurements of maximum platelet aggregation, final platelet aggregation and their correlation with vasodilator-stimulated phosphoprotein in resistant patients. *Thromb Res* 2007; 121:107–15.
79. von Beckerath N, Taubert D, Pogatsa-Murray G, Schömig E, Kastrati A, Schömig A. Absorption, metabolization, and antiplatelet effects of 300-, 600-, and 900-mg loading doses of clopidogrel: results of the ISAR-CHOICE (Intracoronary Stenting and Antithrombotic Regimen: Choose Between 3 High Oral Doses for Immediate Clopidogrel Effect) Trial. *Circulation* 2005; 112:2946–50.
80. Wiviott SD, Trenk D, Frelinger AL, et al. Prasugrel compared with high loading- and maintenance-dose clopidogrel in patients with planned percutaneous coronary intervention: the Prasugrel in Comparison to Clopidogrel for Inhibition of Platelet Activation and Aggregation-Thrombolysis in Myocardial Infarction 44 trial. *Circulation* 2007; 116:2923–32.
81. Wiviott SD, Braunwald E, McCabe CH, et al. Prasugrel versus clopidogrel in patients with acute coronary syndromes. *N Engl J Med* 2007; 357:2001–15.
82. Price MJ, Berger PB, Angiolillo DJ, et al. Evaluation of individualized clopidogrel therapy after drug-eluting stent implantation in patients with high residual platelet reactivity: design and rationale of the GRAVITAS trial. *Am Heart J* 2009; 157:818–24.
83. Virmani R, Burke AP, Farb A, Kolodgie FD. Pathology of the vulnerable plaque. *J Am Coll Cardiol* 2006; 47(8 Suppl):C13–8.
84. Waksman R. Photodynamic therapy. In Virmani R, Narula J, Leon MB, Willerson JT, eds. *The Vulnerable Atherosclerotic Plaque: Strategies for Diagnosis and Management.* Malden, MA: Blackwell Futura, 2007, pp. 321–30.
85. Hecht HS. Applications of multislice coronary computed tomographic angiography to percutaneous coronary intervention: how did we ever do without it? *Catheter Cardiovasc Interv* 2008; 71(4):490–503.
86. van der Giessen WJ, Lincoff AM, Schwartz RS, et al. Marked inflammatory sequelae to implantation of biodegradable and nonbiodegradable polymers in porcine coronary arteries. *Circulation* 1996; 94:1690–7.

87. Tamai H, Igaki K, Kyo E, et al. Initial and 6-month results of biodegradable poly-l-lactic acid coronary stents in humans. *Circulation* 2000; 102(4):399–404.
88. Ormiston J, Serruys PW, Regar E, et al. A bioabsorbable everolimus-eluting coronary stent system for patients with single de-novo coronary artery lesions (ABSORB): a prospective open-label trial. *Lancet* 2008; 371:899–907.
89. Erbel R, Di Mario C, Bartunek J, et al. Temporary scaffolding of coronary arteries with bioabsorbable magnesium stents: a prospective, non-randomised multicentre trial. *Lancet* 2007; 369(9576):1869–75.

4 Predictors of Outcome in Chronic Ischemic Heart Disease

ROBERT J. KIM

OUTLINE

Cardiovascular diseases (CVD) remain the number one killer in the United States (1) and the world (2). Within this group of diseases, coronary heart disease (CHD) accounts for just over 50% of the deaths and was estimated to have caused one of every five deaths in 2004 (1). While the trend in mortality from heart disease has been declining steadily since 1980, any enthusiasm must be tempered by the rising rates of children, adolescents, and adults who are overweight and obese. In addition, in 2005 CVD accounted for 4,036,000 emergency department (ED) visits and 81,836,000 outpatient physician office visits, and also ranked highest among hospital discharges with a staggering estimated total inpatient hospital cost of $71.2 billion dollars. Hospitalizations for acute myocardial infarction (MI) alone resulted in $31 billion of hospital charges. An estimated 80,700,000 (approximately one in every three) Americans have one or more types of CVD, and approximately 16,000,000 have CHD. For 2008, the estimated combined direct and indirect costs related to CVD was $448.5 billion.

This chapter will focus on prognostic indicators of outcome for patients with chronic ischemic heart disease. Despite the stark numbers mentioned above, perhaps the most troubling fact is the realization that these numbers represent only the top layers in the pyramid of patients with coronary artery disease (CAD). Patients may experience silent MIs, sudden cardiac death, or develop incident angina before ever presenting for medical evaluation. In addition to treating established patients with evidence-based therapies, clearly one of the challenges that must be overcome includes improving the identification of patients at high-risk to begin treating more of them in a primary rather than secondary prevention manner.

The predictors of outcome for chronic ischemic heart disease can be categorized as relating primarily to anatomy, physiology, biochemistry, behavior, and from a therapeutic standpoint, pharmacology (Table 4.1). Major anatomical predictors of outcome include ejection fraction (EF), extent of coronary disease (assessed by multiple different methods by different investigators), left ventricular mass, presence of mechanical complications post-MI, and extent of myocardial scar. Physiological predictors include exercise capacity, heart failure class, ischemic burden, lung uptake on thallium-201 scanning, and exercise-induced left ventricular dilatation or dysfunction. Behavioral predictors include most importantly smoking cessation, as well as diet and exercise. Biochemical predictors include levels of LDL and HDL cholesterol, hs-CRP, Lp(a), white blood cell count, troponin, brain natriuretic peptide (BNP), and cystatin C. Finally, the presence of major comorbidities such as diabetes, renal insufficiency, peripheral vascular disease, and hypertension also contributes to increased cardiovascular morbidity and mortality.

Predictors of outcome in chronic ischemic heart disease

	Physiological	Biochemical	Pharmacological	Behavioral
Ejection fraction	Exercise capacity	Lipid levels	ACE inhibitors	Smoking cessation
Scar	Exercise parameters	CRP	Beta-blockers	Exercise
Extent of CAD	Heart failure	Troponin	Antiplatelet agents	Alcohol
LVH	Ischemic burden	BNP	Statins	Diet
		Lp(a)	Omega-3 fatty acids	

BNP, brain natriuretic peptide; CAD, coronary artery disease; CRP, C-reactive protein; LVH, left ventricular hypertrophy; Lp(a), lipoprotein(a).

ANATOMICAL PREDICTORS

Ejection Fraction

The extent and severity of myocardial dysfunction as assessed by wall motion abnormalities and summarized by the overall left ventricular ejection fraction (EF), is perhaps the most powerful predictor of outcomes in chronic ischemic disease. In the Coronary Artery Surgery Study (CASS) Registry, among medically-treated patients with suspected or proven CAD, ejection fraction powerfully predicted survival over the ensuing 12 years. For those with ejection fractions of 50% or greater, 12-year survival was 73% compared to 54% and 21% for those with ejection fractions of 35% to 49%, or <35% respectively (3). This relationship held through subgroups of patients divided into those with one-, two-, and three-vessel disease, with dismal survival rates for patients with three-vessel disease of 58%, 35%, and 10% for the three ejection fraction categories respectively.

Ejection fraction also emerged as the most powerful predictive variable ($\chi^2 = 48.54$) of two-year mortality from a selection of 46 clinical and anatomic variables evaluated in patients undergoing coronary angiography for suspected CAD who were subsequently medically-treated in the Seattle Heart Watch registry (4). Other significantly predictive variables included age, number of diseased vessels with ≥70% stenosis, and the presence of ventricular arrhythmias on resting expand electrocardiogram (ECG). Ejection fraction was also predictive of outcome for surgically-treated patients, although to a lesser degree.

Both of the previous studies used left ventricular angiography to assess left ventricular EF; however, assessment by alternative noninvasive methods has also been found to be predictive of survival. In a more contemporary analysis of post-MI survivors treated with thrombolytics, Burns et al. (5) found ejection fraction to be a stronger predictor of six-month mortality than either end-systolic volume index or even infarct size as assessed by 99mTc sodium pertechnetate radionuclide angiography and 99mTc-sestamibi SPECT imaging, respectively. An important limitation, however, was that of the 2,948 enrolled patients, only 725 (25.5%) patients actually had all three noninvasive imaging tests performed with technically satisfactory and interpretable results.

Among a broader group of 2,686 outpatients referred for myocardial perfusion gated SPECT scans (26% of whom reported a history of MI), Sharir et al. (6) reported a significant, inverse exponential relationship between the annual rate of cardiac death and the ejection fraction as assessed by 99mTc-sestamibi gated SPECT imaging. Of note, patients with nonischemic cardiomyopathies and significant valvular disease were excluded from this study. In those patients with an EF <30%, the rate of cardiac death was high (>4%/year) regardless of the extent of ischemia seen on perfusion imaging.

In another large, heterogeneous group of outpatients with New York Head Association (NYHA) Class II-IV chronic heart failure predominantly from ischemic heart disease, Solomon et al. (7) found that ejection fraction powerfully predicted mortality with a 39% increase in all-cause mortality with every 10% reduction in EF below 45%, as well as a 47% increase in cardiovascular mortality and 48% increase in sudden death. In this population the most common causes of death were sudden cardiac death and heart-failure related death (Figure 4.1). Of note, when the ejection fraction was above 45% it was a poorer predictor of cardiovascular outcomes and no longer useful in risk-stratifying patient outcomes. The majority of patients (79%) in this study underwent quantitative echocardiography to assess their ejection fraction, whereas the remaining 21% underwent RNCA or left ventricular angiography.

Finally, in a different population of chronic stable angina patients without heart failure, Dart et al. (8) found a similar relationship of ejection fraction to all-cause mortality and cardiovascular outcomes. This relationship was curvilinear, with a poorer prognosis noted for those patients with ejection fractions under the range of 45% to 48% by quantitative echocardiography.

Ejection fraction then, as an indicator of global left ventricular function and overall myocardial dysfunction, consistently emerges as a strong and independent predictor of mortality. This relationship holds true regardless of the method of assessment and across a wide variety of patient populations with differing degrees of ischemic heart disease. However, more recently, investigations have examined whether alternative methods of assessing the extent of myocardial damage can prove superior to the traditional assessments of left ventricular EF.

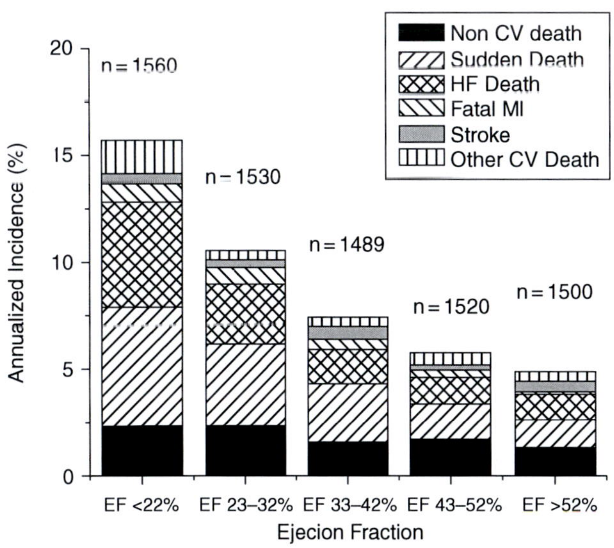

FIGURE 4.1 Annualized mortality by cause and ejection fraction. (From Ref. 7, with permission.)

Delayed-Enhancement Cardiac MRI

Delayed-enhancement cardiac magnetic resonance imaging (DE-CMR) using gadolinium contrast can directly visualize, characterize, and quantify precise amounts of infarcted myocardium as well as peri-infarct zones, thereby providing a more accurate assessment of the extent of myocardial damage. In addition, small subendocardial infarcts may be more readily identified compared to nuclear or echocardiography imaging techniques. This more precise quantification of myocardial damage theoretically has the potential to better risk stratify patients compared with the overall global left ventricular function assessment represented by the ejection fraction. Prior studies using ^{99m}Tc-sestamibi imaging (9) and ^{201}Tl-imaging (10) to quantify infarct size have shown that infarct size can predict subsequent overall- and cardiovascular-related mortality.

To date, only small studies using DE-CMR have compared the abilities of infarct size and ejection fraction to predict subsequent cardiovascular events or all-cause mortality. Wu et al. (11) demonstrated in a small prospective cohort of patients with acute MI undergoing percutaneous coronary intervention (PCI) that an acute infarct size ≥18.5% as assessed by DE-CMR was more strongly associated with an increased risk of major adverse cardiac events compared to acute ejection fraction. However, the number of events was small and predominantly driven by heart failure re-admissions. Roes et al. (12) evaluated 231 stable patients with evidence of myocardial scar on DE-CMR, 84% of whom had a clinical history of myocardial infarction (the remainder had clinically unrecognized MIs). They determined that myocardial infarct size was a stronger predictor of all-cause mortality over a median of 1.7 years compared with LV ejection fraction or volumes. When divided into two groups above and below the median score for extent of scar tissue, the high-risk group had an alarming 20% three-year mortality compared to 2.4% in the low-risk group.

In addition to simply quantifying the extent of myocardial infarcts, DE CMR can provide other potentially useful anatomic findings to help risk-stratify patients. Yan et al. (13) evaluated 144 patients with CAD and abnormal DE-CMR findings and determined that the extent of the peri-infarct zone was superior to EF in predicting mortality over a median follow-up period of 2.4 years. Even after adjustment for age and ejection fraction, the size of the peri-infarct zone maintained strong and independent associations with all-cause and cardiovascular-related mortality.

Finally, Bello et al. (14) reported in a small series of 48 patients with known CAD that infarct surface area and mass were superior to EF in predicting the induction of monomorphic ventricular tachycardia (VT) at electrophysiology (EP) study. The enticing prospect of being able to better predict both all-cause mortality and sudden cardiac death due to arrhythmias using gadolinium contrast DE-CMR is being tested prospectively in the ongoing DETERMINE trial. This trial will randomize patients with evidence of substantial infarct on DE-CMR but a preserved EF >40% to receive or not receive an implantable cardiodefibrillator (ICD). These patients would not otherwise qualify for a defibrillator based on their EF, thus it will be an important trial to determine if DE-CMR has value in identifying patients at increased risk who would otherwise not have been treated.

Extent of Coronary Artery Disease

Another major anatomical predictor of outcome in patients with CAD is the extent of atheromatous disease in the coronary artery tree. In the simplest categorization, patients can be separated into those with one-, two-, and three-vessel coronary disease based on the number of major epicardial vessels with significant coronary artery plaque. In the CASS Registry of medically-treated patients where the definition of clinically significant obstruction was a ≥70% reduction in the internal diameter of the vessel, the 12-year survival of patients with one-, two-, and three-vessel disease was 74%, 59%, and 40%, respectively (3). Stenosis of the left main artery ≥50% was also useful in predicting patient survival; 12-year survival was 60% versus 49% for patients with two-vessel disease without and with left main disease respectively, and 41% and 35% for patients with three-vessel disease. As noted in the previous section, ejection fraction also strongly stratified survival in all three groups.

The number of proximal vessel obstructions was found to separate survival curves within the groups of one-, two-, and three-vessel disease; however, in multivariate analysis this was not found to be significant. The notion of greater myocardium "at jeopardy" from proximal lesions led Califf et al. (15) to test the prognostic power of a so-called "jeopardy score" which weighted proximal lesions more significantly than distal lesions. In a group of 462 nonsurgically treated patients without left main disease, this jeopardy score was found to predict five year survival such that the addition of the actual number of vessels diseased added no prognostic information. It should be noted, however, that ejection fraction did emerge as the most potent predictor of survival, although the jeopardy score did still add a small amount of independent prognostic information.

Similarly, Hammermeister et al. (4) reported that in medically-treated patients from the Seattle Heart Watch registry, the number of diseased vessels was a significant predictive variable for two-year survival; however again, the most powerful predictive variable was the ejection fraction.

A more contemporary analysis of the prognostic significance of the extent of atheromatous disease in the coronary arteries was provided by Min et al. (16) using the technique of cardiac CT angiography (CCTA). In their retrospective cohort of patients presenting with chest symptoms, the extent of CAD was assessed using three different methods: by the number of vessels involved, by a modified Duke prognostic CAD index, and by intuitive clinical "plaque scores" indicating the number of segments stenosed and involved. Their results demonstrated an increased risk of all-cause mortality with increasing amounts of involvement of the coronary artery tree, strikingly similar to findings from the much earlier CASS Registry (3) of medically-treated patients when those patients were additionally separated into categories of no-, mild-, and moderate-CAD (Figure 4.2).

Together these studies demonstrate that the anatomical extent of atheromatous coronary artery plaque, whether assessed by invasive angiography or computed tomography, is a powerful predictor of survival, although typically it remains eclipsed by left ventricular ejection fraction.

Left Ventricular Geometry and Mass

Coronary artery disease can also result in changes in the geometry and mass of the left ventricle, and the specific pattern of these changes and the degree of hypertrophy can predict outcomes. Ghali et al. (17) reviewed the prevalence and significance of four LV geometry patterns—normal, concentric remodeling, eccentric left ventricular hypertrophy, and concentric left ventricular hypertrophy—assessed by echocardiography in patients with and without CAD. In both groups there were increasing rates of both all-cause and cardiac-related deaths among the four patterns, with concentric LVH portending the worst prognosis in both groups, but with CAD patients having nearly double the mortality rates

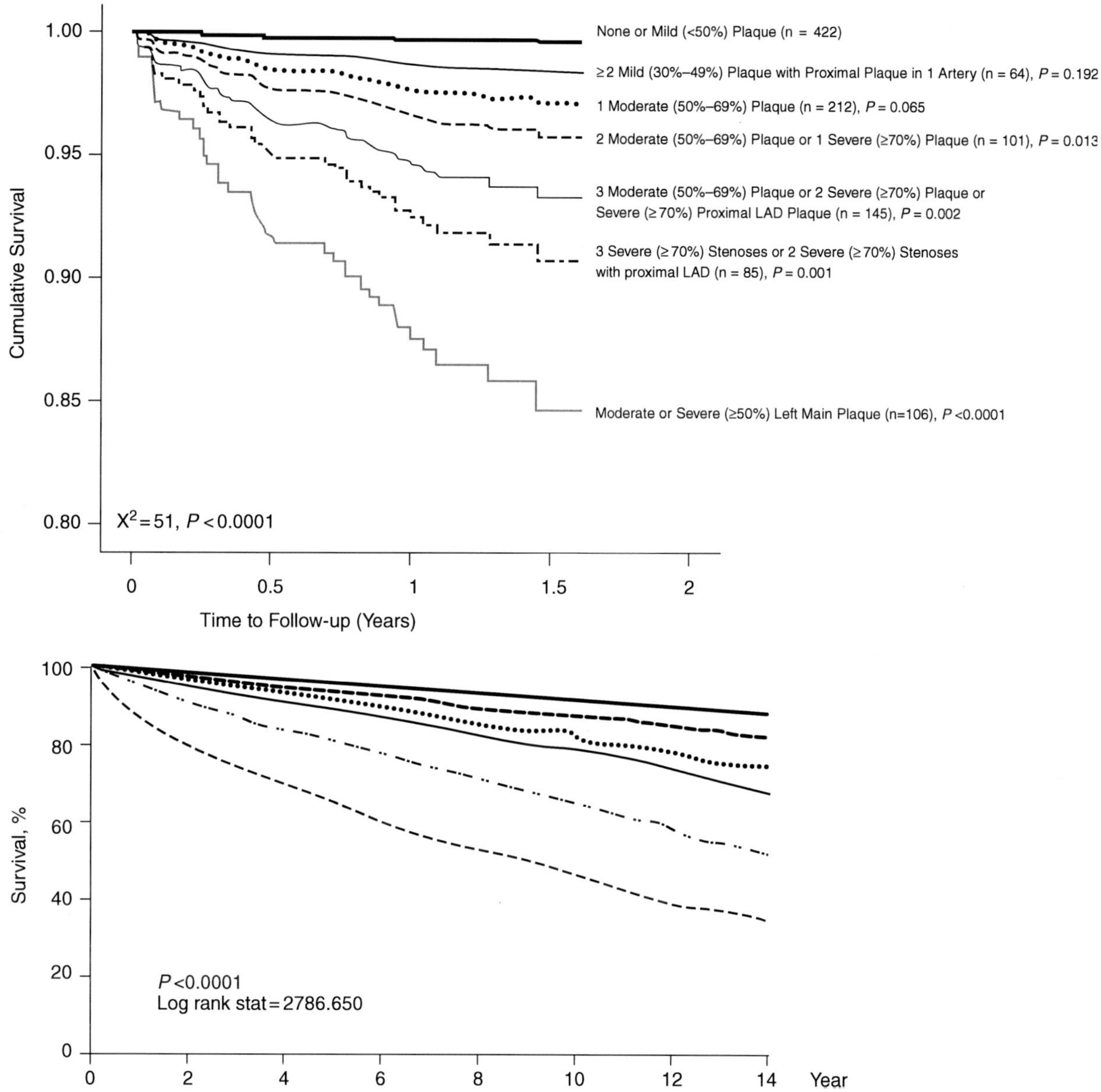

No.	%	No.	%	No.	%	No.	%		DISVES
4,463	100	4,352	98	4,196	95	3,202	91	———	0 (norm)
1,366	100	1,286	96	1,197	91	861	86	- - - -	0 (min)
927	100	790	94	691	86	486	79	••••••••	0 (mod)
4,818	100	2,886	92	2,385	84	1,559	74	———	1
5,286	100	1,897	85	1,410	72	784	59	-·- ·· -	2
6,536	100	1,384	71	917	54	480	40	- - - - -	3

FIGURE 4.2 Comparison of survival curves of patients based on the extent of coronary artery plaque and number of vessels involved. (From Refs. 3 and 16, with permission.) (DISVES, number of diseased vessels)

of those without CAD (7.63 versus 4.19 deaths per 100 patient-years). Of note, patients with an EF <45% were excluded from this study.

Quinones et al. (18) evaluated the interaction of LV mass and EF in patients from the SOLVD trials and registry, a predominantly white (86%), male (80%) population with ischemic (58%) heart failure and LV dysfunction (EF ≤45%). In this population, even after adjustment for EF, ischemic etiology, heart failure class, age, and participation in the Trials or Registry, an increase in LV mass was still significantly associated with an increased risk of all-cause mortality. In addition, there was an interaction between EF and LV mass such that for those patients with an LV mass greater than or equal to the mean (298 g), an EF ≥35% was protective, whereas for those with an LV mass <298 g there was no such effect (Figure 4.3).

Acute Coronary Syndromes

This chapter will not cover the acute coronary syndromes as readers are referred to the accompanying chapter in this text. However, it should be evident that the occurrence of acute plaque rupture and thrombosis has a significant impact on the prognosis of a patient with chronic ischemic heart disease. Cardiogenic shock and mechanical complications such as a ventricular septal defect, free wall rupture, and ischemic mitral regurgitation in particular portend a grave prognosis if these occur during an acute coronary syndrome.

■ PHYSIOLOGICAL PREDICTORS

Exercise Capacity Parameters

Patients with chronic ischemic heart disease may demonstrate varying degrees of endothelial dysfunction and ischemia depending on the status of their endothelium and the presence and robustness of collateral blood supply. From a clinical perspective, this is most easily manifested by the various physiologic parameters of exercise capacity.

Among symptomatic medically-treated patients in CASS, exercise capacity expressed as the final stage achieved during the standard or modified Bruce protocol was a powerful predictor of survival. In the subgroup of patients with three-vessel coronary disease but preserved left ventricular function, four-year survival was 100% for those able to achieve Stage V or greater, whereas survival was only 53% in those only able to achieve stage 1/2 (19). As expected, in the entire

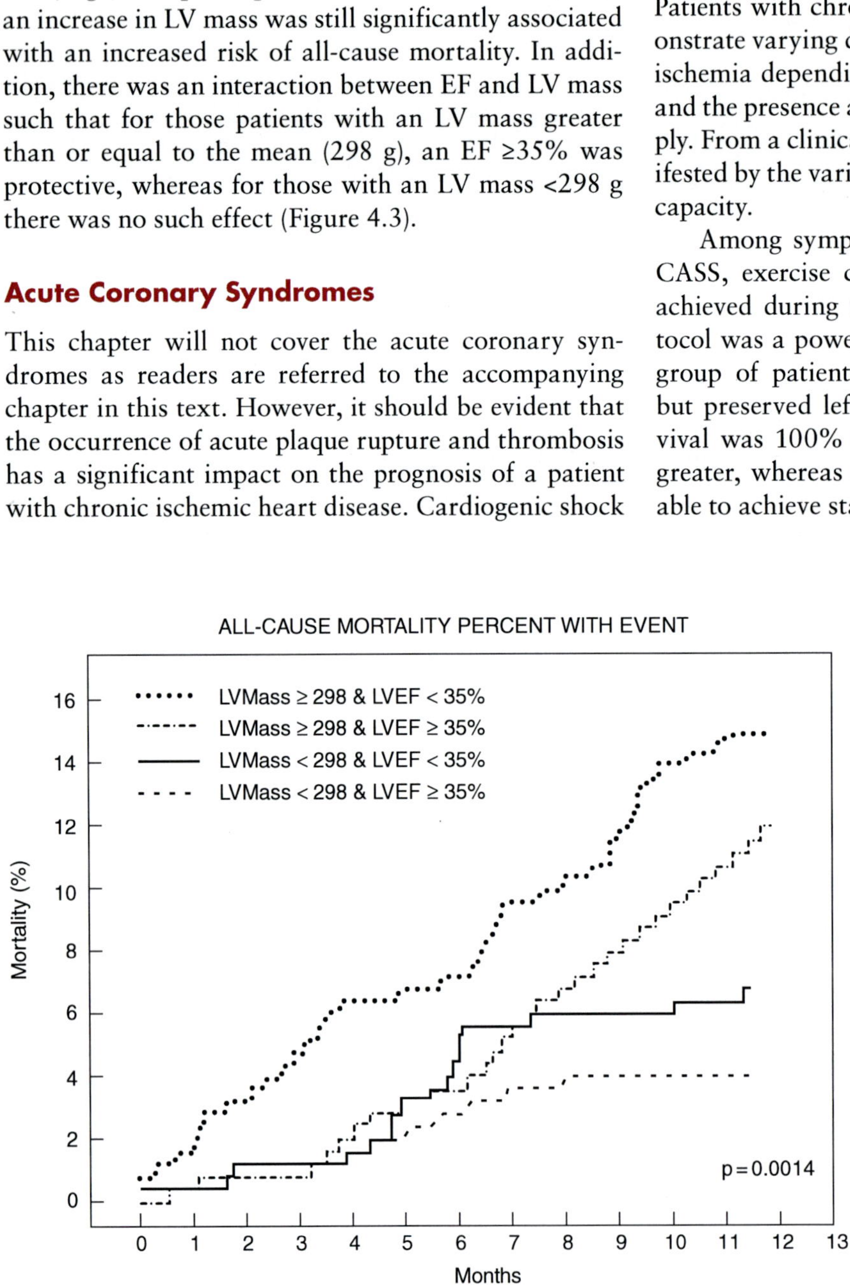

FIGURE 4.3 Interaction of left ventricular mass and ejection fraction in all-cause mortality. (From Ref. 18, with permission.)

population left ventricular function emerged as the overall most significant predictor of survival, followed by the number of diseased vessels.

Mark et al. (20) evaluated the prognostic performance of the Duke Treadmill Score which expanded on total exercise time to also incorporate the presence or absence of angina during exercise and the net magnitude of ST segment deviation. Using this simple additive score, they similarly found that even in patients with three-vessel disease, a very low score (≥+7) resulted in a 5-year survival rate of 93% versus 67% for those with a high-risk score (≤ –11). In their analysis the maximum net ST segment deviation was the most important contributor to the overall score as opposed to the total exercise time.

Myers et al. (21) studied 6,213 men over a mean follow-up of 6.2 years and determined that peak exercise capacity was the strongest predictor of mortality in both normal subjects and those with established CVD. Among patients with known CVD, every 1-MET increase in exercise capacity conferred a 9% improvement in survival. Patients able to exercise to ≥10.7 METs were in the highest quintile and demonstrated the best survival.

Additional exercise testing parameters associated with a poor prognosis have recently been extensively reviewed (22) and include exercise-induced hypotension (23,24), chronotropic incompetence (25,26), impaired heart rate recovery (27,28), and the presence of ventricular arrhythmias either during stress or in recovery (29,30).

Heart Failure Classification

Given the significance of exercise-induced indicators of left ventricular performance, it should come as no surprise that the clinical classification of patients during their daily activities is also correlated with outcome. In the case of those with ischemic cardiomyopathies, the simple classification of patients into the Stages of Heart Failure as outlined by the American Heart Association and American College of Cardiology has also been shown to predict mortality. Ammar et al. (31) sampled a random selection of adults >45 years of age living in Olmstead County, MN and found clear, progressively increasing five-year all-cause mortality rates in the stages proceeding from 0 (no heart failure) to D (severe heart failure). Five-year survival in patients classified as stage 0, A, B, C, or D heart failure was 98.9%, 97.0%, 95.7%, 74.6%, and 20%, respectively. Even though this population was randomly sampled and therefore not restricted to those with chronic ischemic heart disease, 12% of patients had a known history of CAD and 5% had a history of myocardial infarction.

Nuclear Perfusion Imaging

The use of nuclear perfusion imaging in addition to exercise stress testing or as an alternative modality for patients unable to exercise (using pharmacologic agents) can provide important prognostic information for patients with chronic ischemic heart disease.

In stable, medically-treated patients with confirmed CAD, Iskandrian et al. (32) found that the extent of perfusion defect conveyed incremental and independent prognostic information above clinical, exercise, and catheterization data combined. Event-free survival over a period of 28 ± 15 months was 95% in those with a defect <15% of the myocardium versus 75% for those with a >15% defect (P <0.001). Interestingly, combining gender, clinical, and SPECT data appeared to provide equivalent predictive power (chi-square statistic) regardless of whether or not catheterization data was added. As expected, an exercise capacity of >6 METs, an ejection fraction of ≥50%, and a lesser extent of CAD were all also associated with improved survival.

In a broader unselected population referred for nuclear stress testing, Sharir et al. (6) found that the extent of reversible perfusion defect (as expressed by the summed difference score) was the best predictor of subsequent nonfatal myocardial infarction, and was best fit by an exponential curve. Among these patients, 26% had a history of myocardial infarction, and patients with nonischemic cardiomyopathies, valvular disease, or who underwent revascularization within 60 days were excluded. Importantly, even though ejection fraction most powerfully stratified the risk of cardiac death, in patients with an ejection fraction >30% the amount of perfusion defect provided incremental prognostic information. In patients with an ejection fraction of <30%, the rates of cardiac death were high (>4% per year) regardless of the amount of ischemia.

In addition to assessing prognosis in stable patients, nuclear perfusion imaging has been used in a prospective manner to help risk-stratify survivors of acute myocardial infarction. Mahmarian et al. (33) used the extent of total and ischemic perfusion defect size (PDS) on adenosine ^{99m}Technetium sestamibi scans to stratify patients into low-, middle-, and high-risk groups, with subsequent cardiac events occurring in a progressively increasing manner among these groups. For every 10% absolute increment in total or ischemic PDS, the unadjusted relative risk for an adverse event increased by 37% and 64% respectively. In a stepwise logistic regression, the most important independent risk predictors were, in order, total PDS, ischemic PDS, and left ventricular ejection fraction.

Additional findings on nuclear imaging which are predictive of adverse cardiac events include an increased lung-to-heart ratio on either ^{201}Thallium or ^{99m}Technetium imaging following exercise or pharmacologic stress (34), as well as transient ischemic dilation of the left ventricular cavity (35,36).

Dobutamine Echocardiography

Echocardiography provides important prognostic information primarily in two areas: assessment of resting left ventricular function (i.e., ejection fraction), and assessment of provokable ischemia and/or myocardial viability.

As previously discussed, ejection fraction remains the most important prognostic marker, and echocardiography is perhaps the most widely used tool for its assessment. In addition to this finding, however, echocardiography can also assess the functional importance of coronary lesions by evaluating for inducible regional wall motion abnormalities or even global left ventricular dysfunction.

The normal response to stress (i.e., exercise) or infusion of dobutamine is an augmentation of left ventricular contractility. A new wall motion abnormality present with stress but absent at rest suggests inducible ischemia, whereas a fixed abnormality suggests scar. Numerous studies have reported increasing cardiac event rates with inducible ischemia by stress echocardiography. In a group of patients with known or suspected CAD, Marcovitz et al. (37) reported a significant increase in death and myocardial infarction over an average follow-up of 15 months for those patients with a mixed response to dobutamine infusion (i.e., demonstrating both ischemia and fixed defects) as compared to those with a normal response (17% versus 1.4%, $P < 0.001$). Dobutamine was infused at escalating doses in increments of 5 mcg/kg/min starting at 5 mcg/kg/min to an average dose of 25 mcg/kg/min in this study.

In contrast, a stepwise infusion of dobutamine starting at a lower dose (i.e., 2.5 mcg/kg/min) has been used to help identify hibernating myocardium in patients with known CAD and resting left ventricular dysfunction. Specifically, a biphasic response to dobutamine—improvement at a low dose followed by abnormal wall motion at high dose—can help identify areas of dysfunctional myocardium which have a higher likelihood of improving with revascularization. Qureshi et al. (38) studied 34 patients with stable CAD who subsequently underwent successful revascularization (28 patients had angioplasty, 6 underwent bypass surgery) and found that a biphasic response to dobutamine was less sensitive but more specific than ^{201}Thallium SPECT rest-redistribution imaging. Specifically, a biphasic response had a 74% sensitivity and 89% specificity for identifying recovery of function following revascularization compared to a 90% sensitivity and 56% specificity for a maximal ^{201}Thallium uptake of 60% on either rest or redistribution images. In this group of revascularized patients the ejection fraction increased from 39% ± 14% to 43% ± 15% ($P = 0.0002$) at follow-up.

Meluzin et al. (39) correlated the improved ejection fraction following revascularization of a large amount of viable but hibernating myocardium with improved survival in 133 patients with CAD and an EF ≤ 40%. They performed dobutamine echocardiography prior to revascularization (118 bypass surgery, 15 angioplasty) and separated patients into those with a large amount (six segments or more) of viable but hibernating myocardium (defined as an improvement in wall motion of at least one grade in two adjacent segments), a small amount (two to five segments) of viable but hibernating myocardium, and those with irreversibly damaged dysfunctional segments. Ejection fraction was similar in all three groups prior to revascularization. The group with a large amount of viable but hibernating myocardium experienced the greatest increase in EF following revascularization (35 ± 5% to 47 ± 6%) and had the lowest rate of cardiac events over the follow-up period of 20 ± 12 months compared to the other two groups (6.8% versus 30% and 39%). Thus, dobutamine echocardiography can provide prognostic information by identifying those patients who will benefit most from revascularization through the identification of viable but hibernating myocardium.

■ BIOCHEMICAL PREDICTORS

Atherosclerosis is an inflammatory process that begins when circulating leukocytes gain entry into the intimal layer and trigger a cascade of lipid oxidation, smooth muscle cell migration, apoptosis, and cytokine and matrix metalloprotinease production which leads to thickening of the intimal layer and remodeling of the artery (40,41). Accordingly, elevated levels of many of these components to atherosclerosis have been associated with worse prognosis in chronic ischemic heart disease. Perhaps most importantly, hyperlipidemia is a major risk factor for CAD and is strongly associated with outcomes. Additionally, elevated circulating levels of inflammatory markers such as C-reactive protein have been associated with an increased risk of cardiovascular mortality, and even the simple value of the white blood cell count has, in acute coronary syndromes, been associated with an increased risk of subsequent mortality. Biochemical markers thus play an important role in helping to assess the prognosis of patients with chronic ischemic heart disease.

LDL Cholesterol

Since Johann Lobstein first coined the term *arteriosclerosis*, or "hardening of the arteries" in 1833, to the Framingham Study which began in 1948 (42), to the isolation of mevastatin by Akira Endo in 1976 (43), and on to the publication of the Scandinavian Simvastatin Survival Study (4S) in 1994 (44), cholesterol levels have emerged as perhaps the most potent modifiable risk factor in the treatment of chronic ischemic heart disease. Genetic disorders such as homozygous familial hypercholesterolemia where severe atherosclerosis is present by early adolescence have helped clarify the importance of LDL cholesterol in the pathogenesis of atherosclerosis.

Elevated serum cholesterol levels and in particular LDL-cholesterol levels are strongly associated with cardiovascular mortality across the spectrum of epidemiologic studies and pharmacologic intervention studies in primary and secondary prevention trials (Figure 4.4). In the Cholesterol Treatment Trialists' Collaborators meta-analysis of >90,000 patients studied in 14 randomized trials of statin therapy, a reduction in LDL cholesterol of 1 mmol/L (39 mg/dL) was associated with a 12% proportional reduction in all-cause mortality, predominantly driven by a 19% proportional reduction in cardiovascular mortality (45). Among patients with pre-existing heart disease there were 14 fewer deaths per 1000 participants per mmol LDL cholesterol reduction, as well as an approximately 25% reduction in major adverse cardiac events.

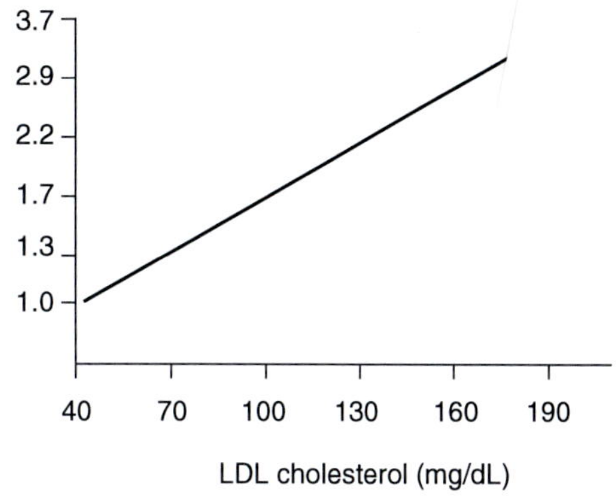

FIGURE 4.4 Log–linear relationship of LDL cholesterol with relative risk for coronary heart disease. (From Ref. 85, with permission.)

Currently, national guidelines support a target LDL cholesterol level of <100 mg/dL or optionally, <70 mg/dL for patients with established CAD. In the PROVE-IT-TIMI 22 trial, Cannon et al. (46) demonstrated that in survivors of acute coronary syndromes, achieving a median LDL of 62 mg/dL with high-dose atorvastatin compared with a median LDL of 95 mg/dL resulted in a statistically significant 16% relative risk reduction in the composite endpoint of death, MI, unstable angina requiring hospitalization, revascularization, or stroke. LaRosa et al. (47) similarly compared low-dose to high-dose atorvastatin in the TNT trial, and found that achieving a mean LDL of 77 mg/dL on 80 mg of atorvastatin, compared to a mean LDL of 101 mg/dL on 10 mg of atorvastatin, resulted in an absolute 2.2% reduction (and 22% relative risk reduction) in the rates of adverse cardiac events. Of note, despite a run-in period where participants with elevated liver function tests (LFTs) or myalgias were excluded, there were a total of five cases of rhabdomyolysis (two in the 80 mg arm and three in the 10 mg arm) and 1.2% of patients assigned 80 mg of atoravastatin developed a persistent LFT abnormality.

Interestingly, in a different cohort of patients 60 years or older with ischemic cardiomyopathies and NYHA Class II or greater systolic heart failure, Kjekshus et al. (48) found in the CORONA trial that 10 mg of rosuvastatin compared to placebo was not effective in reducing death or major cardiovascular outcomes despite achieving a mean LDL of 76 mg/dL compared to 138 mg/dL at three months. Deaths from noncardiac causes were similar between the two groups, as was the incidence of cancer. Muscle-related symptoms and LFT abnormalities were also similar between the two groups, and drug discontinuations for adverse events were actually more common in the placebo group.

Despite the negative results from the CORONA trial, the TNT and PROVE-IT trials support the hypothesis that targeting lower mean LDL cholesterol levels in patients with CAD will result in clinical benefit. The pathophysiologic basis behind this hypothesis is supported by the REVERSAL trial, where Nissen et al. (49) compared the effects of 18 months of therapy with 80 mg of atorvastatin or 40 mg of pravastatin on the percent change in atheroma volume as visualized by intravascular ultrasound. The atorvastatin group achieved a mean LDL cholesterol level of 79 mg/dL compared with 110 mg/dL in the pravastatin group. Intravascular ultrasound demonstrated a lack of progression of atherosclerosis in the atorvastatin group (−0.4%; CI −2.4–1.5%; P = 0.98) compared with a statistically significant progression in the pravastatin group (2.7%; CI 0.2–4.7%; P = 0.001). In patients with established CAD then, it seems most prudent to target the more aggressive goal of an LDL cholesterol level <70 mg/dL in order to try to reduce the risk of major adverse cardiovascular events. It is possible that some patient groups may not derive significant benefit, such as those studied in the CORONA trial; however, it seems unlikely they would suffer adverse events from such therapy.

HDL Cholesterol

In addition to the importance of LDL reduction, HDL cholesterol levels have been associated with coronary atherosclerosis progression and cardiovascular outcomes. In epidemiologic studies a 1 mg/dL increment in HDL cholesterol was associated with a 2% to 3% decrease in cardiovascular outcomes (50). The Third Report of the National Cholesterol Education Program (NCEP) Expert Panel on Detection, Evaluation, and Treatment of High Blood Cholesterol in Adults (ATP III) defined low HDL as <40 mg/dL (51). Nonpharmacologic methods of increasing HDL cholesterol levels include regular aerobic exercise, smoking cessation, weight loss, dietary changes including diets high in omega-3 fatty acids, and mild to moderate alcohol intake (52). These lifestyle changes will be covered in more detail later in this chapter.

HDL cholesterol has also been the target of pharmacologic agents, with increases associated with improved cardiovascular outcomes. In the VA-HIT study by Rubins et al. (53), the use of gemfibrozil in 2,531 men with established CHD with an HDL of 40 mg/dL or less resulted in a 6% increase in HDL cholesterol levels over a median of 5.1 years. This resulted in an absolute risk reduction of 4.4% (relative risk reduction of 22%) in nonfatal MI and death from coronary causes in the absence of differences in LDL cholesterol levels compared to the placebo group. There was additionally a 31% reduction in triglyceride levels, which averaged 160 mg/dL at baseline.

In a long-term follow-up of the Coronary Drug Project, Canner et al. (54) found in 8,341 men with established CHD that treatment with niacin resulted in an 11% relative risk reduction for mortality compared with placebo. Interestingly, despite beneficial effects on HDL cholesterol levels, treatment with estrogen was halted early in this trial for an increase in adverse effects and outcomes (55).

Combination therapy with niacin and a statin has also been shown to produce clinical and angiographic benefits. Brown et al. (56) evaluated the effects of simvastatin in combination with niacin on patients with documented coronary disease in the HATS trial and demonstrated a significant reduction in nonfatal MI or death from cardiovascular causes compared to placebo, albeit with a relatively small number of patients. In the treatment arm, HDL cholesterol increased by 26% over the three years of treatment and was also associated with a slight regression (0.4%) in coronary mean percent stenosis in the proximal arteries by invasive arteriography; the placebo arm experienced a 3.9% increase in stenoses.

Despite the beneficial effects of raising HDL cholesterol levels demonstrated by these trials, it remains a more complex therapeutic target than LDL cholesterol. For example, despite the beneficial effects of estrogen on HDL cholesterol levels, as mentioned previously this was shown to be harmful in men with established CHD and was also found to convey risk to postmenopausal women in the Women's Health Initiative. Despite a mean 7.3% increase in HDL cholesterol levels over a mean follow-up of 5.2 years, there was an increased risk for nonfatal MI or death due to CHD associated with the use of estrogen and progestin (HR 1.24, CI 1.00–1.54) (57). In addition, despite low HDL levels generally being associated with increased cardiovascular risk, a small group of carriers of a genetic variant of apolipoprotein A-I known as ApoA-I Milano have very low levels of HDL (10–30 mg/dL), but a relative absence of evidence of CHD expected for these levels (58). Even more intriguing, in a small study using an intravenous recombinant form of ApoA-I Milano/phospholipid complexes, Nissen et al. (59) demonstrated that five weekly infusions in patients with established CAD resulted in a significant reduction in atheroma volume by intravascular ultrasound (–14.1 mm^3 or a 4.2% decrease from baseline, *P* <0.001 compared to placebo). Further refinement of this recombinant form raises the possibility of a new treatment modality in the near future (60).

Finally, the results of clinical trials with torcetrapib, an inhibitor of cholesterol ester transfer protein (CETP) have once again tempered enthusiasm for novel pharmacologic strategies to translate increased HDL cholesterol levels into beneficial clinical outcomes. In the ILLUMINATE trial, Barter et al. (61) studied 15,067 patients at high cardiovascular risk and demonstrated that despite an astounding increase in HDL cholesterol levels of 72.1% and a 24.9% decrease in LDL cholesterol levels compared with placebo, that torcetrapib was associated with an *increased* risk of cardiovascular events (HR 1.25, CI 1.09–1.44, *P* = 0.001) as well as all-cause mortality (HR 1.58, CI 1.14–2.19, *P* = 0.006). The reason for the increased mortality remains unclear and raised many questions (62,63). Although there was an average increase in systolic blood pressure of 5.4 mmHg, this alone could not account for the overall increased mortality observed in the trial. Further trials with other CETP inhibitors continue, with the hope that the hazard observed with torcetrapib may have been a drug-specific effect and not related to the class of agents.

For now, in patients with established CHD it is recommended to initiate diet and lifestyle changes along with statin therapy to target an LDL of 70 mg/dL or less and then, if the HDL is <40 mg/dL, to consider adding a fibrate or niacin to raise the HDL cholesterol level. Of note, no specific level of HDL was set in the recent ATP III guidelines, further adding to the uncertainty of how to optimally treat low HDL cholesterol levels.

Triglycerides and Lipoprotein(a)

Additional targets of intervention include elevated triglyceride levels (≥200 mg/dL) and elevated lipoprotein(a) (Lp[a]) levels, both of which have been associated with an independent increased risk of CHD (64,65). However, because elevated triglycerides are often associated with other factors conveying coronary risk such as obesity, hypertension, diabetes, and cigarette smoking, treatment focused initially on these problems may ameliorate the elevated triglyceride levels. Nonetheless, because of its independent risk association, the ATP III Guidelines (51) recommend evaluating patients with triglycerides ≥200 mg/dL for "non-HDL" cholesterol levels (due to variability in triglyceride levels) and targeting a level that is 30 mg/dL higher than the LDL cholesterol goal (i.e., non-HDL cholesterol level of 100 mg/dL or less for those with established CAD). Niacin and fibrates are currently the most effective agents to lower triglycerides and therefore are the mainstay of therapy (66).

A causal relationship of elevated Lp(a) levels with increased CHD has not yet been established. Niacin remains the most effective drug to date to decrease Lp(a) levels (67); statins are ineffective. The ATP III Guidelines did not specify Lp(a) as a target for intervention, but some advocates propose counting an elevated Lp(a) as an additional risk factor to help establish the target for LDL cholesterol levels.

C-Reactive Protein

The prognostic utility of measuring high-sensitivity C-reactive protein (hsCRP) in patients with established CAD was demonstrated by Ridker et al. (68) in a subsequent analysis of the PROVE IT-TIMI-22 trial. In this study of survivors of acute coronary syndromes, patients who achieved an LDL cholesterol level of 70 mg/dL or less had a reduced risk of nonfatal MI or death from cardiovascular causes. In addition, those patients who achieved an hsCRP level of <2 mg/L also experienced a risk reduction in the primary endpoint of the same magnitude. Interestingly, the most benefit was derived when both an LDL of <70 mg/dL and a hsCRP level of <2 mg/L was achieved, regardless of the statin given.

Statins have been shown to lower CRP levels by 28% (69) with a strong correlation between the change in LDL cholesterol levels and the change in CRP levels. This link has raised the question as to whether or not CRP levels should be independently targeted in patients with lipid levels that would not otherwise necessitate treatment. Ridker et al. (70) have demonstrated in the JUPITER trial that hsCRP can effectively identify patients who are at increased risk of cardiovascular events and would benefit from statin therapy even when their lipid levels are not considered to necessitate treatment under current guidelines. In their primary prevention trial of 17,802 patients without established heart disease, treatment with 20 mg of rosuvastatin daily compared to placebo resulted in a statistically significant reduction in a combined endpoint of MI, stroke, revascularization, hospitalization for unstable angina or death from cardiovascular causes after a median of only 1.9 years (the trial was stopped early following the first prespecified efficacy evaluation).

Regarding its use in patients with chronic ischemic heart disease, in 2003 the American Heart Association and Centers for Disease Control and Prevention issued a statement detailing the clinical utility of measuring hsCRP levels (71). Because of its consistent association with cardiovascular outcomes in patients with established CHD in both the chronic and acute (i.e., ACS) setting, the statement proposed that hsCRP could be assayed to provide prognostic information regarding the risk for subsequent cardiovascular events. Measurements should be obtained twice, optimally two weeks apart, with levels of <1 mg/L indicating a low-risk for subsequent events, and levels >3.0 mg/L indicating high-risk.

Whether or not reducing hsCRP levels independent of lowering of LDL cholesterol levels will result in clinical benefit will have to await the refinement of specific CRP inhibitors (72).

Additional Biochemical Predictors

Additional biochemical parameters proposed for use in providing prognostic information for patients with chronic ischemic heart disease include troponin I, pro-BNP, cystatin C, macrophage-colony stimulating factor, and the white blood cell count with differential (73–76). In general, the greater the number of abnormal biochemical parameters, the greater the risk for subsequent cardiovascular events—although the relative increase in risk stratification is typically fairly small, potentially limiting the clinical utility of routinely assaying these markers.

■ PHARMACOLOGICAL PREDICTORS

As previously discussed, pharmacologic therapy to modify cholesterol levels including LDL, HDL, and triglycerides, have consistently demonstrated significant clinical benefit in terms of cardiovascular outcomes and mortality. Statin therapy has become a mainstay of medical therapy, and may be primarily responsible for the equipoise achieved in some clinical trials comparing medical to interventional therapy (77). Further optimization of medical therapy for patients with chronic ischemic heart disease includes the use of angiotensin-converting enzyme (ACE) inhibitors, beta-blockers, antiplatelet therapy, and n3 omega-3 fatty acids.

ACE Inhibitors

The benefits of ACE inhibitors in patients with CAD were first established in post-MI patients with left ventricular dysfunction and symptomatic patients with an ejection fraction <35% in the SAVE and SOLVD trials, respectively (78,79). Both demonstrated a substantial reduction in all-cause mortality and cardiovascular outcomes. As a result of these and subsequent trials, oral ACE inhibitors are currently indicated for patients with ACS (without hypotension or other contraindications) and symptoms of heart failure or an ejection fraction of <40% (80–82).

The HOPE trial (83) evaluated the use of ramipril compared to placebo in 9,297 high-risk patients, approximately 80% of whom had a history of CAD, and 38% of whom had diabetes. There was a clear benefit to treatment over a mean of five years, including an absolute risk reduction of 2% in death from cardiovascular causes (6.1% versus 8.1%, RR 0.74, *P* <0.001) and a 2.4% absolute risk reduction in nonfatal MI (9.9% versus 12.3%, RR 0.80, *P* <0.001).

Based on these results treatment with an ACE inhibitor was recommended for patients with CAD and/or diabetes in addition to those indicated by the SAVE and SOLVD trials. The EUROPA trial (84) confirmed the HOPE results by demonstrating that ACE inhibitors were of benefit in the treatment of stable, low-risk patients with CAD as well. A 2% absolute risk reduction in the composite endpoint of cardiovascular mortality, nonfatal MI, and cardiac arrest was achieved using perindopril over a mean of 4.2 years. Patients with clinical heart failure were excluded and ejection fraction was not assessed.

In the PEACE trial (86), the use of trandolapril compared to placebo for 4.8 years in patients with stable CAD and a left ventricular EF of >40% did not show a significant benefit in the primary of death from cardiovascular causes, MI, or coronary revascularization. The investigators note that these patients were at lower risk than previous trials, with a preserved EF (mean 58 ± 9%) and higher rates of treatment with other "standard" therapies (including lipid-lowering agents) such that even the placebo arm had a lower event rate than the active arm from HOPE (10.2% versus 14%) and nearly equivalent rates of the primary outcome from EUROPA (8.6% and 8%). They conclude that low-risk patients on optimal medical therapy with a relatively preserved ejection fraction may not necessarily benefit from adding an ACE inhibitor.

Thus overall it appears that patients with CAD and diabetes, symptomatic heart failure, or an ejection fraction <40% clearly derive benefit from ACE inhibitors. Other patients with stable CAD may also derive benefit from an ACE inhibitor, although the magnitude may diminish if they are at particularly low-risk and already optimized on medical therapy (87).

Beta-blockers

Beta-blockers have been clearly shown to reduce the incidence of all-cause mortality and nonfatal MI in survivors of myocardial infarction (88,89). This effect seems to be more significant in long-term treatment (6–48 months) trials for secondary prevention rather than short-term acute treatment trials as reported in an extensive meta-analysis performed by Freemantle et al. (90). They found a 23% reduction in the odds of death in long term trials with beta-blockers (95% CI 15–31%) but only a 4% reduction in short-term trials (95% CI –8–15%) Underscoring the importance of patient selection in the acute setting, the COMMIT trial investigators (91) reported no overall benefit to the use of metoprolol in patients presenting with acute myocardial infarction. This, however, was the result of an increased hazard for cardiogenic shock in the first 24 hours, counterbalanced by a decreased incidence of recurrent myocardial infarction and ventricular fibrillation in the ensuing days. The applicability of these findings to the U.S. population is somewhat limited since only about half the patients had revascularization and this was only in the form of a fibrinolytic agent. Nonetheless, the importance of assessing the suitability of the patient for initiation of beta-blocker therapy is emphasized by these findings and led to a revision of the ACC/AHA Guidelines in 2007 to outline the specific contraindications to early beta-blockade including signs of heart failure, evidence of a low output state, or patients at an increased risk of cardiogenic shock (80,81).

Beta-blockers also have a role as antianginal therapy in patients with chronic ischemic heart disease. In patients with exertional angina, beta-blockers can limit the heart-rate blood pressure increase during exercise, thereby delaying or even abolishing the onset of angina (92,93). Both symptomatic and asymptomatic episodes of ischemia can be reduced, suggesting added benefits of beta-blockers in controlling ischemia during daily activities (94).

In symptomatic chronic heart failure, beta-blockers are also an essential component of an optimal medical regimen, as demonstrated in several trials (95–98). Currently extended-release metoprolol succinate, carvedilol, and bisoprolol remain the agents of choice for treatment of patients with chronic ischemic heart disease and NYHA Class II–IV symptomatic heart failure.

Thus, beta-blockers are clearly indicated for patients with chronic ischemic heart disease with a history of myocardial infarction, angina, or symptomatic heart failure. There are, however, several subgroups of patients in whom the routine use of beta-blockers is less clear. Patients with no symptoms of heart failure but a reduced EF and CAD are recommended by U.S. Guidelines to be on beta-blocker therapy "although clinical trials are lacking." However, European Guidelines suggest using beta-blockers only if they are also post-myocardial infarction. Patients with evidence of CAD but no symptoms of heart failure and a normal EF are also relatively understudied. Bunch et al. (100) did evaluate a cohort of patients who underwent invasive angiography (many for unstable angina) and found a mortality benefit for patients who were already on a beta-blocker prior to hospitalization. The definition of CAD in this study was at least one coronary artery stenosis of ≥70%, and approximately half underwent revascularization. What remains unclear is whether or not patients with a preserved EF and no symptoms of heart failure who are found to have evidence of subclinical CAD (i.e., coronary calcifications or plaque by cardiac CT) derive benefit from beta-blockade. As these imaging modalities grow in utilization, physicians will increasingly encounter this clinical dilemma. Even the addition of hypertension to this scenario may not help justify the utilization of beta-blockers since it is unclear what degree of subclinical CAD should be considered the equivalent of the "compelling indication" of CHD, especially since the routine use of beta-blockers as first-line therapy for hypertension has recently come into question (101).

Antiplatelet Agents

Aspirin has been proven to be beneficial in patients with chronic ischemic heart disease in lowering the risk of nonfatal myocardial infarction, nonfatal stroke, vascular death, and all-cause mortality (102). Currently it is recommended to administer aspirin at a dose of 162 to 325 mg in the setting of an acute coronary syndrome or during percutaneous intervention, with a decrease to 75 to 162 mg for chronic therapy (80,81). Given that the recommended duration of higher-dose aspirin therapy varies depending on the type of stent used, it may be easiest to simply administer 162 mg of aspirin daily, even though on a practical basis in the United States this may necessitate taking two baby aspirins or splitting a full-strength aspirin in half. For patients with a history of peptic ulcer disease or who experience gastrointestinal upset with aspirin, an 81 mg dose may be sufficient and, if necessary, a proton-pump inhibitor or H2-blocker may be added. Although prospective data is currently lacking, caution is warranted in administering proton pump inhibitors with clopidogrel in patients following an acute coronary syndrome (124,125)

Clopidogrel in addition to aspirin was shown in the CURE trial (103) to reduce the composite endpoint of nonfatal MI, stroke, or death from cardiovascular causes in patients with acute coronary syndromes. In the COMMIT trial (104), clopidogrel in addition to aspirin was similarly shown to reduce the composite endpoint of death, reinfarction, or stroke in patients presenting with ST elevation MI. Importantly, in the CURE trial clopidogrel was administered as a 300 mg loading dose followed by 75 mg a day for a mean duration of nine months and approximately 37% of the patients underwent revascularization (21% underwent PCI, the remainder had bypass surgery). In the COMMIT trial, clopidogrel was administered only as a 75 mg daily dose for a mean duration of 15 days, and just over 50% underwent revascularization solely with a fibrinolytic agent.

Although the addition of clopidogrel to aspirin is clearly indicated for patients with chronic ischemic heart disease presenting with an acute coronary syndrome or who are undergoing percutaneous intervention, the duration of treatment remains unclear (105). Current ACC/AHA recommendations are to continue clopidogrel in addition to aspirin ideally for one year following an acute coronary syndrome, and for *a minimum* of one month following elective implantation of a bare metal stent, and 12 months for a drug-eluting stent. For more detailed discussion on this subject, readers are referred to the related chapter on Medical Therapy in Acute Coronary Syndromes in this book.

Statins

As previously discussed in the LDL cholesterol section, lipid-lowering agents primarily in the form of HMG-CoA reductase inhibitors (i.e., statins) have consistently demonstrated the ability to significantly reduce the incidence of death, myocardial infarction, revascularization, and stroke and are an essential component to the treatment of patients with chronic ischemic heart disease (45).

Omega-3 Fatty Acids

The GISSI-Prevenzione trial (106) evaluated the use of n-3 polyunsaturated fatty acids (i.e., omega-3 fatty acids) in 11,324 patients who had survived a recent (≥3 months) myocardial infarction. After 3.5 years of open-label treatment with one gram daily, there was a small but statistically significant reduction in the primary composite endpoint of all-cause mortality, nonfatal MI, and nonfatal stroke (12.3% versus 14.6% by four-way analysis). Among secondary endpoints, all-cause mortality was reduced by 20%, cardiac death by 35%, and sudden death by 45%. Unfortunately, numerous other trials have been very small with variable results (107). Different study populations, different formulations of fish oil, and methodological problems may have contributed to these disparate results. As a result, in general current guidelines support encouraging increased consumption of omega-3 fatty acids in the form of fish or capsules (one gram/day) for risk reduction, but acknowledge that the evidence base is lacking (80, 81). The ongoing SU.FOL.OM3 Study may help to shed some light on this subject (108).

■ BEHAVIORAL PREDICTORS

Smoking

Exposure to tobacco smoke has been associated with an increased risk of acute myocardial infarction (109). Possible mechanisms include increased platelet adhesion with subsequent thrombosis, and endothelial dysfunction with impaired coronary flow reserve (110). Consistent with these hypotheses has been numerous epidemiologic studies demonstrating a significant decrease in hospital admissions for acute myocardial infarction following the institution of a smoking ban in public places (111,112).

Not surprisingly then, the effect of smoking cessation on the prognosis of patients with chronic ischemic heart disease is substantial. In one meta-analysis by Critchley and Capewell (113), smoking cessation in patients with established CHD resulted in a crude 36% reduction in crude relative risk of all-cause mortality. The crude risk reduction for nonfatal reinfarction was 32%.

Given the disappointing success rates of smoking cessation for individuals, referral to an appropriate smoking cessation program is advised, in addition to encouraging others within the immediate home and work environment who smoke to quit as well. Some pharmacologic options are available including nicotine replacement therapies, as well as bupropion and varenicline, all with odds ratios of successfully quitting compared to placebo of about two (114). Unfortunately, the majority of patients in these trials including those in the active treatment arms were unsuccessful in quitting. This fact coupled with the impressive risk reductions that can be achieved with successful smoking cessation should make it clear that smoking cessation should be addressed at every opportunity both in the acute setting and at every outpatient follow-up visit.

Exercise

As previously discussed, exercise capacity remains a strong predictor of mortality in patients with chronic ischemic heart disease. Perhaps not surprisingly then, regular exercise reflects an important lifestyle habit which has been associated with improved survival. Binjen et al. (115) found that regular exercise in the form of walking or cycling for 20 minutes at least three times per week was associated with a 31% relative risk reduction in cardiovascular death and 29% reduction in all-cause death in a cohort of retired men aged 64 to 84 years at baseline. Kujala et al. (116) studied a Finnish Twin Cohort and determined that exercising at least six times a month for 30 minutes was associated with a hazard ratio of 0.57 (95% CI 0.45–0.74) for all-cause mortality compared to those who were sedentary. Apullan et al. (117) recently related self-reported leisure-time physical activity to long-term survival in 14,021 CASS Registry patients. Over a median follow-up of 14.7 years, both all-cause and cardiovascular mortality increased as patients classified their leisure-time physical activity as strenuous, moderate, mild, or sedentary. Although the hazard ratio for all-cause mortality decreased from 1.63 (95% CI 1.34–1.97, P <0.0001) to 1.23 (95% CI 1.0[illegible]–1.49, P = 0.03), it nonetheless remained significant.

Clearly, regular exercise remains an important lifestyle intervention with significant survival benefit for all patients with chronic ischemic heart disease, and should be encouraged at every opportunity. A minimum of 30 minutes of walking should be prescribed, preferably on a daily basis.

Alcohol

The controversies surrounding the potential risks and benefits of alcohol consumption on cardiovascular health have recently been extensively reviewed (118). As many studies have reported, there appears to be a J-shaped curve relating alcohol consumption with all-cause mortality. In a meta-analysis by Di Castelnuovo et al. (119), the lowest mortality was observed with alcohol consumption of six grams daily (approximately half a drink per day). Maximum protection achieved was similar among men and women (17% and 18% respectively); however, in men, consumption of up to four drinks per day remained protective, whereas for women only up to two drinks per day remained protective. Given concerns over possible adverse effects of encouraging alcohol consumption in nondrinkers and a possible increased cancer risk in women, general recommendations for alcohol consumption are not favored. However, for established drinkers, one to two drinks per day for men and one drink per day in women may convey cardiovascular benefits.

Diet

As previously discussed under pharmacological predictors, fish oil was shown to be beneficial in the GISSI-Prevenzione trial in reducing all-cause and cardiovascular mortality. Increased omega-3 fatty acids are one component of the Mediterranean diet, which has the most substantial evidence for benefit in secondary prevention for patients with chronic ischemic heart disease. As reviewed by Parikh et al. (120), several studies have looked at either the addition of omega-3 fatty acids alone, or the institution of the Mediterranean diet in reducing cardiovascular endpoints in patients with established CHD. Perhaps the most impressive from the dietary standpoint was a follow-up of the Lyon Diet Heart study (121) which evaluated 605 post-MI survivors randomized to a Mediterranean-type diet versus a prudent Western-

ugh the study was halted after 27 of a clear and substantial benefit nean diet, a subsequent follow-up months (122) demonstrated persis- sustained protection against cardiac death and nonfatal MI (14 events versus 44, RR 0.28, 95% CI 0.15–0.53, P = 0.0001). Thus, for patients with chronic ischemic heart disease, a reasonable dietary recommendation would be to have them consume a significant amount of plant foods (fruits, vegetables, breads, seeds, nuts, etc.), minimally processed and locally grown fresh foods, desserts comprised typically of fresh fruits, olive oil as the principal dietary fat, low to moderate amounts of dairy (i.e., yogurts and cheese), more fish and poultry with only rare red meat, up to four eggs per week, and a low to moderate amount of wine with meals.

Alternative diets (e.g., Atkins) may be useful for weight loss; however, the long-term effects on cardiovascular risk are yet to be determined (123).

■ COMORBIDITIES

A review of additional comorbidities that can negatively impact the prognosis of patients with chronic ischemic heart disease is beyond the scope of this chapter. Nonetheless, aggressive management of comorbid conditions such as hypertension, diabetes, atrial fibrillation, renal insufficiency, and peripheral and cerebrovascular disease remain essential to optimizing the treatment of these patients.

■ CONCLUSION

In conclusion, the prognosis of patients with chronic ischemic heart disease can be determined through a variety of invasive and noninvasive tests, measured biochemical and functional parameters, as well as patient-reported symptoms and lifestyle habits. Optimizing the treatment of these patients requires not just pharmacologic interventions but also lasting behavioral changes such as smoking cessation, healthy eating, and regular exercise. Only with this comprehensive approach can we hope to improve the outcomes of patients with chronic ischemic heart disease in the United States and around the world.

■ REFERENCES

1. Rosamond W, Flegal K, Furie K, et al. AHA Statistical Update. Heart Disease and Stroke Statistics—2008 Update. *Circulation* 2008; 117:e25–146.
2. World Health Organization Fact sheet No. 317, February 2007. www.who.int/mediacentre/factsheets/fs317/en/index.html
3. Emond M, Mock MB, Davis KB, et al. Long-term survival of medically treated patients in the Coronary Artery Surgery Study (CASS) Registry. *Circulation* 1994; 90(6):2645–57.
4. Hammermeister KE, DeRouen TA, Dodge HT. Variables predictive of survival in patients with coronary disease. *Circulation* 1979; 59(3):421–30.
5. Burns RJ, Gibbons RJ, Yi Q, et al. The relationships of left ventricular ejection fraction, end-systolic volume index and infarct size to six-month mortality after hospital discharge following myocardial infarction treated by thrombolysis. *J Am Coll Cardiol* 2002; 39(1):30–6.
6. Sharir T, Germano G, Kang X, et al. Prediction of myocardial infarction versus cardiac death by gated myocardial perfusion SPECT: Risk stratification by the amount of stress-induced ischemia and the poststress ejection fraction. *J Nucl Med* 2001; 42(6):831–7.
7. Solomon SD, Anavekar N, Skali H, et al. Influence of ejection fraction on cardiovascular outcomes in a broad spectrum of heart failure patients. *Circulation* 2005; 112(24):3738–44.
8. Dart AM, Otterstad JE, Kirwan BA, et al. Predictive value of local and core laboratory echocardiographic assessment of cardiac function in patients with chronic stable angina: The ACTION study. *Eur J Echocardiogr* 2007; 8:275–83.
9. Miller TD, Christian TF, Hopfenspirger MR, et al. Infarct size after acute myocardial infarction measured by quantitative tomographic 99mTc sestamibi imaging predicts subsequent mortality. *Circulation* 1995; 92(3):334–41.
10. Cerqueira MD, Maynard C, Ritchie JL, et al. Long-term survival in 618 patients from the western Washington streptokinase in myocardial infarction trials. *J Am Coll Cardiol* 1992; 20(7):1452–9.
11. Wu E, Ortiz JT, Tejedor P, et al. Infarct size by contrast enhanced cardiac magnetic resonance is a stronger predictor of outcomes than left ventricular ejection fraction or end-systolic volume index: prospective cohort study. *Heart* 2008; 94(6):730–6.
12. Roes SD, Kelle S, Kaandorp TAM, et al. Comparison of myocardial infarct size assessed with contrast-enhanced magnetic resonance imaging and left ventricular function and volumes to predict mortality in patients with healed myocardial infarction. *Am J Cardiol* 2007; 100(6):930–6.
13. Yan AT, Shayne AJ, Brown KA, et al. Characterization of the peri-infarct zone by contrast-enhanced cardiac magnetic resonance imaging is a powerful predictor of post-myocardial infarction mortality. *Circulation* 2006; 114(1):32–9.
14. Bello D, Fieno DS, Kim RJ, et al. Infarct morphology identifies patients with substrate for sustained ventricular tachycardia. *J Am Coll Cardiol* 2005; 45(7):1104–8.
15. Califf RM, Phillips HR, Hindman MC, et al. Prognostic value of a coronary artery jeopardy score. *J Am Coll Cardiol* 1985; 5(5):1055–63.
16. Min JK, Shaw LJ, Devereux RB, et al. Prognostic value of multidetector coronary computed tomographic angiography for prediction of all-cause mortality. *J Am Coll Cardiol* 2007; 50(12):1161–70.

17. Ghali JK, Liao Y, Cooper RS. Influence of left ventricular geometric patterns on prognosis in patients with or without coronary artery disease. *J Am Coll Cardiol* 1998; 31(7):1635–40.
18. Quinones MA, Greenberg BH, Kopelen HA, et al. Echocardiographic predictors of clinical outcome in patients with left ventricular dysfunction enrolled in the SOLVD Registry and Trials: Significant of left ventricular hypertrophy. *J Am Coll Cardiol* 2000; 35(5):1237–44.
19. Weiner DA, Ryan TJ, McCabe CH, et al. Prognostic importance of a clinical profile and exercise test in medically treated patients with coronary artery disease. *J Am Coll Cardiol* 1984; 3(3):772–9.
20. Mark DB, Hlatky MA, Harrel FE, et al. Exercise treadmill score for predicting prognosis in coronary artery disease. *Ann Intern Med* 1987; 106(6):793–9.
21. Myers J, Prakash M, Froelicher V, et al. Exercise capacity and mortality among men referred for exercise testing. *N Engl J Med* 2002; 346(11):793–801.
22. Kligfield P, Lauer MS. Exercise electrocardiogram testing: Beyond the ST segment. *Circulation* 2006; 114(19) 2070–82.
23. Dubach P, Froelicher VF, Klein J, et al. Exercise-induced hypotension in a male population. Criteria, causes and prognosis. *Circulation* 1998; 78(6):1380–7.
24. Hammermeister KE, DeRouen TA, Dodge HT, et al. Prognostic and predictive value of exertional hypotension in suspected coronary artery disease. *Am J Cardiol* 1983; 51(8):1261–6.
25. Lauer MS, Francis GS, Okin PM, et al. Impaired chronotropic response to exercise stress testing as a predictor of mortality. *JAMA* 1999; 281(6):524–9.
26. Lauer MS, Okin PM, Larson MG, et al. Impaired heart rate response to graded exercise: prognostic implications of chronotropic incompetence in the Framingham Heart Study. *Circulation* 1996; 93(8):1520–6.
27. Cole CR, Foody JM, Blackstone EH, Lauer MS. Heart rate recovery and treadmill exercise score as predictors of mortality in a cardiovascularly healthy cohort. *Ann Intern Med* 2000; 132(7):552–5.
28. Vivekananthan DP, Blackstone EH, Pothier CE, Lauer MS. Heart rate recovery after exercise is a predictor of mortality, independent of the angiographic severity of coronary disease. *J Am Coll Cardiol* 2003; 42(5):831–8.
29. Frolkis JP, Pothier CE, Blackstone EH, Lauer MS. Frequent ventricular ectopy after exercise as a predictor of death. *N Engl J Med* 2003; 348(9):781–90.
30. Jouven X, Zuerik M, Desnos M, et al. Long term outcome in asymptomatic men with exercise-induced premature ventricular depolarizations. *N Engl J Med* 2000; 343(12):826–33.
31. Ammar KA, Jacobsen SJ, Mahoney DW, et al. Prevalence and prognostic significance of heart failure stages. *Circulation* 2007; 115(12):1563–70.
32. Iskandrian AS, Chae SC, Heo J, et al. Independent and incremental prognostic value of exercise single-photon emission computed tomographic (SPECT) thallium imaging in coronary artery disease. *J Am Coll Cardiol* 1993; 22(3):665–70.
33. Mahmarian JJ, Shaw LJ, Filipchuk NG, et al. A multinational study to establish the value of early adenosine technetium-99m sestamibi myocardial perfusion imaging in identifying a low-risk group for early hospital discharge after acute myocardial infarction. *J Am Coll Cardiol* 2006; 48(12):2448–57.
34. Bacher-Stier C, Sharir T, Kavanagh PB, et al. Postexercise lung uptake of 99mTc-sestamibi determined by a new automatic technique: validation and application in detection of severe and extensive coronary artery disease and reduced left ventricular function. *J Nucl Med* 2000; 41(7):1190–7.
35. Weiss AT, Berman DS, Lew AS, et al. Transient ischemic dilation of the left ventricle on stress thallium-201 scintigraphy: a marker of severe and extensive coronary artery disease. *J Am Coll Cardiol* 1987; 9(4):752–9.
36. Mazzanti M, Germano G, Kiat H, et al. Identification of severe and extensive coronary artery disease by automatic measurement of transient ischemic dilation of the left ventricle in dual-isotope myocardial perfusion SPECT. *J Am Coll Cardiol* 1996; 27(7):1612–20.
37. Marcovitz PA, Shayna V, Horn RA, et al. Value of dobutamine stress echocardiography in determining the prognosis of patients with known or suspected coronary artery disease. *Am J Caridol* 1996; 78(4):404–8.
38. Qureshi U, Nagueh SF, Afridi I, et al. Dobutamine echocardiography and quantitative rest-redistribution 201Tl tomography in myocardial hibernation. *Circulation* 1997; 95(3):626–35.
39. Meluzin J, Cerny J, Frelich M, et al. Prognostic value of the amount of dysfunctional but viable myocardium in revascularized patients with coronary artery disease and left ventricular dysfunction. *J Am Coll Cardiol* 1998; 32(4):912–20.
40. Hansson GK. Inflammation, atherosclerosis, and coronary artery disease. *N Engl J Med* 2005; 352(16):1685–95.
41. Libby P, Theroux P. Pathophysiology of coronary artery disease. *Circulation* 2005; 111(25):3481–8.
42. Kannel WB, Dawber TR, Friedman GD, et al. Risk factors in coronary heart disease. An evaluation of several serum lipids as predictors of coronary heart disease; The Framingham Study. *Ann Intern Med* 1964; 61:888–99.
43. Endo A, Kuroda M, Tsujita Y. ML-236A, ML-236B, and ML-236C, new inhibitors of cholesterogenesis produced by Penicillium citrinium. *J Antibiot* 1976; 29(12):1346–8.
44. Scandinavian Simvastatin Survival Study Group. Randomised trial of cholesterol lowering in 4444 patients with coronary heart disease: the Scandinavian Simvastatin Survival Study (4S). *Lancet* 1994; 344(8934):1383–9.
45. Cholesterol Treatment Trialists' (CTT) Collaborators. Efficacy and safety of cholesterol-lowering treatment: prospective meta-analysis of data from 90,056 participants in 14 randomised trials of statins. *Lancet* 2005; 366(9493):1267–78.
46. Cannon CP, Braunwald E, McCabe CH, et al. Intensive versus moderate lipid lowering with statins after acute coronary syndromes. *N Engl J Med* 2004; 350(15):1495–504.
47. LaRosa JC, Grundy SM, Waters DD, et al. Intensive lipid lowering with atorvastatin in patients with stable coronary disease. *N Engl J Med* 2005; 352(14):1425–35.
48. Kjekshus J, Apetrei E, Barrios V, et al. Rosuvastatin in older patients with systolic heart failure. *N Engl J Med* 2007; 357(22):2248–61.
49. Nissen SE, Tuzcu EM, Schoenhagen P, et al. Effect of intensive compared with moderate lipid-lowering therapy on progression of coronary atherosclerosis. *JAMA* 2004; 291(9):1071–80.
50. Gordon DJ, Probstfield JL, Garrison RJ, et al. High-density lipoprotein cholesterol and cardiovascular disease. Four prospective American studies. *Circulation* 1989; 79(1):8–15.
51. Executive Summary of the Third Report of the National Cholesterol Education Program (NCEP) Expert Panel

on Detection, Evaluation, and Treatment of High Blood Cholesterol in Adults (Adult Treatment Panel III). *JAMA* 2001; 285(19):2486–97.
52. Hausenloy DJ, Yellon DM. Targeting residual cardiovascular risk: raising high-density lipoprotein cholesterol levels. *Heart* 2008; 94(6):706–14.
53. Rubins HB, Robins, SJ, Collins D, et al. Gemfibrozil for the secondary prevention of coronary heart disease in men with low levels of high-density lipoprotein cholesterol. *N Engl J Med* 1999; 341(6):410–18.
54. Canner PL, Berge KG, Wenger NK, et al. Fifteen year mortality in Coronary Drug Project patients: long-term benefit with niacin. *J Am Coll Cardiol* 1986; 8(6):1245–55.
55. Coronary Drug Project. Findings leading to discontinuation of the 2.5 mg-day estrogen group. The coronary drug project research group. *JAMA* 1973; 226(6):652–7.
56. Brown BG, Zhao XQ, Chait A, et al. Simvastatin and niacin, antioxidant vitamins, or the combination for the prevention of coronary disease. *N Engl J Med* 2001; 345(22):1583–92.
57. Mason JE, Hsia J, Johnson KC, et al. Estrogen plus progestin and the risk of coronary heart disease. *N Engl J Med* 2003; 349(6):523–34.
58. Sirtori CR, Calabresi L, Franceschini G, et al. Cardiovascular status of carriers of the Apolipoprotein A-I Milano mutant: the Limone sul Garda study. *Circulation* 2001; 103(15) 1949–54.
59. Nissen SE, Tsuonda T, Tuzcu EM, et al. Effect of recombinant ApoA-I Milano on coronary atherosclerosis in patients with acute coronary syndromes. *JAMA* 2003; 290(17):2292–2300.
60. Hunter AK, Suda EJ, Herberg JT, et al. Separation of recombinant apolipoprotein A-I (Milano) modified formed and aggregates in an industrial ion-exchange chromatography unit operation. *J Chromatogr A* 2008; 1204(1):42–7.
61. Barter PJ, Caufield M, Eriksson M, et al. Effects of torcetrapib in patients at high-risk for coronary events. *N Engl J Med* 2007; 357(21):2109–22.
62. Rader DJ. Illuminating HDL—is it still a viable therapeutic target? *N Engl J Med* 2007; 357(21):2180–3.
63. Wild S, Byrne CD. Time to rethink high-density lipoprotein? *Heart* 2008; 94(6):692–3.
64. Austin MA, Hokanson JE, Edwards KL. Hypertriglyceridemia as a cardiovascular risk factor. *Am J Cardiol* 1998; 81(4A):7–12B.
65. Danesh J, Collins R, Peto R. Lipoprotein(a) and coronary heart disease. *Circulation* 2000; 102(10):1082–5.
66. Birjmohun RS, Hutten BA, Kastelein JJP et al. Efficacy and safety of high-density lipoprotein cholesterol-increasing compounds. *J Am Coll Cardiol* 2005; 45(2):185–97.
67. Kosnter K, Gupta S. Niacin: a lipid polypill? *Expert Opin Pharmacother* 2008; 9(16):2911–20.
68. Ridker PM, Cannon CP, Morrow D, et al. C-reactive protein levels and outcomes after statin therapy. *N Engl J Med* 2005; 352(1):20–8.
69. Kinlay S. Low-density lipoprotein-dependent and –independent effects of cholesterol-lowering therapies on C-reactive protein. *J Am Coll Cardiol* 2007; 49(20):2003–9.
70. Ridker PM, Danielson E, Fonseca FAH, et al. Rosuvastatin to prevent vascular events in men and women with elevated c-reactive protein. *N Engl J Med* 2008; 359(21):2195–207.
71. Pearson TA, Mensah GA, Alexander RW, et al. Markers of inflammation and cardiovascular disease. *Circulation* 2003; 107(3):499–511.
72. Casas JP, Shah T, Hingorani AD, et al. C-reactive protein and coronary heart disease: a critical review. *J Intern Med* 2008; 264(4):295–314.
73. Zethelius B, Berglund L, Sundstrom J, et al. Use of multiple biomarkers to improve the prediction of death from cardiovascular causes. *N Engl J Med* 2008; 358(20):2107–16.
74. Sabatine MS, Morrow DA, de Lemos JA, et al. Multimarker approach to risk stratification in non-ST elevation acute coronary syndromes. *Circulation* 2002; 105(15):1760–3.
75. Ikonomidis I, Lekakis J, Revela I, et al. Increased circulating C-reactive protein and macrophage-colony stimulating factor are complementary predictors of long-term outcome in patients with chronic coronary artery disease. *Eur Heart J* 2005; 26(16):1618–24.
76. Horn BD, Anderson JL, John JM, et al. Which white blood cell subtypes predict increased cardiovascular risk? *J Am Coll Cardiol* 2005; 45(10):1638–43.
77. Boden WE, O'Rourke RA, Teo KK, et al. Optimal medical therapy with or without PCI for stable coronary disease. *N Engl J Med* 2007; 356(15):1503–16.
78. Pfeffer MA, Braunwald E, Moye LA, et al. Effect of captopril on mortality and morbidity in patients with left ventricular dysfunction after myocardial infarction. Results of the survival and ventricular enlargement trial. *N Engl J Med* 1992; 327(10):669–77.
79. The SOLVD Investigators. Effect of enalapril on survival in patients with reduced left ventricular ejection fractions and congestive heart failure. *N Engl J Med* 1991; 325(5):293–302.
80. 2007 focused update of the ACC/AHA 2004 guidelines for the management of patients with ST-elevation myocardial infarction: a report of the American College of Cardiology/American Heart Association Task Force on Practice Guidelines. *J Am Coll Cardiol* 2008; 51(2):210–47.
81. Anderson JL, Adams CD, Antman EM, et al. ACC/AHA 2007 guidelines for the management of patients with unstable angina/non-ST-Elevation myocardial infarction: a report of the American College of Cardiology/American Heart Association Task Force on Practice Guidelines. *J Am Coll Cardiol* 2007; 50(7):e1–157.
82. Flather MD, Yusuf S, Kober L, et al. Long-term ACE-inhibitor therapy in patients with heart failure or left-ventricular dysfunction: a systematic overview of data from individual patients. *Lancet* 2000; 355(9215):1575–81.
83. Yusuf S, Sleight P, Pogue J, et al. Effects of an angiotensin-converting-enzyme inhibitor, ramipril, on cardiovascular events in high-risk patients. The Heart Outcomes Prevention Evaluation Study Investigators. *N Engl J Med* 2000; 342(3):145–53.
84. The European trial on reduction of cardiac events with perindopril in patients with stable coronary artery disease investigators. Efficacy of perindopril in reduction of cardiovascular events among patients with stable coronary artery disease: randomized, double-blind, placebo-controlled, multicentre trial (the EUROPA study). *Lancet* 2003; 362(9386):782–8.
85. Grundy SM, Cleeman JI, Merz NB, et al. NCEP Report: implications of recent clinical trials for the National Cholesterol Education Program Adult Treatment Panel III Guidelines. *Circulation* 2004; 110:227–39.
86. The PEACE Trial Investigators. Angiotensin-converting-enzyme inhibition in stable coronary artery disease. *N Engl J Med* 2004; 351(20):2058–68.
87. Remuzzi G, Ruggenenti P. Overview of randomized trials of ACE inhibitors. *Lancet* 2006; 368(9535):555–6.

88. Beta Blocker Heart Attack Research Group. A randomized trial of propranolol in patients with acute myocardial infarction. I. Mortality results. *JAMA* 1982; 247(12):1707–14.
89. The CAPRICORN Investigators. Effect of carvedilol on outcome after myocardial infarction in patients with left-ventricular dysfunction: the CAPRICORN randomised trial. *Lancet* 2001; 357(9266):1385–90.
90. Freemantle N, Cleland J, Young P, et al. Beta-blockade after myocardial infarction: systematic review and meta regression analysis. *BMJ* 1999; 318(7200):1730–7.
91. COMMIT collaborative group. Early intravenous then oral metoprolol in 45,852 patients with acute myocardial infarction: randomized placebo-controlled trial. *Lancet* 2005; 366(9497):1622–32.
92. Frishman WH, Heiman M, Soberman J, et al. Comparison of celiprolol and propranolol in stable angina pectoris. Celiprolol International Angina Study Group. *Am J Cardiol* 1991; 67(8):665–70.
93. Narahara KA. Double-blind comparison of once daily betaxolol versus propranolol four times daily in stable angina pectoris. Betaxolol Investigators Group. *Am J Cardiol* 1990; 65(9):577–82.
94. Fox KM, Mulcahy D, Findlay I, et al. Effects of atenolol, nifedipine SR and their combination on the exercise test and the total ischemic burden in 608 patients with stable angina. The Total Ischaemic Burden European Trial (TIBET). *Eur Heart J* 1996; 17(1):96–103.
95. Foody JM, Farrell MH, Krumholz HM. Beta-blocker therapy in heart failure: Scientific Review. *JAMA* 2002; 287(7):883–9.
96. Hjalmarson A, Goldstein S, Fagerberg B, et al. Effects of controlled-release metoprolol on total mortality, hospitalizations, and well-being in patients with heart failure: the Metoprolol CR/XL Randomized Intervention Trial in congestive heart failure (MERIT-HF): MERIT-HF Study Group. *JAMA* 2000; 283(10):1295–302.
97. Packer M, Coats AJS, Fowler MB, et al. Effect of carvedilol on survival in severe chronic heart failure. *N Engl J Med* 2001; 344(22):1651–8.
98. CIBIS Investigators and Committees. A randomized trial of beta-blockade in heart failure: the Cardiac Insufficiency Bisoprolol Study (CIBIS). *Circulation* 1994; 90(4):1765–73.
99. CIBIS-II Investigators and Committees. The Cardiac Insufficiency Bisoprolol Study II (CIBIS-II). *Lancet* 1999; 353(9146):9–13.
100. Bunch TJ, Muhlestein JB, Bair TL, et al. Effect of beta-blocker therapy on mortality rates and future myocardial infarction rates in patients with coronary artery disease but no history of myocardial infarction or congestive heart failure. *Am J Cardiol* 2005; 95(7):827–31.
101. Cutler JA, Davis BR. Thiazide-type diuretics and beta-adrenergic blockers as first line drug treatments for hypertension. *Circulation* 2008; 117(20):2691–705.
102. Antithrombotic Trialists' Collaboration. Collaborative meta-analysis of randomised trials of antiplatelet therapy for prevention of death, myocardial infarction, and stroke in high risk patients. *BMJ* 2002; 324(7329):71–86.
103. The CURE Investigators. Effects of clopidogrel in addition to aspirin in patients with acute coronary syndromes without ST-segment elevation. *N Engl J Med* 2001; 345(7):494–502.
104. COMMIT collaborative group. Addition of clopidogrel to aspirin in 45,852 patients with acute myocardial infarction: randomized placebo-controlled trials. *Lancet* 2005; 366(9497):1607–21.
105. Grines CL, Bonow RO, Casey DE Jr, et al. Prevention of premature discontinuation of dual antiplatelet therapy in patients with coronary artery stents: a science advisory from the American Heart Association, American College of Cardiology, Society for Cardiovascular Angiography and Interventions, American College of Surgeons, and American Dental Association, with representation from the American College of Physicians. *J Am Coll Cardiol* 2007; 49(6):734–9.
106. GISSI-Prevenzione Investigators (Gruppo Italiano per lo Studio della Sopravvivenza nell'Infarto miocardico). Dietary supplementation with n-3 polyunsaturated fatty acids and vitamin E after myocardial infarction: results of the GISSI-Prevenzione trial. *Lancet* 1999; 354(9177):447–55.
107. Wang C, Harris WS, Chung M, et al. n-3 Fatty acids from fish or fish-oil supplements, but not alpha-linolenic acid, benefit cardiovascular disease outcomes in primary- and secondary-prevention studies: a systematic review. *Am J Clin Nutr* 2006; 84(1):5–17.
108. Galan P, Briancon S, Blacher J, et al. The SU.FOL.OM3 Study: a secondary prevention trial testing the impact of supplementation with folate and B-vitamins and/or Omega-3 PUFA on fatal and nonfatal cardiovascular events, design, methods and participants characteristics. *Trials* 2008; 9:35.
109. Teo KK, Ounpuu S, Hawken S, et al. Tobacco use and risk of myocardial infarction in 52 countries in the INTERHEART study: a case-control study. *Lancet* 2006; 368(9536):647–58.
110. Otsuka R, Watanabe H, Hirata K, et al. Acute effects of passive smoking on the coronary circulation in healthy young adults. *JAMA* 2001; 286(4):436–41.
111. Cesaroni G, Forastiere F, Agabiti N, et al. Effect of the Italian smoking ban on population rates of acute coronary events. *Circulation* 2008; 117(9):1183–8.
112. Juster HR, Loomis BR, Hinman TM, et al. Declines in hospital admissions for acute myocardial infarction in New York state after implementation of a comprehensive smoking ban. *Am J Public Health* 2007; 97(11):2035–9.
113. Critchley JA, Capewell S. Mortality risk reduction associated with smoking cessation in patients with coronary heart disease: a systematic review. *JAMA* 2003; 290(1):86–97.
114. Eisenberg MJ, Filion KB, Yavin D, et al. Pharmacotherapies for smoking cessation: a meta-analysis of randomized controlled trials. *CMAJ* 2008; 179(2):135–44.
115. Bijnen FC, Caspersen CJ, Feskens EJ, et al. Physical activity and 10-year mortality from cardiovascular disease and all causes: The Zutphen Elderly Study. *Arch Intern Med* 1998; 158(14):1499–505.
116. Kujala UM, Kaprio J, Sarna S, et al. Relationship of leisure-time physical activity and mortality: the Finnish twin cohort. *JAMA* 1998; 279(6):440–4.
117. Apullan FJ, Bourassa MG, Tardif JC, et al. Usefulness of self-reported leisure-time physical activity to predict long-term survival in patients with coronary heart disease. *Am J Cardiol* 2008; 102(4):375–9.
118. Kloner RA, Rezkalla SH. To drink or not to drink? That is the question. *Circulation* 2007; 116(11):1306–17.
119. Di Castelnuovo A, Costanzo S, Bagnardi V, et al. Alcohol dosing and total mortality in men and women: an updated

meta-analysis of 34 prospective studies. *Arch Intern Med* 2006; 166(22):2437–45.

120. Parikh P, McDaniel MC, Ashen MD, et al. Diets and cardiovascular disease: an evidence-based assessment. *J Am Coll Cardiol* 2005; 45(9):1379–87.

121. de Lorgeril M, Renaud S, Mamelle N, et al. Mediterranean alpha-linolenic acid-rich diet in secondary prevention of coronary heart disease. *Lancet* 1994; 343(8911):1454–9.

122. de Lorgeril M, Salen P, Martin JL, et al. Mediterranean Diet, traditional risk factors, and the rate of cardiovascular complications after myocardial infarction: final report of the Lyon Diet Heart Study. *Circulation* 1999; 99(6):779–85.

123. Dansinger ML, Gleason JA, Griffith JL, et al. Comparison of the Atkins, Ornish, Weight Watchers, and Zone diets for weight loss and heart disease risk reduction: a randomized trial. *JAMA* 2005; 293(1):43–53.

124. Ho PM, Maddox TM, Wang L, et al. Risk of adverse outcomes associated with concomitant use of clopidogrel and proton pump inhibitors following acute coronary syndrome. *JAMA* 2009;301(9):934–944.

125. Juurlink DN, Gomes T, Ko DT, et al. A population-based study of the drug interaction between proton pump inhibitors and clopidogrel. *CMAJ* 2009;180(7):713–718.

5 Cardiac Resynchronization Therapy

CHRISTOPHER F. LIU
KENNETH M. STEIN

OUTLINE

Cardiac resynchronization therapy (CRT) for systolic congestive heart failure (CHF) represents a new paradigm in cardiology: the use of an electrical therapy (cardiac pacing) to treat a mechanical problem. Multiple randomized clinical trials have proven that resynchronization therapy improves symptoms and functional status, increases quality of life, reduces hospitalizations, and prolongs survival in appropriately selected patients. As a result, this therapy has been quickly established as a standard treatment for patients with severe left ventricular dysfunction, moderate-to-severely symptomatic CHF despite optimal medical therapy, and prolonged QRS duration (1,2).

This chapter will review the results of clinical trials with respect to the outcomes of resynchronization therapy (both functional and structural) and the improvement in survival associated with resynchronization therapy in appropriate patients. The major completed clinical trials of CRT are summarized in Table 5.1. In addition, we will discuss several critical unanswered questions that these trials raise, particularly with respect to the role of resynchronization therapy in minimally symptomatic patients, the role of resynchronization therapy in patients with persistent atrial fibrillation, and the issue of "nonresponders" to resynchronization therapy. Finally, we will review the technical issues with regard to device and lead implantation procedure outcomes and adverse events.

ESTABLISHED CLINICAL OUTCOMES WITH CARDIAC RESYNCHRONIZATION

Functional Capacity and Symptoms

For appropriately selected patients, resynchronization therapy improves exercise capacity and reduces symptoms. The most commonly reported measures of functional capacity include: 6-minute hall walk distance, a measure of the ability to perform activities of daily living (3); peak oxygen consumption during a cardiopulmonary stress test (VO_{2max}); and quality of life, usually assessed using the Minnesota Living with Heart Failure Questionnaire (4). Previous studies had suggested that diminished 6-minute hall walk distance (5) and diminished VO_{2max} (6) are both strong indicators of poor prognosis in advanced heart failure.

In such trials as MUSTIC (7), PATH-CHF (8), MIRACLE (9), CONTAK CD (10), MIRACLE ICD (11), and PATH-CHF II (12), resynchronization therapy consistently improved functional capacity and reduced symptoms. Specifically, resynchronization was associated with a 1% to 23% improvement in 6-minute hall walk distance, a 7% to 10% increase in VO_{2max}, and an 11% to 31% improvement in quality of life scores.

Table 5.1 Randomized multicenter clinical trials of cardiac resynchronization therapy

Trial (Ref.)	Publication Date	N	Entry Criteria	Design	Primary Endpoint(s)/Outcome
MUSTIC (7)	2001	48	LVEF ≤35% LVEDD >60 NYHA III QRS >150 NSR	Single blind, crossover	23% increase in 6MHWD after 3 months (*P* <0.001)
PATH-CHF (8)	2002	41	"Dilated Cardiomyopathy" NYHA III or IV QRS ≥120 PR ≥150 NSR	Single blind, crossover comparison of optimized univentricular (LV only) versus biventricular pacing	No difference between LV only and biventricular pacing in VO_{2max} O_2 uptake at anaerobic threshold or 6MHWD. All parameters improved significantly versus baseline after 12 months.
MIRACLE (9)	2002	453	NYHA III or IV LVEF ≤35% LVEDD ≥55 QRS ≥130 NSR 6MHWD ≤450	Double blind, parallel	Significant improvement in 6MHWD, NYHA class and QoL after 6 months
MUSTIC AF (18)	2002	43	NYHA III LVEF <35% LVEDD >60 Persistent AF with bradycardia requiring permanent ventricular pacing and an RV paced QRS >200 6MHWD <450	Single blind, crossover	No significant difference in 6MHWD
CONTAK-CD (10)	2003	490	NYHA II to IV LVEF ≤35% QRS ≥120 NSR ICD indication	Single blind, originated as a crossover trial but changed midway to a parallel design	No significant change in a composite of mortality, CHF hospitalization, and ventricular tachyarrhythmias requiring device therapy at 3 to 6 months
MIRACLE ICD (11)	2003	369	NYHA III or IV LVEF ≤35% LVEDD ≥55 QRS ≥130 NSR ICD indication	Double-blind, parallel	Significant improvements in quality of life and NYHA class but not 6MHWD after 6 months
PATH-CHF II (12)	2003	69	LVEF ≤30% NYHA II-IV VO_{2max} ≤18 QRS≥120 NSR	Single blind, crossover, stratified by baseline QRS	Significant improvements in V VO_{2max} VO_2 at anaerobic threshold, and 6MHWD after 3 months

Continued

Table 5.1 Randomized multicenter clinical trials of cardiac resynchronization therapy *(Continued)*

Trial (Ref.)	Publication Date	N	Entry Criteria	Design	Primary Endpoint(s)/Outcome
COMPANION (29)	2004	1520	NYHA III or IV LVEF ≤35% QRS ≥120 PR ≥150 NSR CHF hospitalization in the preceding year	Unblinded, parallel comparison of medical therapy, CRT-pacemaker and CRT-Defibrillator (1:2:2)	Significant reduction in the composite of death or hospitalization for any cause
MIRACLE ICD II (19)	2004	186	LVEF ≤35% LVEDD ≥55 NYHA II QRS ≥130 NSR ICD indication	Double blind, parallel	No significant change in VO_{2max} after 6 months
CARE-HF (21)	2005	813	NYHA III or IV LVEF ≤35% LVEDD ≥30 (indexed to height) QRS ≥120 (pts with a QRS interval of 120 to 149 were required to meet 2 of 3 echo criteria for dyssynchrony)	Unblinded parallel	Significant reduction in the composite of death or hospitalization for a major cardiovascular event
PAVE (39)	2005	184	Chronic AF requiring AV node ablation and pacing therapy 6MHWD <450	Single blind, parallel comparison of CRT versus RV-only pacing	Significantly greater increase in 6MHWD with CRT versus RV-only pacing after 6 months
OPSITE (40)	2005	56	Chronic AF and: (1) requiring AV node ablation and pacing therapy OR (2) drug-refractory CHF, depressed LV function, and/or LBBB	Single blind, crossover comparison of biventricular, LV-only and RV-only pacing	Compared with RV pacing, BiV pacing showed a significant improvement in some measures of QoL. BiV pacing and RV-only pacing yielded similar improvements in 6MHWD
RETHINQ (20)	2007	172	NYHA III, LVEF ≤35% QRS duration <130 but with echo evidence of mechanical dyssynchrony (TDI or M-mode) NSR	Double blind, parallel	No significant change in proportion of patients with an increase in VO_{2max} ≥1.0 ml/kg/min after 6 months
REVERSE (33)	2008	610	NYHA I-II, LVEF ≤40%, QRS ≥120 msec	Double-blind, parallel	At 12 months: No significant difference in heart failure clinical composite response endpoint

AF: atrial fibrillation; CHF: congestive heart failure; ICD: implantable cardioverter defibrillator; LBBB: left bundle branch block; LVEDD: left ventricular end diastolic dimension; LVEF: left ventricular ejection fraction; 6MHWD: 6-minute hall walk distance; NSR: normal sinus rhythm; QoL: quality of life; TDI: tissue Doppler imaging.

MUSTIC was designed as a blinded crossover trial comparing active and inactive pacing. After the end of the crossover period, an overwhelming majority of patients (85%) preferred the period of active pacing (7). In MIRACLE, total exercise time during treadmill testing improved by over a minute in patients receiving resynchronization therapy compared with those who did not; this represents a 13% improvement over baseline (9).

Reflecting the impact of these physiologic changes, the data consistently show that resynchronization therapy results in a one New York Heart Association (NYHA) functional class improvement in symptoms—corresponding (on average) to a change from moderate to mild heart failure symptoms. Thus, in MIRACLE 52% of patients improved by one functional class, whereas fewer subjects improved by two functional classes (16%) and the remainder failed to respond to therapy (9). However, it is important to keep in mind the significant placebo effect demonstrated with CRT implant, including the 38% response rate in the placebo (CRT-off) arm of MIRACLE.

MUSTIC, PATH-CHF, MIRACLE, CONTAK CD, MIRACLE ICD, and PATH-CHF II enrolled patients with: (a) moderate to severely symptomatic (NYHA class III–IV) CHF despite optimal medical therapy; (b) severe left ventricular systolic dysfunction (LVEF ≤35%); (c) a wide QRS complex (generally defined as a QRS ≥120–130 msec); and (d) sinus rhythm. As a result, these inclusion criteria have become the standard indications for CRT. The effects in these "conventional indication" trials are robust—indeed, far more robust than the effects observed with conventional pharmacologic therapy of heart failure (Figure 5.1). For instance, improvement in 6-minute hall walk distance was observed in only 2 of 6 trials of ACE-inhibitors, 3 of 17 trials of beta blockers, and 1 of 4 trials of digoxin (13). Trials of both beta-blockers and ACE inhibitors have likewise shown inconsistent results with respect to VO_{2max} (14,15) and quality of life (16,17).

In addition to improving symptoms, randomized clinical trials have also shown that conventionally indicated patients derive objective evidence of beneficial structural changes (often referred to as reverse remodeling) in response to CRT. Resynchronization reduces left ventricular end-systolic (10,18–19) and end-diastolic volumes (10,22,23), and increases left ventricular ejection fraction (10,21,23). The improvements in ejection fraction ranged from 2% to 7% and are noteworthy given that the baseline ejection fractions in these trials were in the range of 21% to 25%. The data from trials reporting sufficient information to determine baseline and treatment versus control ejection fractions is shown in Figure 5.1. A meta-analysis of randomized clinical trials of CRT found the average absolute improvement in ejection fraction to be 3 percentage points (20). The remodeling effects of resynchronization therapy are progressive (22,23) and persist for at least 18 months after the initiation of therapy (21). Resynchronization is also associated with reduced mitral regurgitation (21–23) and with improvements in the neurohumoral milieu as evidenced by lower plasma catecholamine levels (21), increased heart rate variability (22), and striking reductions in N-terminal pro-BNP levels (reductions of 454–567 pg/mL at 12–18 months) (23).

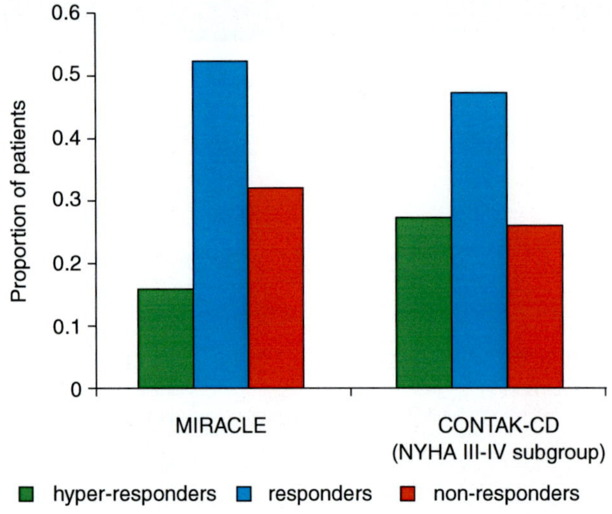

FIGURE 5.1 Proportion of patients from MIRACLE (9) and CONTAK-CD (10) demonstrating varying levels of response in the New York Heart Association (NYHA) functional class with cardiac resynchronization therapy (CRT); hyper-responders improved by two functional classes, responders improved by one functional class, non-responders had no improvement or deterioration in functional status.

CRT and Survival

In addition to improving symptoms, CRT has been demonstrated to improve survival in conventionally indicated populations. Although the early randomized clinical trials of CRT were not large enough to include mortality as a primary endpoint, a meta-analysis of MUSTIC, MIRACLE, MIRACLE ICD, and CONTAK CD concluded that resynchronization therapy, with or without concomitant use of a defibrillator, reduced mortality due to progressive heart failure by 51% (24). comparison of medical therapy, pacing, and defibrillation heart failure (COMPANION) was the first trial adequately powered to analyze total mortality as an independent endpoint (25). In addition to significantly reducing the combined endpoint of hospitalizations and mortality, all-cause mortality was reduced by 24% ($P = 0.06$) in the group receiving CRT-pacemakers, and by 36% ($P = 0.003$) in the group receiving CRT defibrillators. The absolute mortality rate at one year was 19% in the medically treated group (a result that serves to highlight the remarkably poor prognosis for patients with advanced heart failure and prolonged QRS), 15% in the pacemaker group, and 12% in the pacemaker–defibrillator group.

The survival benefit from resynchronization therapy was confirmed in CARE-HF. In this study, which almost exclusively employed CRT-pacemakers (rather than CRT-defibrillators), all-cause mortality was reduced by 36% with resynchronization therapy ($P < 0.002$) (21). The absolute mortality rate in the medical-therapy group was 13% at one year as opposed to 10% in the cardiac resynchronization group. Longer-term evaluation of the CARE-HF cohort shows that the mortality benefit increased in magnitude with longer duration follow-up: mortality at three years was 35% in the medical group and 24% in the CRT group (26). Extensive subgroup analysis was performed in both COMPANION and CARE-HF to attempt to identify which patient groups derive the greatest benefit from the therapy, but neither trial identified any significant heterogeneities according to pre-implant patient characteristics (21,27).

Although resynchronization is proven to prolong survival compared with standard medical therapy of heart failure, it should be noted that there is no direct evidence that resynchronization therapy improves survival when compared with ICD therapy alone (24). It is also curious to note that the addition of resynchronization did not reduce ICD therapies for ventricular tachycardia/ventricular fibrillation in either the CONTAK CD or MIRACLE ICD trials (10,11). It is possible that these observations may reflect the relatively large proportion of secondary prevention patients enrolled in these trials (28), as well as the relatively short duration of follow-up. Indeed, a recent retrospective analysis of the InSync III Marquis trial showed that responders to CRT demonstrated significantly fewer single premature ventricular contractions beats, or PVC runs, and fewer treated episodes of ventricular tachycardia or fibrillation (VT/VF) ($P = 0.050$) than nonresponders by 6 months of follow-up (29).

AREAS OF INCONCLUSIVE EVIDENCE

The available clinical trials regarding CRT provide a wealth of evidence on which to base practice. However, several fundamental questions remain in doubt. Table 5.2 summarizes some of the major ongoing clinical trials of CRT.

Minimally Symptomatic Patients

Perhaps foremost among the unresolved questions concerning resynchronization therapy is whether there is potential benefit for patients with severe left ventricular dysfunction, but minimally symptomatic or asymptomatic heart failure. Many of these patients are candidates for prophylactic ICD implantation (30,31). As noted above, resynchronization therapy results in limited functional improvement for patients who are minimally symptomatic at baseline. In CONTAK CD, there was no improvement in 6-minute hall walk distance, VO_{2max}, quality of life, or NYHA functional status among the NYHA class I and class II patients enrolled in the trial (10). In MIRACLE ICD II, which only enrolled patients in NYHA class II, there was no improvement in the primary outcome (change in VO_{2max}) and there was inconsistent improvement in secondary functional endpoints: a marginally significant improvement in NYHA functional class was observed but there was no change in quality of life score or 6-minute hall walk distance (19).

On the other hand, both CONTAK CD and MIRACLE ICD II showed that resynchronization results in convincing echocardiographic evidence of reverse remodeling in minimally symptomatic patients—less than was observed in more highly symptomatic populations, but nevertheless substantial. In both trials resynchronization led to statistically significant reductions in LV end-systolic and end-diastolic dimensions. MIRACLE ICD II showed a significant increase in ejection fraction; there was also a corresponding trend toward an increase in LVEF in the minimally symptomatic patients in CONTAK CD. The one-year results of the REVERSE trial were recently published (32). REVERSE evaluated 610 patients with a wide QRS and LVEF below 40% who were in NYHA functional class I (with prior history of symptoms) or II, who were randomly assigned to CRT-on versus CRT-off. The investigators found evidence of significant reverse remodeling with CRT as well as a

53% reduction in the incidence of first hospitalization for heart failure. In addition, there was a nonsignificant trend toward a reduction in the rate of worsening CHF as assessed by a clinical composite endpoint (21% versus 16%, $P = 0.10$). Although this study did not reach statistical significance for its primary endpoint, a subset of the REVERSE patients will continue their randomized assignments for a full two years of follow-up.

It is thus clear that there are beneficial structural changes observed with CRT even in minimally symptomatic patients, but because of the reduced baseline severity of their symptoms, significant symptomatic and survival benefits are more difficult to prove. It may be that these effects were not apparent in earlier trials due to the relatively short duration of follow-up or inadequate sample size. The long-term effects of resynchronization therapy in this population are being further evaluated in the MADIT-CRT (33) and Resynchronization/Defibrillation for Ambulatory Heart Failure (34) trials (RAFT).

Atrial Fibrillation

A second fundamental question concerns the role of resynchronization therapy in patients with persistent atrial fibrillation (AF). Atrial fibrillation is common in advanced heart failure (35), but patients with persistent atrial fibrillation were excluded from the majority of randomized clinical trials of resynchronization. Nevertheless, the most recent guidelines classify AF with QRS duration ≥120 msec to be a Class IIa indication for CRT implantation (1). Three multicenter randomized trials of resynchronization therapy have enrolled patients with persistent atrial fibrillation who required permanent pacing. In MUSTIC AF, resynchronization therapy did not result in an improvement in the primary endpoint (improvement in 6-minute hall walk distance) (18). However, when analyzed on an efficacy basis (rather than according to intention-to-treat) the resynchronization therapy group achieved borderline increases in both 6-minute hall walk distance and VO_{2max}. In the post AV nodal ablation evaluation (PAVE) trial, patients receiving CRT (with AV node ablation) experienced a greater improvement in 6-minute hall walk distance than did patients treated with RV-only pacing (36). Furthermore, the resynchronized patients avoided the deterioration in left ventricular ejection fraction that was observed in the RV-paced group. In optimal pacing SITE (OPSITE), biventricular pacing was also associated with a modest improvement in symptoms and a greater improvement in left ventricular ejection fraction when compared with RV-only pacing following AV node ablation for atrial fibrillation (37). Thus, these data suggest that resynchronization therapy is better than conventional RV-only pacing for patients with moderate-to-severely symptomatic heart failure and persistent atrial fibrillation who independently require permanent pacing. This issue is being further evaluated in the ongoing ablation for paroxysmal atrial fibrillation (APAF) and AVERT-AF trials (38,39). The role of resynchronization in the therapy of patients with sinus rhythm who require ventricular pacing is being evaluated in the biventricular versus right ventricular pacing in heart failure patients with atrioventricular block (BLOCK-HF) (40) and prevention of heart failure events with impedance cardiography testing (PREVENT-HF) (41) studies.

Table 5.2 Nonresponders to resynchronization therapy: Potential etiologies

Patient selection	Patients without dyssynchrony (54,55), including those with RBBB (53)
	Patients with transmural lateral myocardial infarction (58)
Device programming	Failure to achieve adequate biventricular capture
	Suboptimal AV interval (63,64)
	Suboptimal LV-RV timing (61)
Lead placement	Failure to place the LV lead in an area leading to adequate resynchronization (73)

PAVE and OPSITE stand out among the published randomized trials of CRT in enrolling patients irrespective of pre-implant ejection fraction. In fact, nearly half of the patients in PAVE had a left ventricular ejection fraction above 45%. Post hoc analysis of PAVE suggests that the majority of the benefit in the trial was confined to the subgroup with a pre-implant ejection fraction of less than 45% (39). However, the opposite pattern was observed in OPSITE. In that trial, the comparative benefit to biventricular pacing was greatest in those patients with normal baseline left ventricular function (40). It is possible that these discordant results reflect the play of chance. A larger trial is necessary to resolve the issue.

Limited nonrandomized data suggest that even without undergoing AV node ablation, patients with atrial fibrillation may derive a benefit from resynchronization that can be comparable to that experienced by patients with sinus rhythm. A recent meta-analysis concluded that patients with AF have similar or even slightly greater improvement in ejection fraction from CRT compared to patients in sinus rhythm (42). However, the functional benefits were somewhat smaller (as measured by NYHA functional class, 6-minute walk, and quality of life score). There appears to be a higher incidence of nonresponders among patients who do not undergo AV node ablation (46%) compared to those who do undergo the procedure (29%) (43). This observation highlights the importance of achieving adequate rate control (sufficient to permit a high percentage of biventricular pacing) in these patients. Other potential causes for smaller benefits in AF include: need to program higher ventricular rates to overcome intrinsic conduction, thereby reducing diastolic filling time; and the higher chance for fusion or pseudofusion beats to cause overestimation of the percentage of biventricular pacing and thus the true effective time of CRT delivery. Truly adequate rate control may be difficult to achieve solely with pharmacologic therapy. In one study, an important 70% of atrial fibrillation patients required AV node ablation in order to achieve adequate (>85%) biventricular pacing (44). It should be noted that although there are numerous anecdotes of patients with persistent AF converting to sinus rhythm following the institution of CRT, this is a rare event and there is no reduction in the incidence of new atrial fibrillation in patients receiving resynchronization for conventional indications (45).

Paced versus Native Left Bundle Branch Block

Most major randomized clinical trials required that a patient's native QRS complex be wide in order to be eligible for resynchronization therapy. However, it has long been recognized that pacing from the right ventricular apex also results in a wide QRS complex with a left bundle-branch block (LBBB) morphology. Substantial data exists showing that chronic RV apical pacing results in intraventricular dyssynchrony (46), a reduction in left ventricular function (47), and poorer outcome in patients with CHF (48,49). Limited observational data suggests that upgrading existing right ventricular pacing systems to biventricular systems can be performed safely with similar implantation success and similar clinical response rates as *de novo* CRT implantation (50). Therefore, the anticipated need for ventricular pacing in the setting of severely reduced LV ejection fraction and moderate-severely symptomatic CHF has become an accepted indication for implant of, or upgrade to, a CRT device (1).

"Nonresponders"

One of the most challenging issues in the field of CRT concerns "nonresponders" (Figure 5.1). A substantial minority of patients receiving resynchronization therapy for conventional indications derive little or no benefit, whether defined on the basis of echocardiographic response (typically a reduction in left ventricular end-systolic volume (LVESV) of at least 15%) or symptomatic improvement (typically improvement by at least 1 NYHA functional class). A closer look at the MIRACLE data is instructive: 52% of patients improved by one functional class and another 16% improved by two or more functional classes (so-called "hyper-responders"). Very few patients experienced a worsening of symptoms with the therapy (2%), but a significant 30% of patients were "nonresponders" (9). Similar proportions were seen in the CONTAK-CD subgroup of patients who were NYHA class III or IV at randomization (10). Three potential explanations might explain "nonresponse" (Table 5.2). First is patient selection: Was the device implanted in a patient who never possibly could have responded? Substantial controversy exists regarding the appropriate QRS width cutoff to determine eligibility for resynchronization. Indeed, controversy exists regarding whether QRS duration should be used at all. As noted above, most resynchronization trials used a QRS duration of greater than 120–130 msec as an enrollment criterion, but this has not been uniform. In MUSTIC, for example, the QRS duration cutoff was 150 msec (7). Even in the trials with more liberal enrollment criteria, the mean QRS width for patients actually enrolled in the trial was quite long: in MIRACLE the mean QRS width in the group eventually randomized to resynchronization was 167 msec and it is estimated that only about one-sixth of patients had a baseline QRS duration less than 145 msec (9). Extrapolation of these results to populations with QRS durations in the 120 s and 130 s is thus difficult.

The PATH-CHF II investigators prospectively stratified patients according to baseline QRS duration (QRS 120–150 versus QRS >150 msec) and found that the benefit of resynchronization was confined to the group with a QRS duration >150 msec (12). There was a nonsignificant tendency toward a similar result in the subgroup analysis of COMPANION (29). The cohort of patients eligible for CRT in trials based on QRS width alone includes the group of patients with right bundle branch block. In these patients, late activation occurs in the right ventricular free wall and there is no a priori reason to expect them to benefit from left ventricular pacing. Indeed, an analysis of pooled data from the MIRACLE and CONTAK CD trials shows that patients with right bundle branch block derive limited benefit from CRT (51).

Growing data show that patients without intraventricular dyssynchrony are unlikely to respond to resynchronization therapy, no matter how wide their QRS (52,53). Two randomized clinical trials have used echocardiographic measurement of dyssynchrony to aid in patient selection for resynchronization therapy. In CARE-HF patients could be enrolled on the basis of QRS duration alone if the QRS was 150 msec or greater. Patients with a QRS of 120–149 msec were required, in addition, to demonstrate two of three echocardiographic criteria for dyssynchrony: an aortic pre-ejection delay >140 msec, an interventricular mechanical delay of >40 msec, and/or delayed activation of the posterolateral LV wall by M-mode or tissue Doppler imaging (54). Perhaps as a result, subgroup analysis of CARE-HF did not show any heterogeneity of response according to pre-implant QRS duration (21). In Resynchronization Therapy in Normal QRS (RETHINQ), patients with a QRS <130 msec were selected for resynchronization if they had echocardiographic evidence of intraventricular dyssynchrony, predominantly on the basis of tissue Doppler imaging. In this trial, patients with a QRS <120 msec experienced no improvement in the primary endpoint (VO_{2max}); however, in the prespecified subgroup of patients with a QRS interval of 120–129 msec, VO_{2max} increased significantly with resynchronization (20). It should be acknowledged, however, that the results of providing regional observations to study predictors of events in the coronary tree (PROSPECT) raise concern regarding the ability of current echocardiographic techniques to reproducibly measure dyssynchrony and to distinguish clinical responders from nonresponders (55).

Data also exist to suggest that patients with transmural myocardial infarctions of the lateral wall are unlikely to improve with lateral left ventricular pacing (56). Echocardiographic substudies of MIRACLE (23) and MUSTIC (22) have shown greater reverse remodeling in patients with nonischemic as opposed to ischemic cardiomyopathies. It is, however, important to recognize that substudy analysis shows no difference in clinical outcomes between patients with ischemic versus nonischemic heart disease (10,21,30).

A second potential cause of "nonresponse" is suboptimal programming, particularly with respect to programming an appropriate AV delay (57,58), but also potentially with respect to programming LV-RV timing (59). In fact, failure to program an optimal AV delay may result in as much as a 10% to 15% decline in cardiac output (60). Although many trials have shown acute hemodynamic benefits with AV optimization, limited data exist to show that systematic optimization results in a long-term improvement in clinical outcome (61,62). The major randomized clinical trials have used wildly different approaches to programming the AV delay: (a) in CONTAK CD a fixed short AV delay was empirically programmed (10), (b) in COMPANION the AV delay was programmed according to a formula taking into account the baseline PR interval and baseline QRS duration (29), and (c) in MIRACLE (9) and CARE-HF (21) echocardiographic imaging of mitral valve inflow was used to determine an "optimum" AV delay. Thus far no large randomized clinical trial has been completed comparing long-term outcomes with various methods of optimizing the programmed AV delay. This issue will be addressed by the future revascularization evaluation in patients with diabetes mellitus: optimal management of multivessel disease (FREEDOM) (63) and SMART-AV trials (according to a personal communication with Boston Scientific).

In addition to AV optimization, it has been proposed that programming sequential rather than simultaneous LV and RV pacing (often referred to as "VV timing") may further improve ventricular performance (64). However, in neither of two randomized clinical trials did VV optimization following AV optimization affect the long-term clinical response to resynchronization therapy (65,66). The effect of other programming choices is unclear. The potential for an improvement in outcome with rate adaptive pacing is particularly interesting. Chronotropic incompetence is common in patients with advanced heart failure (67), and may itself reduce functional capacity as well as limit the use of beta-blockers. Nevertheless, all of the major randomized clinical trials to date used VDD pacing or fixed rate atrial pacing, usually with a rate deliberately programmed low to avoid atrial pacing. The potential effect of rate adaptive pacing in CRT is currently being evaluated in the pacing evaluation atrial support study in cardiac resynchronization therapy (PEGASUS-CRT) trial (68).

A third possible cause of "nonresponse" is failure to place the left ventricular lead in an adequate position. Early data showed that the hemodynamic response to resynchronization was greatest for left ventricular leads placed on the mid-lateral wall of the left ventricle (69). Bearing this in mind, the actual lead positions achieved in clinical trials are striking. For example, in CONTAK CD the left ventricular lead was placed on the mid-lateral wall in only 40% of cases (70). The extent to which precise lead placement affects the response to therapy is controversial. In an animal study, the area yielding 90% of the maximal response to CRT covered only 16% of the left ventricular free wall, but sites yielding 70% of the optimal dP/dtmax covered fully 43% of the free wall (71). In a recently published observational study from the Netherlands (72), patients whose LV lead position was in the same region (concordant) as the site of latest mechanical activation (as determined by speckle tracking radial strain analysis on echocardiography) demonstrated significant reductions in LV end-systolic volume, whereas patients with discordant lead position had no significant echocardiographic improvement. A concordant LV lead position also appeared to predict hospitalization-free survival during 2 years of long-term follow up. This study suggests that the choice of optimum lead position may need to be individualized, although it should be noted that in 69% of the patients in this cohort the site of latest activation was either the lateral wall (33%) or posterior wall (36%).

■ DEVICE IMPLANTATION OUTCOMES

Success of Transvenous LV Lead Implantation

Implantation of a CRT system is performed via the same basic approach as a routine pacemaker or ICD system—via the transvenous approach—except that

A

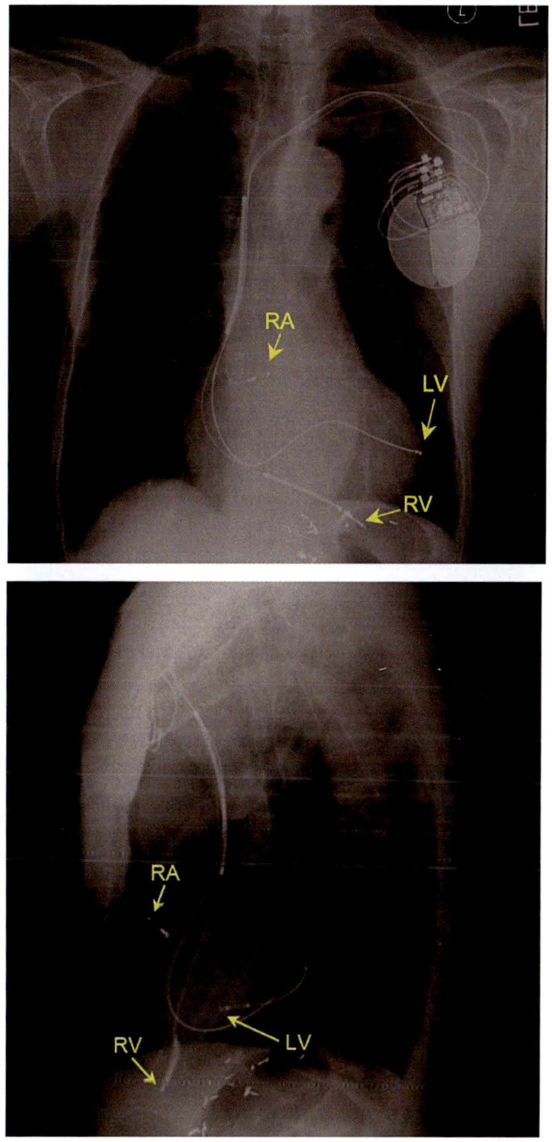

B

FIGURE 5.2 Typical PA and lateral chest X-ray after implantation of CRT-D system. Note the course of the LV lead via the coronary sinus to reach the lateral epicardial wall of the left ventricle, which is posterior as viewed in the lateral projection. (RA, right atrial lead with tip in right atrial appendage; RV, ICD lead with tip in right ventricular apex; LV, left ventricular lead with tip at the mid-lateral wall of the left ventricle.)

a guide sheath is used to direct the LV lead into the coronary sinus; further over-the-wire techniques are used to deliver the lead into the target coronary vein (most commonly a lateral or posterior vein). Figure 5.2 illustrates the typical radiographic appearance of a CRT-defibrillator system after implantation. Some of the potential challenges faced by the implanting physician include: dilation of the right atrium or presence of Thebesian valve resulting in difficulty accessing the coronary sinus; lack of an adequately sized coronary vein reaching the target area (typically the midlateral or posterolateral LV); tortuous venous anatomy; epicardial scar or fat in the target site precluding pacing capture of the LV; and phrenic nerve or direct diaphragmatic stimulation during pacing at the target site.

Successful placement of the LV lead in the target vein has been aided by continuing improvements in the available delivery tools as well as individual operator experience. In CONTAK CD (performed from 1998 to 2000), 79% of attempted implants resulted in successful transvenous implant of the LV lead. In COMPANION (2000 to 2002), the success rate was 89%, with median procedure duration of 2.8 hours. And in CARE-HF (2001–2003), the success rate was 95% (86% on first attempt). Patients who fail to undergo successful transvenous implantation of the LV lead into an optimal target vein have the option to undergo limited thoracotomy for direct implantation of an epicardial LV lead.

Adverse Outcomes

Conceptually, the potential complications of CRT-pacemaker or CRT-defibrillator implantation include the known complications of transvenous pacemaker or ICD implant (bleeding, infection, pneumothorax, vascular injury, cardiac perforation/tamponade, and cardiac decompensation from defibrillation testing) as well as the potential complications of LV lead implant (coronary venous dissection/perforation, contrast nephropathy, and perhaps elevated risk of infection or heart failure exacerbation due to prolonged procedure times). In addition, the passive fixation nature of LV leads raises the rates of post-procedure lead dislodgement. However, the rates of serious adverse events from the implantation procedure reported in the large clinical trials have been low. In MIRACLE, 2 patients (of 571) died as a result of the procedure. Correspondingly, 6% had a dissection or perforation of a coronary vein, but only 3 of those 35 patients required intervention and all recovered without sequelae, pointing to the typically favorable outcome of coronary venous dissection/perforation. The LV lead dislodgement rate was 3.7% in MIRACLE. In COMPANION, 8 deaths (out of 1212 implants) were reported as procedure-related (0.6%).

Diaphragmatic Stimulation

Because of the course of the left phrenic nerve over the anterolateral LV epicardium, there is a relatively large area over which pacing (especially at higher output) can cause stimulation of the phrenic nerve, resulting in stimulation of the diaphragm (experienced by the patient as a hiccup or "jumping" sensation). This is typically avoided by extensive testing during the implantation procedure. However, small shifts in lead position after the procedure can result in closer proximity to the phrenic nerve or higher required output for left ventricular capture—and thus stimulation of the diaphragm. This may be constant or positional (depending on the rotation of the heart while the patient lies on the left or right side). Improvements in device programmability have led to various LV pacing configurations that can be tried in order to still provide CRT pacing while avoiding diaphragmatic stimulation. In the majority of patients, this "electronic repositioning" is successful in precluding the need for invasive lead repositioning. It is possible that the development of multipolar LV leads (≥quadripolar) will further reduce the incidence of diaphragmatic stimulation.

■ SUMMARY

CRT reduces symptoms of CHF and improves cardiac performance in patients with moderate-to-severely symptomatic heart failure, severe left ventricular systolic dysfunction, normal sinus rhythm and a wide QRS complex. Resynchronization therapy significantly reduces hospitalizations in these patients and is highly cost-effective. Perhaps most important, resynchronization therapy for heart failure improves survival for these patients, particularly when employed in conjunction with an implantable defibrillator. However, randomized clinical trials show that a substantial minority of patients are clinical nonresponders. Therefore, critical questions remain with respect to identifying appropriate candidates for CRT, optimal device programming, and left ventricular lead placement.

REFERENCES

1. Epstein AE, DiMarco JP, Ellenbogen KA, et al. ACC/AHA/HRS 2008. Guidelines for device-based therapy of cardiac rhythm abnormalities: a report of the American College of Cardiology/American Heart Association Task Force on practice guidelines. *Circulation* 2008; 117:e350–e408.
2. The Task Force of the European Society of Cardiology. Developed in collaboration with the European Heart Rhythm Association. Cardiac pacing and cardiac resynchronisation therapy. *Eur Heart J* 2007; 28:2256–95.
3. Guyatt GH, Sullivan MJ, Thompson PJ, et al. The 6-minute walk: a new measure of exercise capacity in patients with chronic heart failure. *Can Med Assoc J* 1985; 132:919–23.
4. Rector TS, Kubo SH, Cohn JN. Patients' self-assessment of their congestive heart failure. Part 2: content, reliability and validity of a new measure, the Minnesota Living with Heart Failure Questionnaire. *Heart Failure* 1987; 3:198–209.
5. Bittner V, Weiner DH, Yusuf S, et al. Prediction of mortality and morbidity with a 6-minute walk test in patients with left ventricular dysfunction. *JAMA* 1993; 270:1702–7.
6. Myers J, Gullestad L, Vagelos R, et al. Clinical, hemodynamic, and cardiopulmonary exercise test determinants of survival in patients referred for evaluation of heart failure. *Ann Intern Med* 1998; 129:286–93.
7. Cazeau S, Leclercq C, Lavergne T, et al. Effects of multisite biventricular pacing in patients with heart failure and intraventricular conduction delay. *N Engl J Med* 2001; 344:873–80.
8. Auricchio A, Stellbrink C, Sack S, et al. Long-term clinical effect of hemodynamically optimized cardiac resynchronization therapy in patients with heart failure and ventricular conduction delay. *J Am Coll Cardiol* 2002; 39:2026–33.
9. Abraham WT, Fisher WG, Smith AL, et al. Cardiac resynchronization in chronic heart failure. *N Engl J Med* 2002; 346:1845–53.
10. Higgins SL, Hummel JD, Niazi IK, et al. Cardiac resynchronization therapy for the treatment of heart failure in patients with intraventricular conduction delay and malignant ventricular tachyarrhythmias. *J Am Coll Cardiol* 2003; 42:1454–9.
11. Young JB, Abraham WT, Smith AL, et al. Combined cardiac resynchronization and implantable cardioversion defibrillation in advanced chronic heart failure: the MIRACLE ICD trial. *JAMA* 2003; 289:2685–94.
12. Auricchio A, Stellbrink C, Butter C, et al. Clinical efficacy of cardiac resynchronization therapy using left ventricular pacing in heart failure patients stratified by severity of ventricular conduction delay. *J Am Coll Cardiol* 2003; 42:2109–16.
13. Olsson LG, Swedberg K, Clark AL, Witte KK, Cleland JGF. Six minute corridor walk test as an outcome measure for the assessment of treatment in randomized, blinded intervention trials of chronic heart failure: a systematic review. *Eur Heart J* 2005; 26:778–93.
14. Witte KK, Thackray S, Nikitin NP, Cleland JG, Clark AL. The effects of long-term beta-blockade on the ventilatory responses to exercise in chronic heart failure. *Eur J Heart Fail* 2005; 7:612–7.
15. Williams SG, Cooke GA, Wright DJ, Tan LB. Disparate results of ACE inhibitor dosage on exercise capacity in heart failure: a reappraisal of vasodilator therapy and study design. *Int J Cardiol* 2001; 77:239–45.
16. Reddy P, Dunn AB. The effect of beta-blockers on health-related quality of life in patients with heart failure. *Pharmacotherapy* 2000; 20:679–89.
17. Wolfel EE. Effects of ACE inhibitor therapy on quality of life in patients with heart failure. *Pharmacotherapy* 1998; 18:1323–34.
18. Cleland JGF, Daubert JC, Erdmann E, et al. The effect of cardiac resynchronization on morbidity and mortality in heart failure. *N Engl J Med* 2005; 352:1539–49.
19. Duncan A, wait D, Gibson D, Daubert JC. Left ventricular remodelling and haemodynamic effects of multisite biventricular pacing in patients with left ventricular systolic dysfunction and activation disturbances in sinus rhythm: substudy of the MUSTIC trial. *Eur Heart J*2003; 24:430–41.
20. St. John-Sutton MG, Plappert T, Abraham WT, et al. Effect of cardiac resynchronization therapy on left ventricular size and function in chronic heart failure. *Circulation* 2003; 107:1985–90.
21. McAlister FA, Ezekowitz J, Hooton N, et al. Cardiac resynchronization therapy for patients with left ventricular systolic dysfunction: a systematic review. *JAMA* 2007; 297:2502–14.
22. Braun MU, Rauwolf T, Zerm T, Schulze M, Schnabel A, Strasser RH. Long term biventricular resynchronisation therapy in advanced heart failure: effect on neurohormones. *Heart* 2005; 91:601–5.
23. Adamson PB, Kleckner KJ, VanHout WL, Srinivasan S, Abraham WT. Cardiac resynchronization therapy improves heart rate variability in patients with symptomatic heart failure. *Circulation* 2003; 108:266–9.
24. Fruhwald FM, Fahrleitner-Pammer A, Berger R, et al. Early and sustained effects of cardiac resynchronization therapy on N-terminal pro-B-type natriuretic peptide in patients with moderate to severe heart failure and cardiac dyssynchrony. *Eur Heart J* 2007; 28:1592–7.
25. Bradley DJ, Bradley EA, Baughman KL, et al. Cardiac resynchronization and death from progressive heart failure: a meta-analysis of randomized controlled trials. *JAMA* 2003; 289:730–40.
26. Bristow MR, Saxon LA, Boehmer J, et al. Cardiac-resynchronization therapy with or without an implantable defibrillator in advanced chronic heart failure. *N Engl J Med* 2004; 350:2140–50.
27. Cleland JG, Daubert JC, Erdmann E, et al. Longer-term effects of cardiac resynchronization therapy on mortality in heart failure). *Eur Heart J* 2006; 27:1928–32.
28. Wilkoff BL, Hess M, Young J, Abraham WT. Differences in tachyarrhythmia detection and implantable cardioverter defibrillator therapy by primary or secondary prevention indication in cardiac resynchronization therapy patients. *J Cardiovasc Electrophysiol* 2004; 15:1002–9.
29. Moss AJ, Zareba W, Hall WJ, et al. Prophylactic implantation of a defibrillator in patients with myocardial infarction and reduced ejection fraction. *N Engl J Med* 2002; 346:877–83.
30. Markowitz SM, Lewen JM, Wiggenhorn CJ, et al. Relationship of reverse anatomical remodeling and ventricular arrhythmias after cardiac resynchronization. *J Cardiovasc Electrophysio.* Published Online: 31 Oct. 2008.
31. Moss AJ, Zareba W, Hall WJ, et al. Prophylactic implantation of a defibrillator in patients with myocardial infarction and reduced ejection fraction. *N Engl J Med* 2002; 346:877–83.
32. Bardy GH, Lee KL, Mark DB, et al. Amiodarone or an implantable cardioverter-defibrillator for congestive heart failure. *N Engl J Med* 2005; 352:225–37.

33. Linde C, Abraham WT, Gold MR, et al. Randomized trial of cardiac resynchronization in mildly symptomatic heart failure patients and in asymptomatic patients with left ventricular dysfunction and previous heart failure symptoms. *J Am Coll Cardiol* 2008; 52:1834–43.
34. MADIT-CRT: Automatic Defibrillator Implantation With Cardiac Resynchronization Therapy, ClinicalTrials.gov, http://www.clinicaltrials.gov/ct2/show/NCT00180271, accessed January 22, 2008.
35. Resynchronization/Defibrillation for Ambulatory Heart Failure Trial (RAFT), ClinicalTrials.gov, http://www.clinicaltrials.gov/ct2/show/NCT00251251, accessed January 22, 2008.
36. Wang TJ, Larson MG, Levy D, et al. Temporal relations of atrial fibrillation and congestive heart failure and their joint influence on mortality: the Framingham Heart Study. *Circulation* 2003; 107:2920–5.
37. Doshi RN, Daoud EG, Fellows C, et al. Left ventricular-based cardiac stimulation post AV nodal ablation evaluation (the PAVE study). *J Cardiovasc Electrophysiol* 2005; 16:1160–5.
38. Brignole M, Gammage M, Puggioni E, et al. Comparative assessment of right, left, and biventricular pacing in patients with permanent atrial fibrillation. *Eur Heart J* 2005; 26:712–22.
39. National Institutes of Health. www.clinicaltrials.gov/ct2/show/NCT00111527, accessed January 31, 2008.
40. National Institutes of Health.http://www.clinicaltrials.gov/ct2/show/NCT00547794, accessed January 31, 2008.
41. National Institutes of Health.http://www.clinicaltrials.gov/ct2/show/NCT00267098, accessed January 31, 2008.
42. National Institutes of Health.http://www.clinicaltrials.gov/ct2/show/NCT00170326, accessed March 5, 2008.
43. Upadhyay GA, Choudhry NK, Auricchio A, Ruskin J, Singh JP. Cardiac resynchronization in patients with atrial fibrillation. *J Am Coll Cardiol* 2008; 52:1239–46.
44. Molhoek SG, Bax JJ, Bleeker GB, et al. Comparison of response to cardiac resynchronization therapy in patients with sinus rhythm versus chronic atrial fibrillation. *Am J Cardiol* 2004; 94:1506–9.
45. Gasparini M, Auricchio A, Regoli F, et al. Four-year efficacy of cardiac resynchronization therapy on exercise tolerance and disease progression: the importance of performing atrioventricular junction ablation in patients with atrial fibrillation. *J Am Coll Cardiol* 2006; 48:734–43.
46. Hoppe UC, Casares JM, Eiskjaer H, et al. Effect of cardiac resynchronization on the incidence of atrial fibrillation in patients with severe heart failure. *Circulation* 2006; 114:18–25.
47. Prinzen FW, Peschar M. Relation between the pacing induced sequence of activation and left ventricular pump function in animals. *Pacing Clin Electrophysiol* 2002; 25(pt 1):484–98.
48. Nahlawi M, Waligora M, Spies SM, Bonow RO, Kadish AH, Goldberger J. Left ventricular function during and after right ventricular pacing. *J Am Coll Cardiol* 2004; 44:1883–8.
49. Sweeney MO, Hellkamp AS, Ellenbogen KA, et al. Adverse effect of ventricular pacing on heart failure and atrial fibrillation among patients with normal baseline QRSd in a clinical trial of pacemaker therapy for sinus node dysfunction. *Circulation* 2003; 23:2932–7.
50. The DAVID Trial Investigators. Dual-chamber pacing or ventricular backup pacing in patients with an implantable defibrillator: the Dual Chamber and VVI Implantable Defibrillator (DAVID) Trial. *JAMA* 2002; 288:3115–23.
51. Duray GZ, Israel CW, Pajitnev D, Hohnloser SH. Upgrading to biventricular pacing/defibrillation systems in right ventricular paced congestive heart failure patients: prospective assessment of procedural parameters and response rate. *Europace* 2008; 10:48–52.
52. Egoavil CA, Ho RT, Greenspon AJ, Pavri BB. Cardiac resynchronization therapy in patients with right bundle branch block: analysis of pooled data from the MIRACLE and Contak CD trials. *Heart Rhythm* 2005; 2:611–5.
53. Yu C-M, Fung J W-H, Zhang Q, et al. Tissue doppler imaging is superior to strain rate imaging and postsystolic shortening on the prediction of reverse remodeling in both ischemic and nonischemic heart failure after cardiac resynchronization therapy circulation 2004; 110:66–73.
54. Bax JJ, Bleeker GB, Marwick TH, et al. Left ventricular dyssynchrony predicts response and prognosis after cardiac resynchronization therapy. *J Am Coll Cardiol* 2004; 44:1834–40.
55. Cleland JGF, Daubert JC, Erdmann E, et al. The CARE-HF study (CArdiac REsynchronisation in Heart Failure study): rationale, design and end-points. *Europ J Heart Failure* 2001; 3:481–9.
56. Chung ES, Leon AR, Tavazzi L, et al. Results of the predictors of response to CRT. *Circulation* 2008; 117:2608–16.
57. Bleeker GB, Kaandorp TAM, Lamb HJ, et al. Effect of posterolateral scar tissue on clinical and echocardiographic improvement after cardiac resynchronization therapy. *Circulation* 2006; 113:969–76.
58. Auricchio A, Stellbrink C, Block M, et al. Effect of pacing chamber and atrioventricular delay on acute systolic function of paced patients with congestive heart failure. *Circulation* 1999; 99:2993–3001.
59. Auricchio A, Ding J, Spinelli JC, et al. Cardiac resynchronization therapy restores optimal atrioventricular mechanical timing in heart failure patients with ventricular conduction delay. *J Am Coll Cardiol* 2002; 39:1163–9.
60. Vernooy K, Verbeek XAAM, Cornelussen RNM, et al. Calculation of effective VV interval facilitates optimization of AV delay and VV interval in cardiac resynchronization therapy. *Heart Rhythm* 2007; 4:75–82.
61. Kerlan JE, Sawhney NS, Waggoner AD, et al. Prospective comparison of echocardiographic atrioventricular delay optimization methods for cardiac resynchronization therapy. *Heart Rhythm* 2003; 3:148–54.
62. Sawhney NS, Waggoner AD, Garhwal S, Chawla MK, Osborn J, Faddis MN. Randomized prospective trial of atrioventricular delay programming for cardiac resynchronization therapy. *Heart Rhythm* 2004; 1:562–7.
63. Morales M-A, Startari U, Panchetti L, Rossi A, Piacenti M. Atrioventricular delay optimization by doppler-derived left ventricular dP/dt improves 6-month outcome of resynchronized patients. *PACE* 2006; 29:564–8.
64. National Institutes of Health. www.clinicaltrials.gov/ct2/show/NCT00418314, accessed January 31, 2008.
65. Sogaard P, Egeblad H, Pedersen AK, et al. Sequential versus simultaneous biventricular resynchronization for severe heart failure: evaluation by tissue Doppler imaging. *Circulation* 2002; 106:2078–84.
66. Rao RK, Kumar UN, Schafer J, Viloria E, Delurgio D, Foster E. Reduced ventricular volumes and improved systolic function

with cardiac resynchronization therapy: a randomized trial comparing simultaneous biventricular pacing, sequential biventricular pacing, and left ventricular pacing. *Circulation* 2007; 115:2136–44.

67. Boriani G, Müller CP, Seidl KH, et al. Randomized comparison of simultaneous biventricular stimulation versus optimized interventricular delay in cardiac resynchronization therapy. The Resynchronization for the HemodYnamic Treatment for Heart Failure Management II implantable cardioverter defibrillator (RHYTHM II ICD) study. *Am Heart J* 2006; 151:1050–8.
68. Colucci WS, Ribeiro JP, Rocco MB, et al. Impaired chronotropic response to exercise in patients with congestive heart failure. Role of postsynaptic β-adrenergic desensitization. *Circulation* 1989; 80:314–23.
69. Martin DO, Stolen KQ, Brown S, et al. Pacing evaluation-atrial support study in cardiac resynchronization therapy (PEGASUS CRT): design and rationale. *Am Heart J* 2007; 153:7–13.
70. Auricchio A, Klein H, Tockman B, et al. Transvenous biventricular pacing for heart failure: can the obstacles be overcome? *Am J Cardiol* 1999; 83(5B):136D–42D.
71. CONTAK CD study clinical report. Date data courtesy of Guidant.
72. Helm RH, Byrne M, Helm PA, et al. Three-dimensional mapping of optimal left ventricular pacing site for cardiac resynchronization. *Circulation* 2007; 115:953–61.
73. Ypenburg C, van Bommel RJ, Delgado V, et al. Optimal left ventricular lead position predicts reverse remodeling and survival after cardiac resynchronization therapy. *J Am Coll Cardiol* 2008; 52:1402–9.

6 Catheter Ablation of Atrial Fibrillation

ANDY LIN
STEVEN M. MARKOWITZ

OUTLINE

EPIDEMIOLOGY AND BACKGROUND

Atrial fibrillation (AF) is the most common cardiac arrhythmia in the United States, affecting greater than 2.2 million Americans (1). In the largest U.S. study reported to date, the Anticoagulation and Risk Factors in Atrial Fibrillation (ATRIA) study, the prevalence in persons aged <55 years was 0.1%, while AF was documented in 9% of persons aged ≥80 years (2). The latter estimate is consistent with earlier results from the Framingham Heart Study, which found a prevalence of 8.8% in persons aged ≥80 years (3). Current estimates are that approximately 75% of patients with AF are aged ≥65 years (2). The number of patients diagnosed with AF is expected to rise more than 2.5-fold over the next 50 years in the United States, driven primarily by the expected aging of the population (2). Estimated lifetime risks for development of AF in the Framingham population are one in every four men and women 40 years of age and older (4). Lifetime risks for AF are high (one in every six), even in the absence of antecedent congestive heart failure or myocardial infarction (4).

In addition to advanced age, other well-recognized risk factors for AF include hypertension, diabetes mellitus, valvular heart disease (in particular, of the mitral valve) and congestive heart failure (5). While alcohol binge drinking has been described as a trigger for acute episodes of transient AF, only heavy alcohol use (≥35 drinks/week) has been associated with an increased risk for AF in men, after adjusting for hypertension, coronary artery disease and congestive heart failure (6,7). A recent prospective community-based study identified obesity as an independent risk factor for AF, possibly mediated by left atrial dilatation (8). Additionally, while obstructive sleep apnea (OSA) has been strongly associated with AF recurrence, it is not clear whether OSA is a risk factor for AF or is merely a surrogate for other risk factors such as obesity and hypertension. Long term endurance exercise has also been associated with an increased risk of AF in men (9). The trends of increasing incidence and prevalence of AF are due to multiple factors. Although an aging population is a significant contributor, the increasing prevalence of traditional cardiovascular risk factors and obesity appears to play an important role in the growing epidemic of AF (10).

African American ethnicity was found to be associated with a lower risk of AF in the Cardiovascular Health Study, although African Americans constituted only 5% of the study cohort (11). There is an overall dearth of much needed population-based data on the prevalence, incidence and risk factors for AF in nonwhite populations. Monogenic forms of AF have been found to be caused by mutations in potassium channel genes. However, the patients in these studies were enrolled mostly from referral centers, and common AF is known to be genetically heterogeneous. To date, two large-population studies have clearly demonstrated a genetic component to common AF in the general population. A prospective cohort study within the Framingham study revealed that in patients <75 years, AF in at least one parent increased the risk of offspring AF with an odds ratio of 3.23 (12). In another population-based study conducted in Iceland, first-degree relatives of AF patients were 1.77-fold more likely to have AF than the general population (13). In patients diagnosed with AF before the age of 60, first-degree relatives were five times more likely to develop AF than the general population. New methodologies such as genome-wide association studies are currently underway to identify genetic determinants of common acquired AF in the general population (10).

■ LONE ATRIAL FIBRILLATION

While the vast majority of patients with AF are >60 years of age and have associated hypertension, valvular heart disease, cardiomyopathy, or diabetes mellitus, there is a subset of patients with AF who are <60 years of age and have normal physical examination, laboratory testing, echocardiography and exercise stress testing. These patients are considered to have lone AF, or AF without "overt" structural heart disease, and are thought to be at low risk for thromboembolism and do not require anticoagulation (14). Recent evidence suggests that while most AF is due to substrate related changes (diseased and dilated atria due to stretch and fibrosis), lone AF is probably more related to electrophysiological phenomena (triggers) in structurally normal atria (15). Paroxysmal lone AF rarely progresses to persistent or permanent AF. Although lone AF has a generally benign course, regular follow-up of patients with lone AF is important because risk factors such as advanced age, hypertension, heart failure, and diabetes mellitus may develop, changing prognosis. A recent study of the 30-year long term natural history of lone AF in an Olmsted County, Minnesota population showed a very low incidence of truly "lone" AF (2%) and among these patients, a low risk of progression to permanent AF, mortality, congestive heart failure, and stroke/transient ischemic attack (16). Also important was the finding that increased thromboembolic complications in patients with lone AF compared to control subjects occurred only after 25 years of follow-up at a time when a significant number of these patients had reached advanced age and developed hypertension. Taken together, these findings demonstrate that comorbidities significantly modulate the progression and complications of lone AF.

Several clinical and experimental studies have provided novel insights into the pathogenesis of lone AF, and modern diagnostic techniques have revealed previously unappreciated abnormalities. Thus in some patients with "lone" AF, there may be underlying abnormalities that are either occult or have yet to be discovered. In some patients with lone AF, occult hypertension may be present but masked by the antihypertensive effects of medications used for rate control. Several epidemiological associations of AF include obesity, sleep apnea, diabetes, metabolic syndrome, increased alcohol consumption, anger and hostility, increased pulse pressure, and subclinical atherosclerosis (assessed by carotid intima-media thickness) (17). Most patients with lone AF are male and young and present with paroxysmal AF triggered by sleep, exercise, alcohol use and eating. These triggers may play an important role in the progression of lone AF to permanent AF through fluctuations in autonomic tone that lead to electrophysiological but not structural changes in the atria. Modern echocardiographic techniques have shown that left ventricular diastolic dysfunction relates to left atrial dilatation and stretch as well as to the development of AF in patients age >65 years (18). Left atrial volume has been shown to be a predictor of cardiovascular events in young male patients with lone AF (19). Furthermore, traditional two-dimensional (2-D) echocardiography in the anteroposterior dimension has been shown to underestimate the true left atrium (LA) size in patients with lone paroxysmal AF. It is unclear whether these concomitant structural changes represent a cause and/or consequence of the arrhythmia, or whether they confer any increased risk for thromboembolic events.

■ CLASSIFICATION OF ATRIAL FIBRILLATION

Various classification systems have been proposed for AF. The ACC/AHA/ESC 2006 guidelines for the management of patients with AF have classified the arrhythmia as paroxysmal, persistent (including long-standing persistent) or permanent (20). First-detected episodes of AF should be noted because of the importance of recognizing the uncertainty about the actual duration of the episode and about previous undetected episodes. After two or more episodes, AF is considered recurrent. AF is classified as paroxysmal if episodes terminate spontaneously within seven days. Persistent AF is defined as AF which is sustained beyond seven days or necessitates pharmacologic or electrical cardioversion. Long-standing persistent AF is defined as persistent AF lasting longer than one year, and permanent AF is applied to situations in which cardioversion has failed or has been foregone. The HRS/EHRA/ECAS expert consensus statement on catheter and surgical ablation of AF does not recognize permanent AF in patients undergoing catheter and/or surgical ablation as it refers to a group of patients where a decision has been made not to pursue restoration of sinus rhythm by any means, including catheter or surgical ablation (21). It is worth noting that the aforementioned AF categories are not mutually exclusive, and that it is practical to categorize patients by their most frequent presentation.

■ SYMPTOMS AND MORBIDITIES OF ATRIAL FIBRILLATION

Atrial fibrillation can cause incapacitating symptoms and reduced exercise tolerance due to uncontrolled and irregular rates, as well as loss of atrial contribution to cardiac output. An irregular sequence of ventricular contractions has been shown to reduce cardiac output independent of heart rate (22,23). AF increases the long-term risk of embolic stroke and has been implicated in one third of strokes in patients older than 60 years (24). Analysis of nearly 1,200 Danish patients diagnosed with acute stroke showed a rising incidence of AF with increasing age. Patients with stroke and concomitant AF also had a markedly poorer prognosis due to initially more severe strokes (25). The annual risk of stroke attributable to AF was 1.5% in patients aged 50 to 59 years and 23.5% in those aged 80 to 89 years. The rate of ischemic stroke among patients with nonvalvular AF in the Framingham Heart Study averaged 5% per year, two to seven times that of people without AF (3). In patients with rheumatic heart disease and AF, stroke risk was increased 17-fold compared with age-matched controls (26), and attributable risk was five times greater than in those with nonrheumatic AF (3).

AF is also associated with increased heart failure and all-cause mortality, especially in women (27). Analysis of the natural history of AF in a Canadian population supports the finding that AF independently increases the risk for stroke, heart failure and total mortality (28). In large heart failure trials (COMET and Val-HeFT), AF was a strong independent risk factor for morbidity and mortality (29,30). AF and heart failure frequently occur together, and recent data from the Framingham Health Study has shown that heart failure promotes AF, AF aggravates heart failure, and patients with either condition who develop the alternate condition share a poor prognosis (31). Furthermore, AF conveys an increased risk of mortality independent of structural heart disease. The mortality related to AF may be due to heart failure, stroke, drug toxicity, and ventricular arrhythmias.

■ RATE VERSUS RHYTHM CONTROL

It has been estimated that between 14% and 24% of patients with paroxysmal AF eventually progress to persistent AF (20). In a 30-year follow-up study of the previously characterized Olmsted County population, 31% of patients with paroxysmal or persistent AF progressed to permanent AF, with most doing so within the first 15 years after diagnosis (16). Furthermore, conversion of AF to sinus rhythm becomes increasingly difficult as the duration of AF increases because of changes in atrial structure and function, an array of processes known as atrial remodeling (32). Because it appears that ongoing AF facilitates disease progression, it would seem preferable to strive for rhythm control whenever possible. However, attempts to prove that a strategy to maintain sinus rhythm has a favorable effect on survival have remained elusive. The Atrial Fibrillation Follow-up Investigation of Rhythm Management (AFFIRM) study compared a rate control versus rhythm control study in a large group of patients with AF and high risk for stroke. In an intention-to-treat analysis, there was no mortality benefit observed for either strategy, and there was a lower risk of adverse drug effects with the rate control strategy (33). Subgroup analysis from the AFFIRM study demonstrated that younger patients (<65 years of age) and those with a history congestive heart failure responded more favorably to rhythm control than did older patients and those without heart failure (34). It has been postulated that the absence of a benefit on survival with rhythm control reflects the incomplete suppression of AF and/or the negative impact of cardiac and noncardiac side effects of current antiarrhythmic therapies. In a post-hoc analysis of the AFFIRM study, the risk of death decreased dramatically for patients who remained in sinus rhythm, but antiarrhythmic drug use was associated with increased mortality (35). Four other randomized clinical trials have failed to show a benefit of rhythm control with antiarrhythmic drugs over rate control in terms cardiovascular mortality or combined endpoints of morbidity and mortality (36–38).

In contrast to the results of prospective randomized trials, post-hoc analyses of other studies have shown that rhythm control is associated with reduced mortality, including patients with structural heart disease. The Danish Investigations of Arrhythmia and Mortality ON Dofetilide (DIAMOND) study showed that restoration of sinus rhythm with dofetilide in patients with AF and left ventricular dysfunction was associated with improved survival (39). In the veterans affairs Congestive Heart Failure Survival Trial of Antiarrhythmic Therapy (CHF-STAT), patients with AF who converted to sinus rhythm on amiodarone had a significantly lower mortality rate compared to patients who did not convert to sinus rhythm (40).

Several caveats must be considered in interpreting the rhythm versus rate control trials. The prospective trials generally enrolled older patients with risk factors for stroke or mortality. For example, the mean age of patients in AFFIRM was 70 years. Also, enrolled patients were asymptomatic or minimally symptomatic and could thus tolerate a rate control strategy. Thus, these trials do not necessarily apply to younger, more symptomatic patients. Importantly, strokes in AFFIRM frequently occurred when patients stopped anticoagulation in the rhythm control arm, implying that continuation of anticoagulation after cardioversion might improve the outcomes in patients attempting maintenance of sinus rhythm.

While the true impact of rhythm control on mortality remains to be determined, current data suggest that the restoration and maintenance of sinus rhythm in patients with AF may impart other important clinical benefits, such as improvements in symptoms, exercise tolerance, ability to perform activities of daily living and quality of life (41). In the Rate Control versus Electrical Cardioversion (RACE) study, patients with AF who converted to sinus rhythm had a significant reduction in atrial size and improvement in left ventricular function (36). Despite efforts to enroll patients who would tolerate rate-controlled AF, the AFFIRM Functional Status Substudy showed that AF was associated with poorer New York Heart Association (NYHA) functional capacity and rhythm control was associated with a modest improvement in six-minute walk distance compared to rate control (42).

Several factors may explain the failure to detect benefits with conventional antiarrhythmic drugs in randomized trials. Despite randomization to antiarrhythmic drugs, AF recurred frequently in these patients, with 37% of patients in AFFIRM having recurrent AF at five years. Other factors include toxicity of antiarrhythmic drugs and the possibility that AF may be a marker of poor prognosis rather than the direct cause of morbidity or mortality. As a result, ablation therapy is currently being evaluated as an alternative to rhythm control strategy to pharmacologic antiarrhythmic therapy.

PATHOPHYSIOLOGY OF ATRIAL FIBRILLATION

In the early 1900s, Sir Thomas Lewis made several important observations on AF and suggested reentry as the likely mechanism for this arrhythmia. However, Scherf subsequently performed a series of experiments that suggested the mechanism of AF was due to a rapidly firing ectopic focus which resulted in possible reentry waves of excitation which he called "fibrillatory conduction" (43). This was overshadowed by the work of Moe et al. in the 1950s (183), who described fractionation of grossly irregular wave fronts as they divided around islets or strands of refractory tissue into daughter wavelets. The concept of coexisting randomly wandering wavelets, with local excitation limited by the heterogeneous distribution of refractory periods throughout the atria became known as the multiple wavelet hypothesis and remained the dominant mechanistic model for AF for the next 50 years. While supporting reentry as the major mechanism of AF, Moe et al. also concluded that the irregular activation of the atria could be produced by several factors including a single rapidly discharging ectopic focus, multiple rapidly discharging foci, or rapidly circulating circus movement. Following publication of the multiple wavelet hypothesis, it became generally accepted that AF was the result of the random propagation of multiple wavelets across the atria, a process that was thought to be independent of the initiating event.

Experimental support for the multiple wavelet hypothesis developed out of work done by Allessie et al. in 1985. They were able to map the spread of excitation in the atria of a dog heart during rapid pacing-induced AF in the presence of acetylcholine, and provided the first demonstration in vivo of multiple propagating wavelets giving rise to turbulent atrial activity (44). They estimated that maintenance of AF would require a critical number of four to six wavelets. In a canine sterile pericarditis model of paroxysmal AF, unstable reentrant circuits of very short cycle length have been shown to be critical for maintenance of AF (45). In addition, pharmacological experiments have further shown that termination of AF by class IC antiarrhythmic drugs is preceded by a decrease in the mean number of wavelets (46,47).

However, the classic Lewis idea that fibrillation results from the activity of a small number of rapidly firing reentrant circuits that give rise to wavefront fractionation and fibrillatory conduction has been revived. Experimental models have identified localized rotors due to functional reentrant activity, and the rapidly succeeding wavefronts emanating from it propagate throughout the cardiac muscle and interact with anatomical and/or functional obstacles, causing fragmentation and new wavelet formation—that is, fibrillatory conduction (48). Optical mapping studies of AF in sheep hearts point to a primary local generator, consisting of either a single small reentry circuit or an ectopic focus (49). A left atrium-right atrium frequency gradient during AF supports the hypothesis that this arrhythmia is the result of high-frequency periodic sources in the LA, with fibrillatory conduction away from such sources (50).

The pulmonary veins (PVs) play a central role in initiating paroxysmal AF. As originally described by Haissaguerre et al. in 1998, PV potentials, located 2 to 4 cm within the veins, precede the onset of AF and appear to drive the initiating beats of AF (Figure 6.1) (51). The underlying basis of PV activity remains poorly understood. Myocardial tissue in the sleeves around the proximal ends of pulmonary veins can generate spontaneous action potentials (52), and the rate of pulmonary vein activity can be greatly increased by adrenergic stimulation (53). The PV-atrial junction also demonstrates anisotropic conduction and repolarization heterogeneity allowing reentrant conduction to occur (54). Distal PVs have been shown to have shorter refractory periods and thus may be capable of supporting high frequency drivers (55). Using high-resolution optical mapping in an atrial-PV preparation, both spontaneous impulse generation and reentry within the PV antrum have been demonstrated (56). Furthermore, myocyte arrangement immediately beneath the venous walls has revealed complex arrangements of myocardial fibers with abrupt changes in fiber direction, which might facilitate reentry and arrhythmias associated with ectopic activity (57). While the pulmonary veins are the main source of focal activity, other thoracic veins and anatomic sites associated with focal activity include the ostium of the coronary sinus, ligament of Marshall, crista terminalis, vena cavae, mitral valve and less commonly the interatrial septum, as well as the atrial free wall (58).

AUTONOMIC EFFECTS IN ATRIAL FIBRILLATION

It has been postulated that one possible trigger for AF is the autonomic nervous system (ANS). In humans

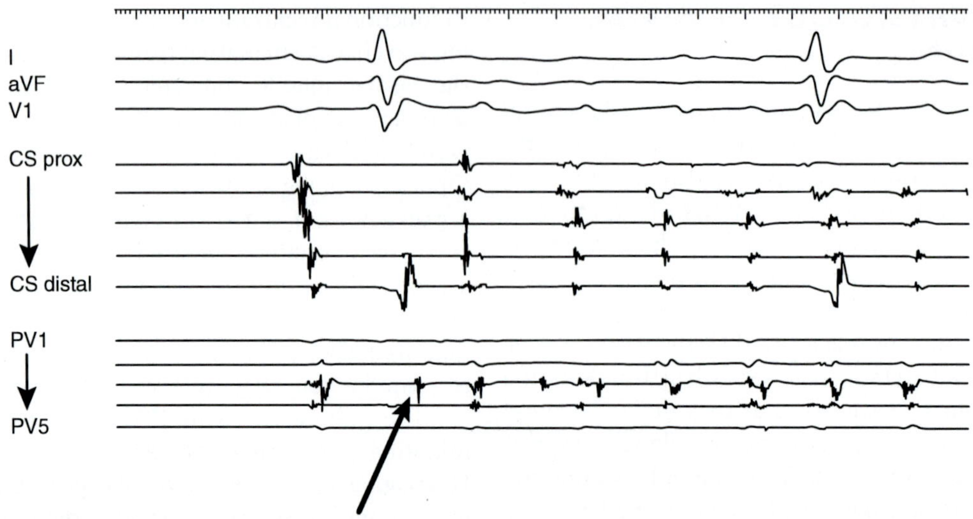

FIGURE 6.1 Initiation of atrial fibrillation (AF) with ectopic beats arising from the left superior pulmonary vein (PV). Shown are three surface leads (I, aVF, and V1), five intracardiac electrograms form the coronary sinus (CS prox to CS distal) and five electrograms from a catheter in the left superior PV (PV1 through PV5). After a sinus beat, a premature PV potential appears on PV3, which initiates AF (arrow).

with lone AF, situations of high vagal tone such as sleep or postprandial states commonly stimulate AF. Parasympathetic activation mediated by acetylcholine abbreviates atrial action potential duration through activation of the outward potassium current I_{KACh} and produces heterogeneous effects on atrial refractory periods, thus providing the electrophysiological conditions for leading circle reentry, multiple wavelet reentry, and fibrillatory conduction (59). Conversely, sympathetic stimulation can also provoke AF in some animal models. For example, in dogs with chronic rapid pacing, sympathetic stimulation can lead to rapid repetitive activations in isolated canine PV and vein of Marshall preparations (53). Simultaneous parasympathetic and sympathetic activation may be particularly arrhythmogenic. Sympathetic stimulation induced delayed afterdepolarizations are capable of triggering extrasystoles in PV myocytes, which in the setting of parasympathetic stimulation allows the induction of AF (60–62).

The PV–LA junction is rich in autonomic innervation (63). Human autonomic nerve density is high in the anterosuperior segments of both superior veins and inferior segments of both inferior veins, highest in the left atrium within 5 mm of the PV–LA junction, and higher in the epicardium than endocardium. A significant proportion (30%) of ganglion cells express dual adrenocholinergic phenotypes (64). In human hearts, gradients of nerve density exist, with the highest concentration of neural inputs occurring at the PV–LA junction, fanning out towards the distal pulmonary vein and anterior wall of the left atrium (65). High-frequency electrical stimulation (HFS) of ganglionated plexi in the PVs of dogs may induce ectopic beats that result in AF (66). Other work in canines has shown that stimulation of epicardial fat pads that contain clusters of ganglionated plexi may facilitate the induction of AF with atrial premature stimuli (67). In addition, radio frequency ablation of ganglionated plexi has been shown to reverse the refractory period change and abolish the ability of right superior and left superior pulmonary vein premature stimuli to induce AF (68).

■ ATRIAL REMODELING IN ATRIAL FIBRILLATION

Left atrial remodeling refers to a time-dependent adaptive regulation of cardiac myocytes in order to maintain homeostasis against external stressors. It occurs either as a result of underlying systemic disease affecting cardiac tissue, maladaptive processes resulting from cardiac disease, or gradual fibrosis from senescence. Remodeling occurs at the tissue and subcellular level, and creates a suitable environment for both the spontaneous induction and maintenance of AF. The most common stressors of atrial myocytes include tachycardia with high rates of cell depolarization, and volume/pressure overload such as in heart failure. Diastolic dysfunction, ischemia, and valvular disease impose excess pressure and/or volume load on the LA, which responds with a range of adaptive as well as maladaptive processes. These include myocyte growth, hypertrophy, necrosis and apoptosis; alterations in the composition of extracellular matrix; recalibration of energy production and expenditure; changes in the expression of cellular ionic channels and atrial hormones; and reversal to a fetal gene program. These changes promote a cascade of reactions, which lead to left atrial remodeling with structural, functional, electrical, metabolic, and neurohormonal consequences (69). Under acute or chronic stress injury, the LA stretches and stiffens resulting in extensive interstitial fibrosis and myocyte hypertrophy. Early changes in cellular ultrastructure including mitochondria and sarcoplasmic reticulum occur without signs of cellular degeneration (70). Additional changes include altered cellular calcium handling, cellular myolysis, and decreased release of systolic calcium. There is also evidence for spatially heterogeneous reductions in atrial expression of connexin 40 (71). Adaptation to chronic overload results in a shift in gene expression resulting in dedifferentiation to a fetal-like phenotyope. The intra- and extracellular changes contribute to alterations in electrical make-up rendering the LA more vulnerable to AF development.

AF, once initiated, alters atrial electrophysiological properties in a way that favors the ease of induction and maintenance of the arrhythmia, a process called electrical remodeling (Figure 6.2). Increased atrial rates lead to progressive cytosolic calcium loading and inefficient calcium handling which threatens cell viability. Cellular adaptive responses to reduce intracellular calcium levels include short-term voltage-dependent and intracellular calcium-concentration-dependent inactivation of L-type calcium channels (I_{Ca}) and long term down-regulation of I_{Ca} gene expression (72,73). Because I_{Ca} accounts for a large part of the action potential plateau, reduced I_{Ca} decreases action potential duration (APD), reduces refractory period, and promotes the induction and maintenance of AF by multiple circuit reentry. Several distinct types of electrical remodeling have been associated with AF. Atrial tachycardia-induced remodeling is associated with shortening of the atrial effective refractory period (ERP) and reduction of its physiological rate adaptation, leading to the concept that "AF begets AF" (74). In contrast, electrical remodeling in the aging heart and during heart failure (HF) is associated with prominent fibrosis, producing heterogeneous slowing of conduction velocity and prolongation of the action potential duration at faster heart rates (75,76). In HF models, inward I_{Ca} is reduced much less than in atrial tachycardia remodeling. Meanwhile, outward $I_{Ks,}$ which is unaffected by AF, is decreased by about 30% and inward Na^{+}–Ca^{2+} exchange (NCX) is increased (76). Thus, HF-induced remodeling does not reduce action potential duration; rather, the increased NCX promotes afterdepolarization-related atrial ectopic firing and AF (77).

Tissue fibrosis is a hallmark of arrhythmogenic structural remodeling. It results from an accumulation of fibrillar collagen deposits, occurring most commonly as a reparative process to replace degenerating myocardial parenchyma with concomitant reactive fibrosis, which causes interstitial expansion (78). Atrial fibrosis involves multi-factorial processes that result from complex interactions among neurohormonal and cellular mediators (79). Increased collagen deposition has been documented in lone AF patients compared with sinus rhythm control subjects (80), and in patients with AF secondary to mitral valve disease versus those in sinus rhythm (81). Dense and disorganized collagen fibrils physically separate myocytes and create potential barriers to impulse propagation. This leads to localized regions of conduction slowing and increased conduction heterogeneity, providing an AF substrate. Conduction abnormalities provide a basis for unidirectional conduction block and macroreentry; however, there is also evidence for focal atrial tachyarrhythmias (82,83). Fibrosis also interferes with inter-myocyte coupling. Hypophosphorylation of connexins and their redistribution to lateral cell borders have been correlated with fibrosis (84).

Increases in atrial natriuretic peptide (ANP), brain natriuretic peptide (BNP), angiotensin II (Ang-II), aldosterone, transforming growth factor-β_1 and sympathetic hyperinnervation have been described as neurohormonal disturbances in LA remodeling (69). The vasoconstriction caused by angiotensin II, increasing cardiac afterload and promoting left ventricular hypertrophy, is indirectly proarrhythmic by increasing atrial pressure and stretch (85). Experimental HF results in a rapid, sustained increase in atrial angiotensin II, and

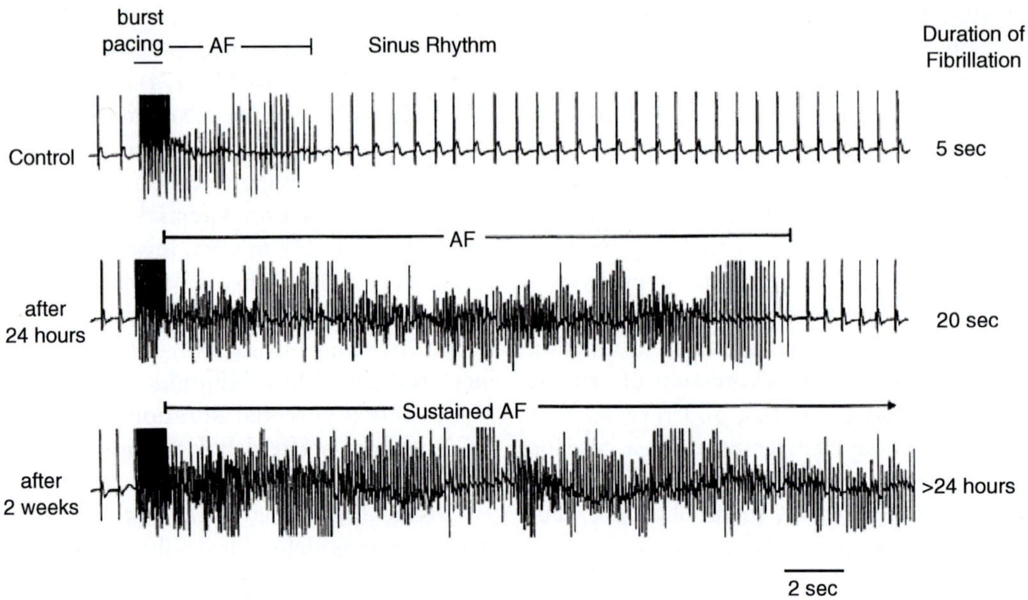

FIGURE 6.2 Electrical remodeling in a goat model of atrial fibrillation (AF). Atrial burst pacing is applied repetitively to simulate AF. There is prolongation of the duration of episodes of electrically induced AF after maintaining AF for respectively 24 hours and 2 weeks. The three tracings show a single atrial electrogram recorded from the same goat during induction of AF by a 1-s burst of stimuli (50 Hz, 4 × threshold). In the upper tracing the goat has been in sinus rhythm all the time and atrial fibrillation self-terminated within 5 s. The second tracing was recorded after the goat had been connected to the fibrillation pacemaker for 24 hours showing a clear prolongation of the duration of AF to 20 s. The third tracing was recorded after 2 weeks of electrically maintained atrial fibrillation. After induction of AF this episode became sustained and did not terminate. (From Ref. 74, with permission.)

ACE inhibition and angiotensin receptor blockade have both been shown to attenuate fibrosis and AF maintenance (79). Downstream mediators of angiotensin II include transforming growth factor β_1 and mitogen activated protein kinases. Aldosterone infusion also results in atrial fibrosis independent of changes in wall stress or arterial hypertension in small animal models, and antagonism by spironolactone prevents fibrotic remodeling in the heart. The most direct clinical evidence for a role of aldosterone in AF comes from a study that showed that patients with primary hyperaldosteronism have a 12-fold increased relative risk of developing AF compared with blood pressure-matched controls (86). The TRACE trial first demonstrated the benefit of inhibiting angiotensin II signaling with the ACE inhibitor trandolapril in human subjects with AF (87). A meta-analysis of 11 trials trials studying ACE inhibitors or angiotensin receptor blockers for heart failure, hypertension, after myocardial infarction, and after cardioversion of AF demonstrated a 28% reduction in the relative risk of AF, but the benefit appeared limited to patients with systolic left ventricular dysfunction or hypertrophy (88). A randomized study in patients with lone AF has shown a reduction in AF recurrences with ramipril (89).

Importantly, left atrial remodeling is reversible. Studies have shown that LA size and function can improve with certain medications, after restoration of sinus rhythm from AF and after repair of the mitral valve in the case of severe mitral regurgitation. Direct evidence of reversing LA remodeling on cardiovascular outcomes remains to be seen, but the evidence indirectly suggests that the risk of AF can be significantly reduced.

■ HISTORY OF CATHETER ABLATION IN ATRIAL FIBRILLATION

The original surgical MAZE procedure was introduced by James Cox in 1987 and was designed to preclude the development of macroreentry in the atria (90).

Subsequent realization that only a limited number of left atrial sites are capable of sustaining such circuits led to modification of the procedure to the Cox MAZE III operation, which is now acknowledged to be the gold standard for surgical treatment of AF. Previous data demonstrate that the MAZE procedure with concomitant cardiac surgery achieves successful restoration of sinus rhythm in 70% to 96% of patients, although monitoring technologies were not as sensitive as they are today (91–93). Specifically, the five lesions of the standard MAZE III procedure include an encircling lesion around the pulmonary veins, septal lesion, left atrial isthmus lesion between the inferior pulmonary veins and the mitral annulus, cryolesion on the coronary sinus and left atrial appendage lesion (94). A lesion in the isthmus between the coronary sinus and the tricuspid valve is also made to disable a critical limb of the macroreentrant circuit sustaining typical right atrial flutter. Surgical excision of the left atrial appendage with cut-and-sew techniques is an integral component of the MAZE procedure and contributes to the low risk for stroke after the MAZE procedure. In the largest series to date, Cox et al. noted a single late stroke at a mean follow-up of 5 years in 300 patients who had a classic MAZE procedure (95). Taken together, these maneuvers are critical to the efficacy of the MAZE procedure in restoration of sinus rhythm and reduction of the risk of thromboembolism (96). The MAZE III procedure requires considerable surgical skill and operation time, between 45 and 60 minutes of cardiopulmonary bypass and cardiac arrest. Therefore, cardiac surgeons are now deploying a reduced set of scars in the left atria, and using radiofrequency, cryotherapy, microwave, high intensity focused ultrasound, or laser sources to create endocardial and epicardial lesions.

In 1982, Scheinman et al. (97) used direct current energy to ablate the atrioventricular node in patients with supraventricular arrhythmias. Radiofrequency energy has replaced direct current energy as a source of energy for catheter ablation of arrhythmias. Catheter ablation techniques aimed at curing AF rather than simply controlling the ventricular response target the triggers of AF. Curative catheter ablation techniques initially attempted to mimic the linear lesions created by the surgical MAZE III procedure. Haissaguerre and colleagues described focal firing as an important source of ectopic beats, which could lead to AF, and reported that these foci respond to radiofrequency ablation (98). This changed the emphasis of catheter ablation away from linear lesions compartmentalizing the atria to treating focal sources. Original experience with mapping paroxysmal AF demonstrated that as many as 94% of such triggers originate from the pulmonary veins, and that focal ablation within the PVs could eliminate these triggers (51). As catheter ablation progressed from treating patients with paroxysmal AF to long-lasting persistent AF, the importance of treating the left atrial substrate became apparent. Catheter ablation is now a realistic therapeutic option in most patients with paroxysmal and long-lasting AF, including patients with moderate-to-severe left ventricular dysfunction (99). In fact, there is evidence to suggest that restoration and maintenance of sinus rhythm by catheter ablation may lead to improved outcomes in these patients (100).

■ INDICATIONS FOR CATHETER ABLATION OF ATRIAL FIBRILLATION

Historically, most patients having catheter ablation had paroxysmal AF, were relatively young and had little or no structural heart disease. With improved experience and techniques, the indications for AF ablation have expanded. Now, AF ablations are performed with reasonable success and low complication rates in older patients and those with persistent AF, structural heart disease, and left atrial dilatation (100). The ACC/AHA/ESC 2006 Practice Guidelines for the management of AF state that "catheter ablation is a reasonable alternative to pharmacological therapy to prevent recurrent AF in symptomatic patients with little or no LA enlargement" (Class 2A recommendation, level of evidence C) (20). For maintenance of sinus rhythm treatment, catheter ablation is considered second-line therapy after antiarrhythmic therapy for all categories of patients, according to these guidelines. An expert consensus statement endorsed by three professional electrophysiology societies considers AF ablation to be indicated in symptomatic patients who failed at least one class I or III antiarrhythmic drug (21). In some circumstances, ablation may be considered appropriate as first-line therapy, particularly in relatively young patients who do not wish to take antiarrythmic drugs and fully understand the risks and benefits of this procedure. In patients with advanced age, significant left atrial dilatation and long duration of AF, catheter ablation is less likely to be successful. These patients are also at higher risk for complications including myocardial perforation and thromboembolism.

■ TECHNIQUES OF CATHETER ABLATION IN ATRIAL FIBRILLATION

Pulmonary Vein Isolation

The identification of triggers that initiate AF within the PVs led to prevention of AF recurrences by ablation at the site of origin of the trigger. Direct catheter ablation of the triggers was limited by the infrequency with which AF initiation could be reproducibly triggered during an ablation procedure. A further limitation of this approach is that multiple sites of triggering foci were commonly observed (101) and ablation of individual triggering foci was associated with high rates of AF recurrence. It was also subsequently appreciated that PV stenosis could result from extensive ablation within a vein (102). Because discrete electrical connections between the LA and the PVs can be identified, an ablation approach was introduced which was designed to electrically isolate the PV myocardium by targeting these PV-atrial connections (103). This segmental PV isolation technique involves insertion of a circular mapping catheter into the PVs and a series of segmental lesions are then created at the PV ostium until isolation of the vein could be demonstrated by disappearance of the potentials within the vein (Figure 6.3). Segmental isolation typically requires the delivery of RF energy to 30% to 80% of the circumference of the PVs. Segmental PV isolation has been shown to have a higher rate of recurrence than circumferential techniques (101,103–105). Occasionally, individual pulmonary veins may be identified as the triggers of AF in a given patient, and it may seem prudent to isolate only the veins identified as harboring triggers in these cases. Failure to isolate all the pulmonary veins, however, yields a lower long-term success rate (106,107).

Wide Area Circumferential Ablation

Wide area circumferential PV ablation around individual PVs or two ipsilateral veins using three-dimensional (3-D) electroanatomical mapping was initially described by Pappone et al. (108,109). This technique represented a shift in strategy from one that assumed most of the arrhythmogenic activity responsible for AF to be confined within the PVs to one that assumed that the atrial tissue adjacent to the orifice of the PVs is involved in the mechanisms responsible for AF. In the original description of this technique, electrical isolation of areas surrounded by the ablation line was not mandatory as long as significant abatement of local potential and/or consistent local conduction delay was achieved. Initially, the lesion set was limited to wide (>0.5 cm outside PV ostia) circumferential lesions around and outside the PV ostia, but over time it was modified with wider (1–2 cm outside PV ostia) circumferential lesions, and additional linear ablation lines in the posterior wall connecting the PVs, and in the mitral isthmus in order to increase the amount of substrate ablated and to prevent recurrences

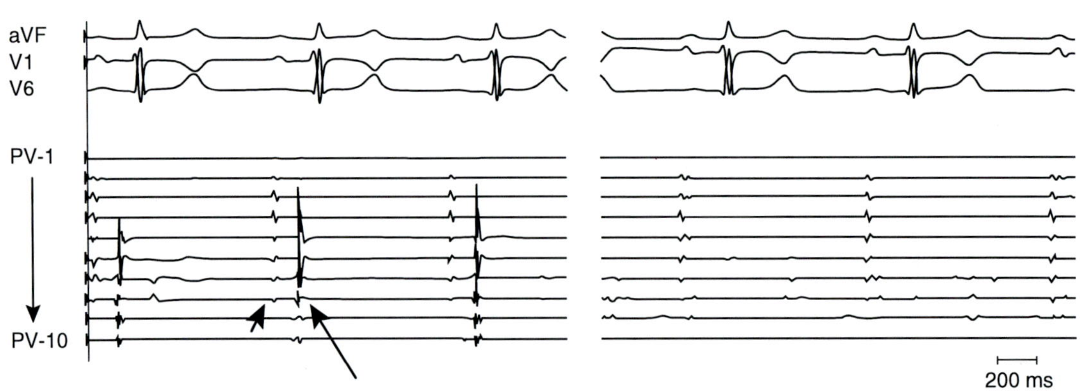

FIGURE 6.3 Pulmonary vein (PV) isolation. Left panel shows three sinus beats with surface leads aVF, V1, and V6, and ten intracardiac electrograms from the left superior PV (PV-1 through PV-10) before PV isolation. Low amplitude potentials represent atrial activity (small arrow) followed by high amplitude PV potentials (large arrow). Right panels shows elimination of PV potentials after encircling radiofrequency ablation.

of atrial tachycardia (110). Successful lesion creation at each point is verified when the local bipolar voltage has decreased by 90% or to less than 0.05 mV. The same ablation schema can be used when ablating paroxysmal, persistent, and long-lasting AF, as similar results have been reported for all different AF types (111).

Pulmonary Vein Antral Isolation

Although it is known that most triggers of AF arise from the muscular sleeves of the PVs, the junction of the PVs and the LA is not a discrete ostium. Instead, PV triggers often exist proximally in this junction (112). As the atrial walls expand during the early embryologic stages, the smooth tissue of the PVs becomes incorporated into the walls of the left atrium, which later become the posterior wall and some of the roof of the left atrium. This incorporated portion of the LA along with the PVs defines the PV antra (113). Studies of PV anatomy from pathologic specimens and 3-D CT have shown that the PV is funnel shaped, with a tube that fans out into a proximal "cup" that blends into the posterior atrial wall. To avoid stenosis, increase success rate, and achieve complete isolation of the PV, ablation lesions have been deployed in more proximal locations around the PV antrum and not the tubular ostium (114). This understanding has shaped the development of catheter ablation for AF from a distal ablation procedure isolating the PVs at the ostium, what is commonly known as PV isolation (PVI), to a more proximal isolation of the entire PV antrum, referred to as PV antrum isolation (PVAI). In contrast to selective PV angiography, intracardiac echocardiography (ICE) can accurately define the proximal edge of the PV antrum. The PV antra isolated by this technique encompasses the PVs and portions of the LA roof, posterior wall, and interatrial septum anterior to the right PVs. The endpoint is either amplitude reduction within the ablated area, elimination (or dissociation) of the PV potentials recorded from the ipsilateral PVs, and/or exit block from the PV (21).

Linear Ablation in Atrial Fibrillation

Linear ablation that accomplishes complete electrical block disrupts large macroreentrant circuits capable of sustaining AF. A number of studies have shown that the addition of linear lesions to PVI improves outcomes. The most common sites are the LA "roof" connecting the superior aspects of the left and right upper PVI lesions, the region of tissue between the mitral annulus and the ostium of the left inferior PV (the mitral isthmus), and anteriorly between the roof line near the left or right circumferential lesion and the mitral annulus. Prospective studies of adding ablation in the mitral isthmus and/or LA roof to PVI show improvement in maintenance of sinus rhythm compared to PVI alone (115–119). Linear lesions have been reported to be associated with conversion of AF either directly to sinus rhythm or to atrial tachycardia, demonstrating that such lesions may modify the substrate for AF. In many patients, conversion to a macro-reentrant atrial tachycardia is observed during the ablation process, requiring linear lesions for termination. One study showed that among patients with persistent AF, 96% ultimately required a roof line and 86% a mitral isthmus line for termination of AF or to treat macroreentant atrial tachycardias (120). The goal of linear lesions is the achievement of bidirectional block. This may be more difficult to achieve along the mitral isthmus compared to the roof of the left atrium due to thicker atrial myocardium, the presence of numerous recesses and cavities, as well as epicardial muscular connections necessitating ablation within the coronary sinus (115).

The importance of electrically isolating the posterior left atrial wall was highlighted in a study of patients undergoing cardiac surgery, which showed that isolation of the posterior wall can control AF, and the isolated posterior wall can sustain spontaneous or induced AF (121). Areas of functional conduction delay can be demonstrated in the posterior LA with marked anisotropic conduction that is exacerbated in the setting of left atrial disease, specifically congestive heart failure and mitral regurgitation (122). In general, the lesion sets that incorporate the largest extent of left atrial-pulmonary venous tissue have the theoretical advantage of addressing the greatest amount of arrhythmogenic tissue, but the disadvantage of requiring longer linear lesions. One such ablation strategy is the posterior "box" lesion set (123). Similar to the surgical "mini-maze" procedure, this lesion set involves ablation along the anterior aspects of both sets of PVs connected by a roof line and an inferior line. Together, these joining linear lesions electrically isolate the PVs and complete posterior LA wall *en masse*.

Complex Fractionated Electrograms

During AF, it is possible to record complex electrical activity in some areas of the atria. Nademanee et al.

advanced the concept of targeting sites with complex fractionated atrial electrograms (CFAEs) to abolish AF (124). In exclusively targeting CFAEs in both the left and right atria in patients with paroxysmal and persistent AF, they achieved maintenance of sinus rhythm of 91% at one year, with an average of 1.2 procedures per patient. CFAE areas are presumed to correspond to key regions of the AF substrate, based on intraoperative observations indicating that CFAEs localize at areas of conduction block or at pivot points for reentrant wave activity (125). They are typically identified in the PV ostia, interatrial septum, anterior LA and base of the LA appendage, inferior LA, and coronary sinus. CFAEs are electrograms with highly fractionated potentials or with a very short cycle length, and are usually low-voltage multiple potential signals between 0.06 and 0.25 mV (Figure 6.4). Multiple definitions for CFAEs have been proposed, including electrograms with two or more deflections and/or baseline perturbation with continuous activity over a 10-s recording period, and electrograms with a mean cycle length <120 msec over a 10-s recording period. For CFAE-based ablation, the primary endpoints are either complete elimination of the areas with CFAEs, conversion of AF to sinus rhythm (either directly or first to an atrial tachycardia), and/or noninducibility of AF. In patients with long-lasting persistent AF, the long-term success rate of CFAE ablation was 71%, as monitored by symptoms and annual Holter monitoring (100). There is, however, a discrepancy in results between different groups using a defractionation only strategy. In a separate study, CFAE-based ablation resulted in only 33% of patients maintaining sinus rhythm without antiarrhythmic medication at a mean of 14 months follow-up, rising to 57% when a repeat ablation was performed (126).

Ganglionated Plexi

The ANS is known to play a role in the generation of AF, with increased sympathetic and parasympathetic activity preceding pulmonary vein firing, and shortening the atrial refractory period. Autonomic ganglionated plexi are present in epicardial fat pads (superior left, inferior left, superior right, and inferior right) at the border of the PV antrum, and can be identified by endocardial high-frequency stimulation (HFS). High-

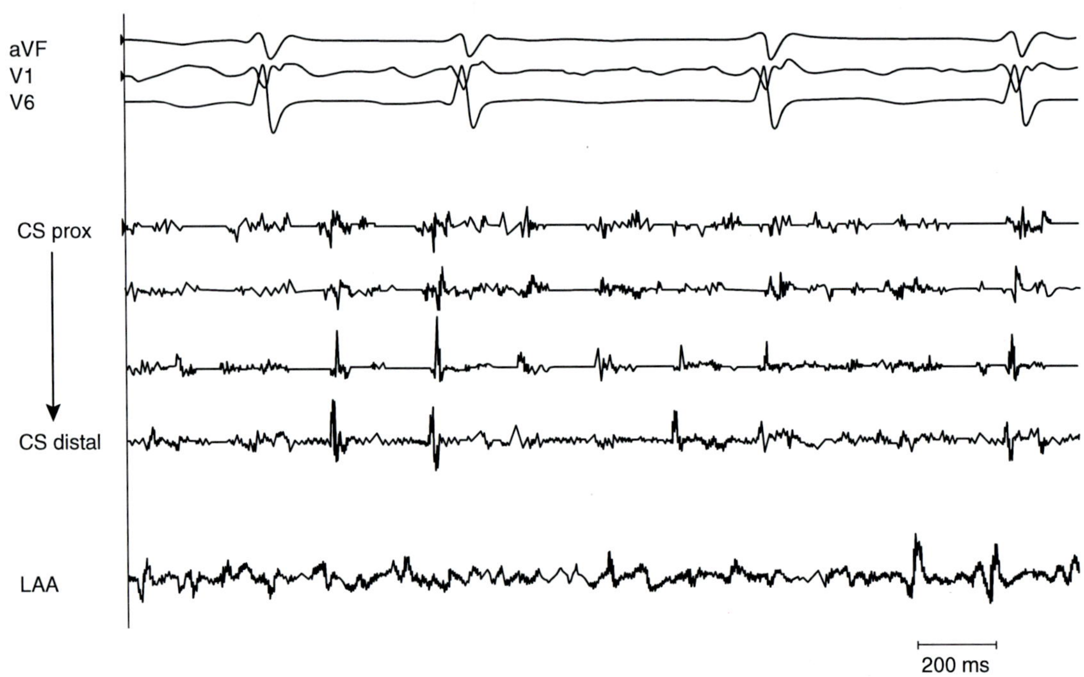

FIGURE 6.4 Complex fractionated electrograms. Tracing is from a patient with persistent atrial fibrillation (AF), showing surface leads aVF, V1, and V6, followed by recordings from the coronary sinus (CS prox through distal) and a mapping catheter at the base of the left atrial appendage (LAA). During AF, complex fractionated electrograms are recorded on the mapping catheter, identified by low amplitude, multicomponent signals.

frequency stimulation (cycle length 50 msec, 12 V, 1–10 msec pulse width) delivered by a mapping catheter in the LA at these sites leads to induction of AF and/or bradycardia or AV block due to increased vagal tone. The ganglionated plexi are usually located within areas of CFAEs during AF (127). Vagal reflexes can be observed during radiofrequency ablation near the PV ostia, and abolition of inducible vagal reflexes has been proposed as an endpoint of ablation on the basis of experimental data in dogs (128). Encircling PV lesions and both the LA roof line and the mitral isthmus line incorporate the locations of known vagal ganglia, with the highest density of cardiac autonomic nerves occurring within 5 mm of the LA-PV junction. Although it is feasible to map and locate individual vagal ganglia with HFS, this is not routinely performed clinically, nor may it be necessary given the overlap between the PV ostia and the vagal ganglia. In a study of patients with drug refractory paroxysmal AF, the abolition of evoked vagal responses seen during circumferential PV ablation rendered 99% of patients free of AF at 12 months, compared with 85% in those in whom vagal responses could not be evoked (129). However, it is currently unclear whether an independent effect of ablation at sites of ganglionic plexi is due to a neural affect compared to the effect on local atrial tissue (130).

Staged Ablation in Atrial Fibrillation

Pulmonary vein isolation is associated with lower success in patients with persistent and chronic AF compared to paroxysmal AF, implicating atrial disease beyond PV activity as the driver for fibrillation in these patients (131). The mechanisms of initiating, maintaining, or perpetuating AF are varied, complex and multifactorial, so that different techniques may be better suited to individual patients. The poor efficacy of PVI in patients with chronic AF has prompted the evolution of ablation strategies to target the atrial myocardium beyond the PV–LA junction in an effort to identify other sites critical for maintenance of the fibrillatory process. The supplementary targets which have emerged in treating persistent AF include LA linear lesions to interrupt reentrant wavelets, CFAEs, areas of short cycle length activity, sites of dominant frequency, and cardiac autonomic denervation (132). A stepwise or tailored approach in which several ablation strategies are combined to target multiple atrial areas has resulted in higher success in maintaining sinus rhythm in the medium term with recovery of atrial mechanical function (133,134). In addition to PV electrical disconnection and demonstrable complete block across the roof and mitral isthmus (when performed), ablation is performed at sites displaying continuous electrical and complex fractionated activity, with the endpoint of local organization, as well as at sites displaying electrograms consistent with focal sources driving AF in the left or right atria or coronary sinus. Stepwise ablation is accompanied by a cumulative increase in the AF cycle length prior to termination of AF by conversion either directly to sinus rhythm or to an atrial tachycardia, which is then mapped conventionally and ablated. With this approach, termination of AF occurred in 87%, resulting in freedom from AF at one year of 95%, with 38% of patients requiring more than one procedure (134). Furthermore, the order of ablation targets has been shown to be irrelevant, suggesting that all of the targets contributed to the maintenance of AF.

The 2007 Task Force consensus guidelines endorsed by three professional organizations recommend that ablation strategies that target the PVs and/or PV antra should be the cornerstone for most AF ablation procedures with a goal of complete electrical isolation. Careful identification of the PV ostia is mandatory to avoid ablation within the PVs, which can lead to pulmonary stenosis. If a focal trigger is identified outside a PV at the time of an AF ablation procedure, it should be targeted. If linear lesions are applied, line completeness should be confirmed with mapping or pacing maneuvers. Ablation of the cavotricuspid isthmus is recommended in patients with a history of typical atrial flutter or inducible cavotricuspid isthmus-dependent atrial flutter. Finally, if patients with longstanding persistent AF are approached, ostial PVI alone may not be sufficient (21).

■ RADIOFREQUENCY ABLATION AND CRYOTHERAPY IN ATRIAL FIBRILLATION

Successful AF ablation depends upon achieving lesions that are reliably transmural (135,136). Radiofrequency energy consists of alternating electrical current which can be delivered to the myocardial tissue through a transvenous electrode catheter. The tissue resistivity results in dissipation of RF energy as heat, which conducts passively to deeper tissue layers. Most tissues exposed to temperatures of 50°C or higher for more than several seconds will show irreversible coagulation necrosis and evolve into nonconducting myocardial scar. High power delivery and good electrode-tissue contact promote the formation of larger lesions and improve procedure efficacy. The ablation electrode temperature is dependent on the opposing effects of heating from the tissue and cooling by the blood flowing around the electrode. At any given electrode temperature, the RF power delivered to the tissue is significantly reduced in areas of low blood flow, such as dilated and poorly contracting atria seen in AF. Two approaches have been developed to increase electrode cooling to allow RF power to be maintained in a desirable range in areas of low blood flow. One approach is to increase the electrode surface area exposed to the blood by increasing electrode circumference and length (8–10 mm) to increase convective cooling for a given level of blood flow. The second approach is fluid irrigation of the electrode either by circulating fluid within the electrode (closed loop system) or flushing saline through openings in the electrode (open irrigation system). This allows sustained RF power, even at sites with low blood flow, to produce deeper lesions.

Cryoenergy causes adherence of the catheter tip to the underlying tissue during energy delivery, ensuring catheter stability in lesion creation (137). Cryoenergy also has the ability to create reversible loss of function, allowing the prediction of the effectiveness and safety of a lesion. It preserves the extracellular matrix and endothelial integrity, and thus has not been associated with PV stenosis, esophageal perforation, or thromboembolic events during the treatment of AF (138–140). In a study of patients with recent-onset paroxysmal AF and no structural heart disease, PV cryoisolation utilizing a focal strategy was shown to be effective in 82% of patients during long-term follow-up of 33 months, including 49% with complete success (no recurrent AF and no antiarrhythmic drugs) (141).

■ MAPPING SYSTEMS AND IMAGING FOR ATRIAL FIBRILLATION ABLATION

Catheter ablation of AF is facilitated by 3-D electroanatomic mapping systems, which allow for nonfluoroscopic catheter manipulation, activation and voltage mapping, and precise identification and tagging of ablation sites (Figure 6.5) (142,143). This technology allows for superimposition of electrical information onto the 3-D map reconstructed by the spatial locations of the endocardium sampled by a roving catheter. An advance in the use of electroanatomic mapping systems is the ability to "register" preacquired magnetic resonance (MR), computed tomography (CT), or rotational angiography images to the real time mapping space during AF ablation procedures (Figure 6.6). The process of image integration allows for visualization of the mapping catheter within the registered 3-D MR/CT images. CT/MR facilitates AF ablation by providing important preprocedural information regarding variability of PV morphologies including supernumerary right PVs, early branching of right inferior PVs, and common ostia of left or right PVs resulting in broad PV–LA junctions (144). CT/MR also facilitates localization of the true PV–LA junction, the LA appendage and the ridge between PV and LA appendage. Potential sources of error which may influence the accuracy of the integration process include differences in patient volume status, respiratory phase between the CT/MR image and the electroanatomic map, cardiac rhythm differences, as well as the registration algorithm.

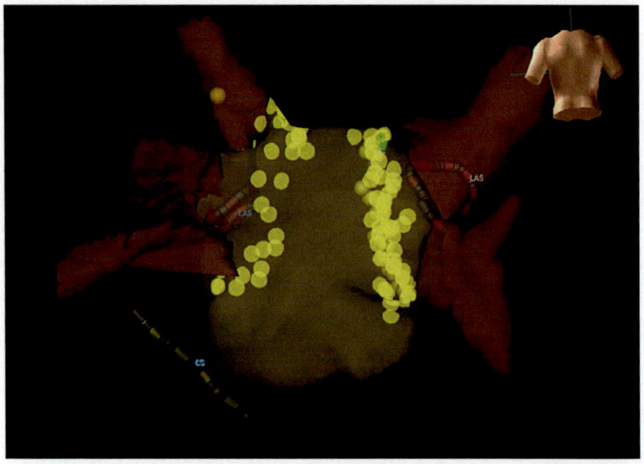

FIGURE 6.5 Pulmonary vein (PV) isolation guided by electroanatomical mapping. A posteroanterior view of the left atrium is displayed with locations of the PVs indicated by brown tubes. Yellow tags show locations of radiofrequency lesion around the left and right PVs. (From Ref. 182, with permission.)

During ablative procedures, fluoroscopy is unable to identify key anatomic structures such as the fossa ovalis, the PVs, the LA appendage, the valve apparatus, and extracardiac structures. ICE is able to provide real time anatomic information without the drawbacks of transesophageal echocardiography (TEE). A phased-array, catheter-mounted ultrasound transducer provides high resolution 2-D images with a penetration ranging from 2 to 12 mm. This allows imaging of the LA with

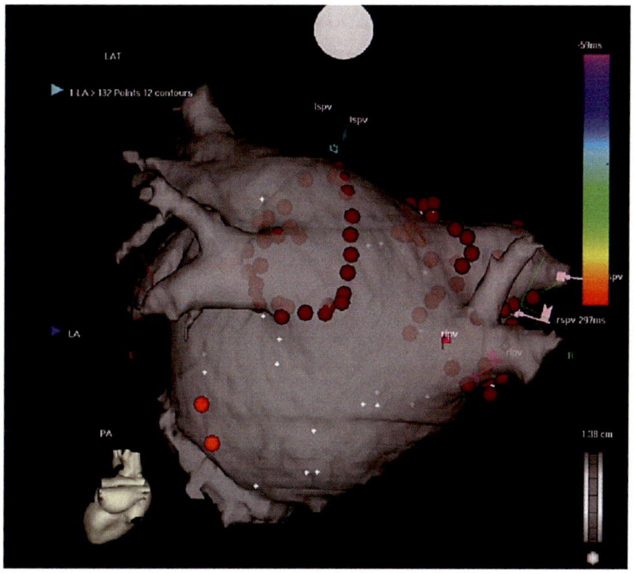

FIGURE 6.6 Computed tomographic angiogram of left atrium demonstrates pulmonary vein anatomy. and is merged with an electroanatomical mapping system to guide locations of ablation lesions (red tags).

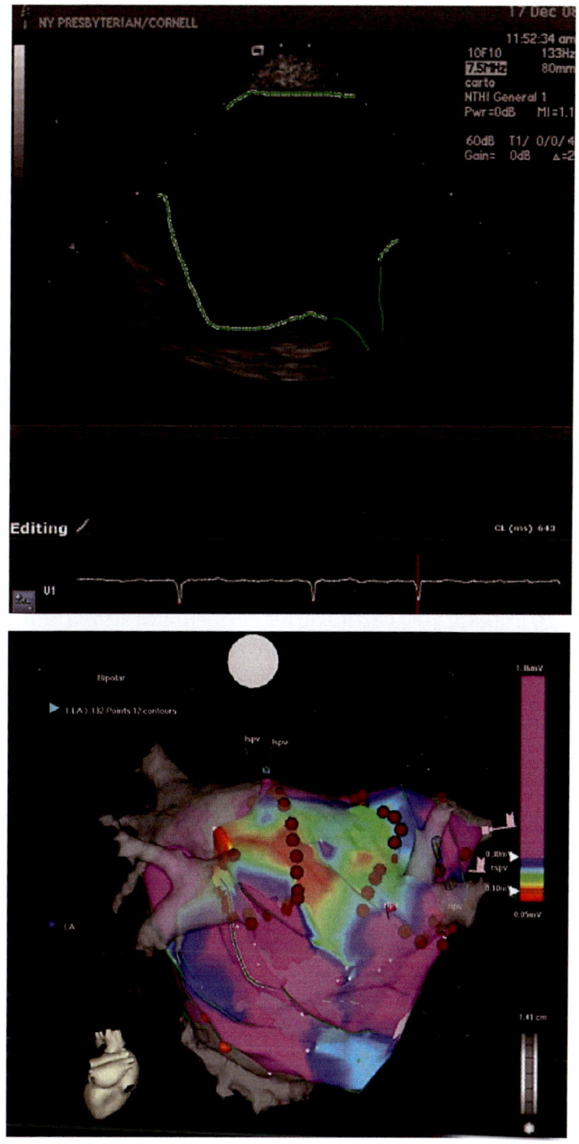

FIGURE 6.7 Intracardiac ultrasound (A) shows the left atrium (LA) imaged from a phased array transducer in the right atrium. A contour of the LA is incorporated into an electroanatomical map (B) and also merged with a preacquired Computed tomographic angiogram.

the ICE probe placed in the right atrium (Figure 6.7). During catheter ablation of AF, ICE facilitates transseptal puncture especially in the presence of anatomic variants or specific clinical conditions such as large septal aneurysm, lipomatous hypertrophy of the septum, previous cardiac surgery with distorted anatomy, or prior surgical or device closure of an atrial septal defect. ICE can visualize the location of the PV ostia to guide catheter placement and verify catheter contact with the endocardium during ablation. ICE may decrease the risk of complications by identifying pericardial effusions, intracardiac thrombi, and the location of the esophagus behind the posterior LA wall. ICE has also been incorporated into an electroanatomical mapping system that allows integration of 3-dimensional maps and real-time ultrasound (Cartosound, Biosense Webster, Diamond Bar, CA).

■ OUTCOMES OF ATRIAL FIBRILLATION ABLATION

Procedural success rates for AF ablation depend on numerous factors, including type of AF (paroxysmal, persistent, or long-lasting persistent), clinical and anatomic considerations, ablation technique, and definition of success. Recurrences of AF and atrial tachycardia within weeks after ablation are common and do not necessarily predict long-term failure. In one study, early recurrences of AF were reported in approximately 35% of patients with paroxysmal and persistent AF within two weeks after segmental PVI (145). These early recurrences were associated with a lower long-term success rate although approximately 30% of these patients had no further symptomatic AF during long-term follow-up.

Currently, most studies include a "blanking period" of one to three months in reporting freedom from AF. In addition, success rates are clearly affected by the intensity of rhythm monitoring after ablation, as clinically asymptomatic AF is known to occur postablation as with medical therapy for AF. A study of patients with paroxysmal AF who underwent PVI compared patients' perception of clinical AF with episodes detected by event recorder and found a sensitivity of 75% and a specificity of 92% (146). Another study which compared daily event monitoring with "routine" follow-up consisting of ECGs and Holter monitors demonstrated higher recurrences in patients followed with intensive monitoring, and one half of patients were asymptomatic during at least one recurrence (147). These results suggested that reliance on perception of AF by patients after PVI results in an underestimation of recurrence of the arrhythmia. In contrast, a prospective analysis of patients with symptomatic AF and prior pacemaker/implantable cardioverter defibrillator implantation showed that none of patients with recurrent AF remained completely asymptomatic, suggesting that simple symptomatic follow-up of highly symptomatic patients after catheter ablation of AF might be adequate (148). Leadless implantable loop recorders may in the future offer constant surveillance in patients without preexisting dual chamber devices. Such data would assist in predicting the risk for future thromboembolic events in patients postablation. Finally, protocols for postablation treatment also differ in the use of antiarrhythmic drugs and success may be reported with or without concomitant drug therapy.

For paroxysmal AF, single procedure success rates are generally 70% or greater, whereas higher success rates have been reported for multiple procedures. The first prospective randomized multicenter clinical trial of patients with paroxysmal AF treated with either antiarrhythmic therapy or catheter ablation showed that 63% of patients randomized to the antiarrhythmic arm had at least one AF recurrence compared with 13% of patients treated with catheter ablation at one year of follow-up (149). Including the latter, a total of three randomized studies of circumferential PV ablation for paroxysmal AF reported success rates of 86% to 89% at one year following a single procedure, with higher success rates attainable with second procedures (149–151). Comparable success rates in the antiarrhythmic drug arms of these trials were 22% to 37%. For persistent AF, early experience yielded success rates of ≤30% for single procedures, and multiple procedure success rates were highly variable at 50% or greater (21). A randomized trial for persistent AF using wide circumferential ablation as adjunctive therapy to amiodarone and cardioversions demonstrated freedom from AF in 74% in patients after one year, compared with 58% who did not undergo ablation (110). In the Catheter Ablation for the Cure of Atrial Fibrillation study (CACAF), patients with both paroxysmal and persistent AF undergoing circumferential PV ablation had an AF-free rate of 56% after one year, compared with 9% in the drug-treated patients (152). With more intensive ablation techniques that involve the addition of substrate modification and staged ablation, success rates of ≥90% at almost one year have been reported (134). A meta-analysis of published trials comparing circumferential pulmonary vein ablation to antiarrhythmic drug therapy for the management of AF found that recurrence-free survival during a 12-month follow-up period was observed in 76% of patients following ablation versus only 19% of patients treated with antiarrhythmic drugs (153). In addition, fewer adverse events were reported in the former group compared with the latter. Current treatment guidelines recommend ablation therapy as second-line therapy after failure of at least 1 antiarrhythmic medication (21). It remains to be determined whether circumferential PV ablation as a first-line treatment of AF is a reasonable approach for most patients.

A number of studies have incorporated some measure of quality of life into their study design. In particular, two randomized but nonblinded clinical trials have demonstrated greater improvements in quality of life and severity of symptoms after catheter ablation based on health surveys in patients with paroxysmal and persistent AF (110,149). Because AF can be viewed in part as a rate-related atrial cardiomyopathy that results from electrical and structural remodeling of the atria, some studies have examined the possibility that catheter ablation may effect reverse remodeling of the atria, consistently demonstrating a 10% to 20% decrease in the dimensions of the LA following ablation (154–156). While this may be due to reverse remodeling, it is not clear what contribution atrial scar formation contributes to the reduction in atrial size. The impact of catheter ablation of AF on LA transport function has been investigated in two studies with conflicting results. One study of patients with paroxysmal and chronic AF undergoing left atrial circumferential ablation demonstrated a partial return of LA function in patients with chronic AF, but a significant decrease in LA ejection fraction (EF) from 32% to 21% in patients with paroxysmal AF (157), raising concerns whether the impairment in LA function after catheter ablation was severe enough to predispose to LA thrombi despite elimination of AF. A second study of patients with paroxysmal and persistent AF undergoing PV antrum isolation demonstrated postablation improvement in LA EF from 17% to 22% (158). To date, only observational data are available regarding survival benefits after AF ablation. Pappone et al. reported that survival among 589 patients who underwent AF ablation exceeded that of 582 control patients treated with antiarrhythmic drugs, with a hazard ratio of 0.46 (mean follow-up 2.5 years) (159). In Kaplan–Meier analysis, freedom from AF at 3 years was 78% among those treated with ablation versus 37% among those in the medically treated group.

ATRIAL FIBRILLATION AND CONGESTIVE HEART FAILURE

Atrial fibrillation is present in 10% to 50% of patients with HF. AF and HF can form a vicious cycle in which AF leads to HF, which in turn causes atrial remodeling that perpetuates AF. An excessive ventricular rate, loss of atrial contraction, and an irregular ventricular filling time that is associated with AF all have negative clinical consequences in patients with HF. Heart failure patients with AF have a worse prognosis and higher mortality than those in whom sinus rhythm is maintained and that the presence of AF is an independent risk factor for death. In light of these data, the restoration and maintenance of sinus rhythm with electrical cardioversion and antiarrhythmic drugs are often attempted. Data from multiple trials do not support a routine strategy of rhythm control in patients with AF. These findings were corroborated by data from the multicenter, randomized Atrial Fibrillation and Congestive Heart Failure (AF-CHF) trial, which found no significant difference in the rate of death or worsening heart failure between patients treated with rhythm versus rate control strategies (160). However, these results are confounded by multiple factors, including lack of efficacy in maintaining sinus rhythm with cardioversion or antiarrhythmic agents as well as the significant toxicities of antiarrhythmic drugs. The role and appropriate lesion set for catheter ablation in patients with AF and left ventricular (LV) dysfunction is the focus of ongoing research. Several studies have demonstrated marked improvements in LV function in patients undergoing successful catheter ablation. In one study of 58 patients with predominantly chronic AF and (LV) dysfunction, 78% remained in sinus rhythm after 12 months, with a second procedure required in 50% (99). Left ventricular EF normalized or improved by an absolute 20% or greater in 72% of patients. The improvement in ejection fraction was observed in all subgroups including patients with adequate rate control and ischemic or valvular heart disease. Significant improvements were also demonstrated in LV dimensions, quality of life and exercise capacity. In another study of 40 patients with LV dysfunction, circumferential PV ablation with a mitral isthmus line achieved sinus rhythm in 87% at a mean follow-up of 14 months, and there were improvements in LV function, symptoms, and quality of life (161). These studies suggest that catheter ablation for AF is successful in the majority of patients and associated with substantial improvements in LV function. The recovery of LV function is apparent in the setting of adequate rate control, strengthening the argument for detrimental effects on ventricular function beyond a tachycardia mediated mechanism. The PABA-CHF trial compared a catheter-based rhythm control strategy versus optimal rate control strategy by randomizing patients with heart failure and either paroxysmal or persistent AF to pulmonary vein isolation or AV node ablation with biventricular pacing (162). Freedom from AF was demonstrated in 72% of patients in the PVI group at six months with statistically significant improvement in the primary composite endpoint of LV EF, exercise capacity and quality of life. The findings indicate superiority of successful rhythm control with PVI versus optimal rhythm control with AV node ablation and biventricular pacing. Despite the initial conclusions from AFFIRM, if sinus rhythm can be successfully and safely restored, there are likely to be substantial improvements in quality of life and left ventricular function (163). Whether this translates to a survival advantage is the center of ongoing multicenter trials.

COMPLICATIONS OF ATRIAL FIBRILLATION ABLATION

In a worldwide survey of AF ablation, major complications were reported in 6% of patients, including cardiac tamponade in 1.2%, stroke in 0.28% and transient ischemic attacks in 0.66% of left sided procedures (164). Periprocedural mortality was reported in 0.05%, Most thromboembolic strokes occur within two weeks of the ablation procedure (165). To reduce the risk of stroke, anticoagulation is often instituted prior to ablation, particularly in patients with CHADS-II risk factors (congestive heart failure or left ventricular dysfunction, hypertension, age >75, diabetes, and prior thromboembolic phenomena). Screening with a transesophageal echocardiogram is effective in detecting existing left atrial thrombi. Cardiac computed tomography has been shown to have a high sensitivity in detecting left atrial thrombi, which manifest as contrast filling defects (166). Task Force recommendations from 2007 are to use warfarin for at least two months postablation and continue warfarin long term in patients with a CHADS score of ≥2 (21).

Pulmonary vein stenosis occurred with higher frequency earlier in the history of AF ablation, when energy was applied within the pulmonary veins rather than the antral region. The rate of PV occlusion was found to be 0.8% among patients treated from 1999 to 2004 using a variety of ablation techniques (167). Patients with single PV occlusion are often asymptomatic, but patients with concomitant ipsilateral PV stenosis or occlusion have required pulmonary interventions to restore pulmonary flow and prevent associated lung disease. Esophageal injury is a potentially serious complication of radiofrequency ablation in the posterior wall of the LA (168). The distance of the LA endocardium to the esophagus may be as small as <5 mm, within the lesion depth of radiofrequency induced necrosis (169). Left atrial-esophageal fistulae are rare but are associated with high mortality if not recognized and treated early. Other esophageal complications include ulceration and interruption of periesophageal vagal efferent fibers which result in gastroparesis (170). Techniques to minimize esophageal injury include minimizing power and duration of ablation in the posterior wall; imaging the esophagus with ultrasound, contrast barium swallow, or catheter/gastric tube placement; and monitoring esophageal temperature. Other potential complications are femoral arterial pseudoaneurysm, arteriovenous fistula, and phrenic nerve injury.

Linear lesions deployed during AF ablation may be proarrhythmic, giving rise to atrial tachycardias, especially if complete line of block is not obtained. Some atrial tachycardias that occur early after ablation (within five months) may resolve and do not require early reablation (171), but persistent atrial tachycardias remain a common reason for retreatment. One mechanism of organized atrial tachycardias after AF ablation is macroreentry, and common circuits include perimitral reentry ("mitral flutter") and reentry around ipsilateral pulmonary veins involving the LA roof (Figure 6.8) (171–173). Gaps in the PVI lines may give rise to complex reentrant circuits involving the PV antrum (174). Focal atrial tachycardias also occur after AF ablation and often arise adjacent to previous ablation lesions. Convincing evidence suggests that many of these focal tachycardias are due to localized reentry ("microreentry") (175,176). Atrial tachycardias that complicate AF ablation can be ablated with high success rates.

Fluoroscopic radiation exposure is another potential source of morbidity, particularly for complex or lengthy procedures. Peak skin doses of radiation during AF ablation procedures have been measured in the range of 0.5 to 2.0 Gy, (with average values of 1.0 and 1.5 Gy in the right and left anterior oblique projections) (177). At these dose levels, the estimated lifetime risk of excess fatal malignancies is estimated in the range 0.1% (177,178).

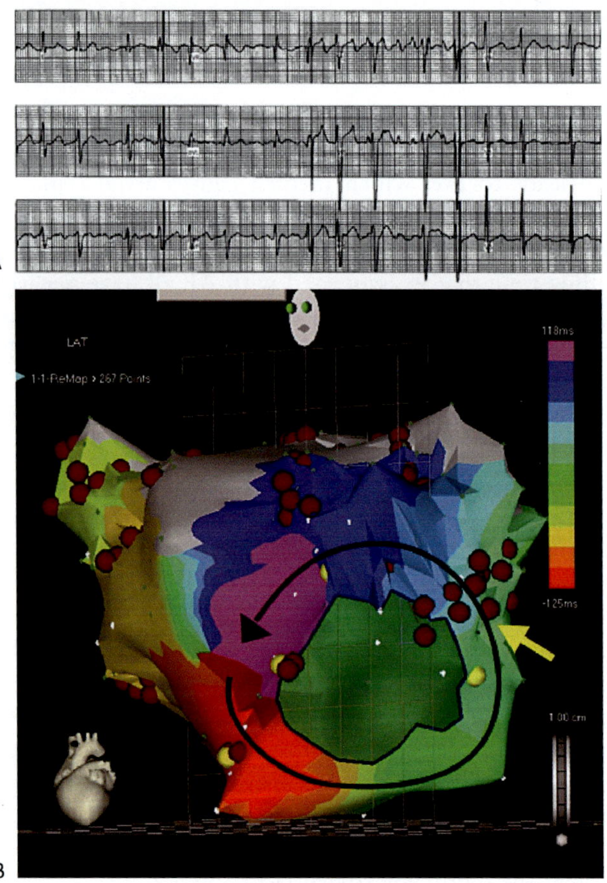

A
B

FIGURE 6.8 Atrial tachycardia after wide encircling pulmonary vein (PV) isolation. During ablation of persistent atrial fibrillation, the arrhythmia organized into a regular atrial tachycardia (A). Shown is an electroanatomical map of the left atrium, constructed during mapping of the atrial tachyardia (B). Red region indicates areas of early action, and purple are areas of late activation. A counterclockwise circuit around the mitral annulus is identified, which was eliminated with a linear ablation lesion between the mitral annulus and left inferior PV ("mitral isthmus," yellow arrow).

■ NOVEL TECHNOLOGIES FOR ATRIAL FIBRILLATION ABLATION

New catheter technology is intended to simplify the ablation procedure and improve long term efficacy. To achieve efficient PVI, catheters that encircle the PV ostia have been designed to deliver circumferential ablative energy. A circular ablation catheter and a mesh catheter employ phased radiofrequency energy and enable operators to target specific segments of the PV ostia (179,180). Balloon catheters that utilize cryotherapy have also demonstrated efficacy in achieving PVI in clinical trials (181). Investigational energy sources for ablation include high focused ultrasound, microwave, and laser.

Robotic and magnetic navigation have been developed to remotely maneuver intracardiac catheters. The robotic technology (Sensei, Hansen Medical, Mountain View, CA) utilizes a deflectable sheath that can be manipulated from a control console and accommodates a variety of ablation catheters. The magnetic technology (Niobe, Stereotaxis, St. Louis, MO) uses an external magnetic field to deflect a mapping catheter with a ferromagnetic tip within the applied field. Both technologies can be integrated with electroanatomical mapping systems and have the potential for fully automated ablation procedures.

■ CONCLUSIONS AND FUTURE DIRECTIONS

Catheter ablation has provided insights into the pathophysiology of AF, prompting paradigm shifts in the understanding of both paroxysmal and persistent AF. Further study of AF mechanisms should produce insights that will refine the targets of AF ablation. Combined with technological evolution of safe and efficient energy sources, these advances have the potential to improve outcomes of catheter ablation.

Interventional approaches have an established role in the treatment of symptomatic patients with drug-refractory AF. Randomized trials will assess catheter ablation as first line therapy as an alternative to antiarrhythmic drug therapy, with emphases on efficacy, safety, and survival (Table 6.1). The Radiofrequency Ablation versus Antiarrhythmic Drugs for Atrial Fibrillation Treatment (RAAFT) study is a multicenter, randomized trial designed to assess the efficacy and

Table 6.1 Randomized trials of atrial fibrillation ablation

Author (Ref.)	Acronym	Year	N	AF population	Design	Freedom from AF at 12 month (ablation versus control)
Wazni et al. (149)	RAAFT pilot	2005	70	Paroxysmal	PVI versus AAD	87% versus 37%
Pappone et al. (150)	APAF	2006	198	Paroxysmal	CPVA versus AAD	86% versus 22%
Jais et al. (151)	A4	2008	112	Paroxysmal	PVI versus AAD	89% versus 23%
Oral et al. (110)		2006	146	Persistent	CPVA + amio + CV versus amio + CV	74% versus 58%
Stabile et al. (152)	CACAF	2006	137	Paroxysmal (92) Persistent (45)	CPVA versus AAD	56% versus 9%

Abbreviations: A4, atrial fibrillation ablation versus antiarrhythmic drugs; AAD, antiarrhythmic drug; APAF, ablation for paroxysmal atrial fibrillation; CACAF, catheter ablation for the cure of atrial fibrillation; CPVA, circumferential pulmonary vein ablation; PVI, pulmonary vein isolation; RAAFT, radiofrequency ablation versus antiarrhythmic drugs for atrial fibrillation treatment.

safety of catheter ablation as first line therapy for AF, with a primary endpoint of recurrent AF and secondary endpoint quality-of-life measures. The Catheter Ablation versus Antiarrhythmic Drug Therapy for Atrial Fibrillation (CABANA) study is a large, randomized, multicenter trial which also tests the role of AF ablation as first line therapy for AF, with an endpoint of overall mortality. Such studies are imperative to determine if ablation impacts the natural history of AF and reduces the long-term risk of stroke, in addition to providing symptomatic relief.

■ REFERENCES

1. Feinberg WM, Blackshear JL, Laupacis A, Kronmal R, Hart RG. Prevalence, age distribution, and gender of patients with atrial fibrillation. Analysis and implications. *Arch Intern Med* 1995; 155:469–73.
2. Go AS, Hylek EM, Phillips KA, et al. Prevalence of diagnosed atrial fibrillation in adults: national implications for rhythm management and stroke prevention: the AnTicoagulation and Risk Factors in Atrial Fibrillation (ATRIA) Study. *JAMA* 2001; 285:2370–5.
3. Wolf PA, Abbott RD, Kannel WB. Atrial fibrillation as an independent risk factor for stroke: the Framingham Study. *Stroke* 1991; 22:983–8.
4. Lloyd-Jones DM, Wang TJ, Leip EP, et al. Lifetime risk for development of atrial fibrillation: the Framingham Heart Study. *Circulation* 2004; 110:1042–6.
5. Benjamin EJ, Levy D, Vaziri SM, D'Agostino RB, Belanger AJ, Wolf PA. Independent risk factors for atrial fibrillation in a population-based cohort. The Framingham Heart Study. *JAMA* 1994; 271:840–4.
6. Mukamal KJ, Tolstrup JS, Friberg J, Jensen G, Gronbaek M. Alcohol consumption and risk of atrial fibrillation in men and women: the Copenhagen City Heart Study. *Circulation* 2005; 112:1736–42.
7. Spodick DH. The role of alcohol in new-onset atrial fibrillation. *Arch Intern Med* 1984; 144:862–3.
8. Wang TJ, Parise H, Levy D, et al. Obesity and the risk of new-onset atrial fibrillation. *JAMA* 2004; 292:2471–7.
9. Molina L, Mont L, Marrugat J, et al. Long-term endurance sport practice increases the incidence of lone atrial fibrillation in men: a follow-up study. *Europace* 2008; 10:618–23.
10. Chen LY Shen WK. Epidemiology of atrial fibrillation: a current perspective. *Heart Rhythm* 2007; 4:S1–6.
11. Psaty BM, Manolio TA, Kuller LH, et al. Incidence of and risk factors for atrial fibrillation in older adults. *Circulation* 1997; 96:2455–61.
12. Fox CS, Parise H, D'Agostino RB Sr, et al. Parental atrial fibrillation as a risk factor for atrial fibrillation in offspring. *JAMA* 2004; 291:2851–5.
13. Arnar DO, Thorvaldsson S, Manolio TA, et al. Familial aggregation of atrial fibrillation in Iceland. *Eur Heart J* 2006; 27:708–12.
14. Kopecky SL, Gersh BJ, McGoon MD, et al. The natural history of lone atrial fibrillation. A population-based study over three decades. *N Engl J Med* 1987; 317:669–74.
15. Schoonderwoerd BA, Smit MD, Pen L, Van Gelder IC. New risk factors for atrial fibrillation: causes of 'not-so-lone atrial fibrillation.' *Europace* 2008; 10:668–73.
16. Jahangir A, Lee V, Friedman PA, et al. Long-term progression and outcomes with aging in patients with lone atrial fibrillation: a 30-year follow-up study. *Circulation* 2007; 115:3050–6.
17. Korantzopoulos P, Liu T, Milionis HJ, Li G, Goudevenos JA. 'Lone' atrial fibrillation: hunting for the underlying causes and links. *Int J Cardiol* 2009; 131:180–5.
18. Tsang TS, Gersh BJ, Appleton CP, et al. Left ventricular diastolic dysfunction as a predictor of the first diagnosed nonvalvular atrial fibrillation in 840 elderly men and women. *J Am Coll Cardiol* 2002; 40:1636–44.
19. Sitges M, Teijeira VA, Scalise A, et al. Is there an anatomical substrate for idiopathic paroxysmal atrial fibrillation? A case-control echocardiographic study. *Europace* 2007; 9:294–8.
20. Fuster V, Ryden LE, Cannom DS, et al. ACC/AHA/ESC 2006 guidelines for the management of patients with atrial fibrillation—executive summary: a report of the American College of Cardiology/American Heart Association Task Force on Practice Guidelines and the European Society of Cardiology Committee for Practice Guidelines (Writing Committee to Revise the 2001 Guidelines for the Management of Patients With Atrial Fibrillation). *J Am Coll Cardiol* 2006; 48:854–906.
21. Calkins H, Brugada J, Packer DL, et al. HRS/EHRA/ECAS expert consensus statement on catheter and surgical ablation of atrial fibrillation: recommendations for personnel, policy, procedures and follow-up. A report of the Heart Rhythm Society (HRS) Task Force on Catheter and Surgical Ablation of Atrial Fibrillation developed in partnership with the European Heart Rhythm Association (EHRA) and the European Cardiac Arrhythmia Society (ECAS), in collaboration with the American College of Cardiology (ACC), American Heart Association (AHA), and the Society of Thoracic Surgeons (STS). Endorsed and approved by the governing bodies of the American College of Cardiology, the American Heart Association, the European Cardiac Arrhythmia Society, the European Heart Rhythm Association, the Society of Thoracic Surgeons, and the Heart Rhythm Society. *Europace* 2007; 9:335–79.
22. Daoud EG, Weiss R, Bahu M, et al. Effect of an irregular ventricular rhythm on cardiac output. *Am J Cardiol* 1996; 78:1433–6.
23. Clark DM, Plumb VJ, Epstein AE, Kay GN. Hemodynamic effects of an irregular sequence of ventricular cycle lengths during atrial fibrillation. *J Am Coll Cardiol* 1997; 30:1039–45.
24. Risk factors for stroke and efficacy of antithrombotic therapy in atrial fibrillation. Analysis of pooled data from five randomized controlled trials. *Arch Intern Med* 1994; 154:1449–57.
25. Jorgensen HS, Nakayama H, Reith J, Raaschou HO, Olsen TS. Acute stroke with atrial fibrillation. The Copenhagen Stroke Study. *Stroke* 1996; 27:1765–9.
26. Wolf PA, Dawber TR, Thomas HE Jr, Kannel WB. Epidemiologic assessment of chronic atrial fibrillation and risk of stroke: the Framingham study. *Neurology* 1978; 28:973–7.
27. Stewart S, Hart CL, Hole DJ, McMurray JJ. A population-based study of the long-term risks associated with atrial fibrillation: 20-year follow-up of the Renfrew/Paisley study. *Am J Med* 2002; 113:359–64.

28. Krahn AD, Manfreda J, Tate RB, Mathewson FA, Cuddy TE. The natural history of atrial fibrillation: incidence, risk factors, and prognosis in the Manitoba Follow-Up Study. *Am J Med* 1995; 98:476–84.
29. Poole-Wilson PA, Swedberg K, Cleland JG, et al. Comparison of carvedilol and metoprolol on clinical outcomes in patients with chronic heart failure in the Carvedilol Or Metoprolol European Trial (COMET): randomised controlled trial. *Lancet* 2003; 362:7–13.
30. Maggioni AP, Latini R, Carson PE, et al. Valsartan reduces the incidence of atrial fibrillation in patients with heart failure: results from the Valsartan Heart Failure Trial (Val-HeFT). *Am Heart J* 2005; 149:548–57.
31. Wang TJ, Larson MG, Levy D, et al. Temporal relations of atrial fibrillation and congestive heart failure and their joint influence on mortality: the Framingham Heart Study. *Circulation* 2003; 107:2920–5.
32. Schoonderwoerd BA, Van Gelder IC, Van Veldhuisen DJ, Van den Berg MP, Crijns HJ. Electrical and structural remodeling: role in the genesis and maintenance of atrial fibrillation. *Prog Cardiovasc Dis* 2005; 48:153–68.
33. Wyse DG, Waldo AL, DiMarco JP, et al. A comparison of rate control and rhythm control in patients with atrial fibrillation. *N Engl J Med* 2002; 347:1825–33.
34. Curtis AB, Gersh BJ, Corley SD, et al. Clinical factors that influence response to treatment strategies in atrial fibrillation: the Atrial Fibrillation Follow-up Investigation of Rhythm Management (AFFIRM) study. *Am Heart J* 2005; 149:645–9.
35. Corley SD, Epstein AE, DiMarco JP, et al. Relationships between sinus rhythm, treatment, and survival in the Atrial Fibrillation Follow-Up Investigation of Rhythm Management (AFFIRM) Study. *Circulation* 2004; 109:1509–13.
36. Hagens VE, Van Veldhuisen DJ, Kamp O, et al. Effect of rate and rhythm control on left ventricular function and cardiac dimensions in patients with persistent atrial fibrillation: results from the RAte Control versus Electrical Cardioversion for Persistent Atrial Fibrillation (RACE) study. *Heart Rhythm* 2005; 2:19–24.
37. Carlsson J, Miketic S, Windeler J, et al. Randomized trial of rate-control versus rhythm-control in persistent atrial fibrillation: the Strategies of Treatment of Atrial Fibrillation (STAF) study. *J Am Coll Cardiol* 2003; 41:1690–6.
38. Opolski G, Torbicki A, Kosior DA, et al. Rate control vs rhythm control in patients with nonvalvular persistent atrial fibrillation: the results of the Polish How to Treat Chronic Atrial Fibrillation (HOT CAFE) Study. *Chest* 2004; 126:476–86.
39. Pedersen OD, Bagger H, Keller N, Marchant B, Kober L, Torp-Pedersen C. Efficacy of dofetilide in the treatment of atrial fibrillation-flutter in patients with reduced left ventricular function: a Danish investigations of arrhythmia and mortality on dofetilide (DIAMOND) substudy. *Circulation* 2001; 104:292–6.
40. Deedwania PC, Singh BN, Ellenbogen K, Fisher S, Fletcher R, Singh SN. Spontaneous conversion and maintenance of sinus rhythm by amiodarone in patients with heart failure and atrial fibrillation: observations from the veterans affairs congestive heart failure survival trial of antiarrhythmic therapy (CHF-STAT). The Department of Veterans Affairs CHF-STAT Investigators. *Circulation* 1998; 98:2574–9.
41. Cohen M, Naccarelli GV. Pathophysiology and disease progression of atrial fibrillation: importance of achieving and maintaining sinus rhythm. *J Cardiovasc Electrophysiol* 2008; 19:885–90.
42. Chung MK, Shemanski L, Sherman DG, et al. Functional status in rate- versus rhythm-control strategies for atrial fibrillation: results of the Atrial Fibrillation Follow-Up Investigation of Rhythm Management (AFFIRM) Functional Status Substudy. *J Am Coll Cardiol* 2005; 46:1891–9.
43. Prystowsky EN. The history of atrial fibrillation: the last 100 years. *J Cardiovasc Electrophysiol* 2008; 19:575–82.
44. Allessie MA, Lammers WJ, Bonke IM, Hollen J. Intra-atrial reentry as a mechanism for atrial flutter induced by acetylcholine and rapid pacing in the dog. *Circulation* 1984; 70:123–35.
45. Kumagai K, Khrestian C, Waldo AL. Simultaneous multisite mapping studies during induced atrial fibrillation in the sterile pericarditis model. Insights into the mechanism of its maintenance. *Circulation* 1997; 95:511–21.
46. Wang Z, Page P, Nattel S. Mechanism of flecainide's antiarrhythmic action in experimental atrial fibrillation. *Circ Res* 1992; 71:271–87.
47. Wang J, Bourne GW, Wang Z, Villemaire C, Talajic M, Nattel S. Comparative mechanisms of antiarrhythmic drug action in experimental atrial fibrillation. Importance of use-dependent effects on refractoriness. *Circulation* 1993; 88:1030–44.
48. Vaquero M, Calvo D, Jalife J. Cardiac fibrillation: from ion channels to rotors in the human heart. *Heart Rhythm* 2008; 5:872–9.
49. Mandapati R, Skanes A, Chen J, Berenfeld O, Jalife, J. Stable microreentrant sources as a mechanism of atrial fibrillation in the isolated sheep heart. *Circulation* 2000; 101:194–9.
50. Mansour M, Mandapati R, Berenfeld O, Chen J, Samie FH, Jalife J. Left-to-right gradient of atrial frequencies during acute atrial fibrillation in the isolated sheep heart. *Circulation* 2001; 103:2631–6.
51. Haissaguerre M, Jais P, Shah DC, et al. Spontaneous initiation of atrial fibrillation by ectopic beats originating in the pulmonary veins. *N Engl J Med* 1998; 339:659–66.
52. Cheung DW. Electrical activity of the pulmonary vein and its interaction with the right atrium in the guinea-pig. *J Physiol* 1981; 314:445–56.
53. Chen YJ, Chen SA, Chang MS, Lin CI. Arrhythmogenic activity of cardiac muscle in pulmonary veins of the dog: implication for the genesis of atrial fibrillation. *Cardiovasc Res* 2000; 48:265–73.
54. Kumagai K, Ogawa M, Noguchi H, Yasuda T, Nakashima H, Saku K. Electrophysiologic properties of pulmonary veins assessed using a multielectrode basket catheter. *J Am Coll Cardiol* 2004; 43:2281–9.
55. Chen SA, Hsieh MH, Tai CT, et al. Initiation of atrial fibrillation by ectopic beats originating from the pulmonary veins: electrophysiological characteristics, pharmacological responses, and effects of radiofrequency ablation. *Circulation* 1999; 100:1879–86.
56. Arora R, Verheule S, Scott L, et al. Arrhythmogenic substrate of the pulmonary veins assessed by high-resolution optical mapping. *Circulation* 2003; 107:1816–21.
57. Hocini M, Ho SY, Kawara T, et al. Electrical conduction in canine pulmonary veins: electrophysiological and anatomic correlation. *Circulation* 2002; 105:2442–8.
58. Wit AL, Boyden PA. Triggered activity and atrial fibrillation. *Heart Rhythm* 2007; 4:S17–23.

59. Olshansky B. Interrelationships between the autonomic nervous system and atrial fibrillation. *Prog Cardiovasc Dis* 2005; 48:57–78.
60. Sharifov OF, Fedorov VV, Beloshapko GG, Glukhov AV, Yushmanova AV, Rosenshtraukh LV. Roles of adrenergic and cholinergic stimulation in spontaneous atrial fibrillation in dogs. *J Am Coll Cardiol* 2004; 43:483–90.
61. Patterson E, Po SS, Scherlag BJ, Lazzara R. Triggered firing in pulmonary veins initiated by in vitro autonomic nerve stimulation. *Heart Rhythm* 2005; 2:624–31.
62. Chen PS, Tan AY. Autonomic nerve activity and atrial fibrillation. *Heart Rhythm* 2007; 4:S61–4.
63. Kawashima T. The autonomic nervous system of the human heart with special reference to its origin, course, and peripheral distribution. *Anat Embryol (Berl)* 2005; 209:425–38.
64. Tan AY, Li H, Wachsmann-Hogiu S, Chen LS, Chen PS, Fishbein MC. Autonomic innervation and segmental muscular disconnections at the human pulmonary vein-atrial junction: implications for catheter ablation of atrial-pulmonary vein junction. *J Am Coll Cardiol* 2006; 48:132–43.
65. Chevalier P, Tabib A, Meyronnet D, et al. Quantitative study of nerves of the human left atrium. *Heart Rhythm* 2005; 2:518–22.
66. Schauerte P, Scherlag BJ, Patterson E, et al. Focal atrial fibrillation: experimental evidence for a pathophysiologic role of the autonomic nervous system. *J Cardiovasc Electrophysiol* 2001; 12:592–9.
67. Scherlag BJ, Nakagawa H, Jackman WM, et al. Electrical stimulation to identify neural elements on the heart: their role in atrial fibrillation. *J Interv Card Electrophysiol* 2005; 13 Suppl 1:37–42.
68. Pokushalov E. The role of autonomic denervation during catheter ablation of atrial fibrillation. *Curr Opin Cardiol* 2008; 23:55–9.
69. Casaclang-Verzosa G, Gersh BJ, Tsang TS. Structural and functional remodeling of the left atrium: clinical and therapeutic implications for atrial fibrillation. *J Am Coll Cardiol* 2008; 51:1–11.
70. Ausma J, Litjens N, Lenders MH, et al. Time course of atrial fibrillation-induced cellular structural remodeling in atria of the goat. *J Mol Cell Cardiol* 2001; 33:2083–94.
71. van der Velden HM, Ausma J, Rook MB, et al. Gap junctional remodeling in relation to stabilization of atrial fibrillation in the goat. *Cardiovasc Res* 2000; 46:476–86.
72. Yue L, Feng J, Gaspo R, Li GR, Wang Z, Nattel S. Ionic remodeling underlying action potential changes in a canine model of atrial fibrillation. *Circ Res* 1997; 81:512–25.
73. Courtemanche M, Ramirez RJ, Nattel S. Ionic mechanisms underlying human atrial action potential properties: insights from a mathematical model. *Am J Physiol* 1998; 275:H301–21.
74. Wijffels MC, Kirchhof CJ, Dorland R, Allessie MA. Atrial fibrillation begets atrial fibrillation. A study in awake chronically instrumented goats. *Circulation* 1995; 92:1954–68.
75. Li D, Fareh S, Leung TK, Nattel S. Promotion of atrial fibrillation by heart failure in dogs: atrial remodeling of a different sort. *Circulation* 1999; 100:87–95.
76. Li D Melnyk P, Feng J, Wang Z, Petrecca K, Shrier A, Nattel S. Effects of experimental heart failure on atrial cellular and ionic electrophysiology. *Circulation* 2000; 101:2631–8.
77. Nattel S. New ideas about atrial fibrillation 50 years on. *Nature* 2002; 415:219–26.
78. Silver MA, Pick R, Brilla CG, Jalil JE, Janicki JS, Weber KT. Reactive and reparative fibrillar collagen remodelling in the hypertrophied rat left ventricle: two experimental models of myocardial fibrosis. *Cardiovasc Res* 1990; 24:741–7.
79. Burstein B, Nattel S. Atrial fibrosis: mechanisms and clinical relevance in atrial fibrillation. *J Am Coll Cardiol* 2008; 51:802–9.
80. Frustaci A, Chimenti C, Bellocci F, Morgante E, Russo MA, Maseri A. Histological substrate of atrial biopsies in patients with lone atrial fibrillation. *Circulation* 1997; 96:1180–4.
81. Boldt A, Wetzel U, Lauschke J, et al. Fibrosis in left atrial tissue of patients with atrial fibrillation with and without underlying mitral valve disease. *Heart* 2004; 90:400–5.
82. Fenelon G, Shepard RK, Stambler BS. Focal origin of atrial tachycardia in dogs with rapid ventricular pacing-induced heart failure. *J Cardiovasc Electrophysiol* 2003; 14:1093–102.
83. Nattel S, Li D, Yue L. Basic mechanisms of atrial fibrillation—very new insights into very old ideas. *Annu Rev Physiol* 2000; 62:51–77.
84. Akar FG, Nass RD, Hahn S, et al. Dynamic changes in conduction velocity and gap junction properties during development of pacing-induced heart failure. *Am J Physiol Heart Circ Physiol* 2007; 293:H1223–30.
85. Ehrlich, JR, Hohnloser, SH Nattel, S. Role of angiotensin system and effects of its inhibition in atrial fibrillation: clinical and experimental evidence. *Eur Heart J* 2006; 27:512–18.
86. Milliez P, Girerd X, Plouin PF, Blacher J, Safar ME, Mourad JJ. Evidence for an increased rate of cardiovascular events in patients with primary aldosteronism. *J Am Coll Cardiol* 2005; 45:1243–8.
87. Pedersen OD, Bagger H, Kober L, Torp-Pedersen C. Trandolapril reduces the incidence of atrial fibrillation after acute myocardial infarction in patients with left ventricular dysfunction. *Circulation* 1999; 100:376–80.
88. Healey JS, Baranchuk A, Crystal E, et al. Prevention of atrial fibrillation with angiotensin-converting enzyme inhibitors and angiotensin receptor blockers: a meta-analysis. *J Am Coll Cardiol* 2005; 45:1832–9.
89. Belluzzi F, Sernesi L, Preti P, Salinaro F, Fonte ML, Perlini S. Prevention of recurrent lone atrial fibrillation by the angiotensin-II converting enzyme inhibitor ramipril in normotensive patients. *J Am Coll Cardiol* 2009; 53:24–9.
90. Cox JL, Schuessler RB, Cain ME, et al. Surgery for atrial fibrillation. *Semin Thorac Cardiovasc Surg* 1989; 1:67–73.
91. McCarthy PM, Gillinov AM, Castle L, Chung M, Cosgrove D 3rd. The Cox-Maze procedure: the Cleveland Clinic experience. *Semin Thorac Cardiovasc Surg* 2000; 12:25–9.
92. Prasad SM, Maniar HS, Camillo CJ, et al. The Cox maze III procedure for atrial fibrillation: long-term efficacy in patients undergoing lone versus concomitant procedures. *J Thorac Cardiovasc Surg* 2003; 126:1822–8.
93. Schaff HV, Dearani JA, Daly RC, Orszulak TA, Danielson GK. Cox-Maze procedure for atrial fibrillation: Mayo Clinic experience. *Semin Thorac Cardiovasc Surg* 2000; 12:30–7.
94. Cox JL. Surgical treatment of atrial fibrillation: a review. *Europace* 2004; 5(Suppl 1):S20–9.
95. Cox JL, Ad N, Palazzo T. Impact of the maze procedure on the stroke rate in patients with atrial fibrillation. *J Thorac Cardiovasc Surg* 1999; 118:833–40.
96. Gillinov AM, Saltman AE. Surgical approaches for atrial fibrillation. *Med Clin North Am* 2008; 92:203–15, xii.

97. Scheinman MM, Morady F, Hess DS, Gonzalez R. Catheter-induced ablation of the atrioventricular junction to control refractory supraventricular arrhythmias. *JAMA* 1982; 248:851–5.
98. Haissaguerre M, Marcus FI, Fischer B, Clementy J. Radiofrequency catheter ablation in unusual mechanisms of atrial fibrillation: report of three cases. *J Cardiovasc Electrophysiol* 1994; 5:743–51.
99. Hsu LF, Jais P, Sanders P, et al. Catheter ablation for atrial fibrillation in congestive heart failure. *N Engl J Med* 2004; 351:2373–83.
100. Nademanee K, Schwab MC, Kosar EM, et al. Clinical outcomes of catheter substrate ablation for high-risk patients with atrial fibrillation. *J Am Coll Cardiol* 2008; 51:843–9.
101. Hocini M, Haissaguerre M, Shah D, et al. Multiple sources initiating atrial fibrillation from a single pulmonary vein identified by a circumferential catheter. *Pacing Clin Electrophysiol* 2000; 23:1828–31.
102. Robbins IM, Colvin EV, Doyle TP, et al. Pulmonary vein stenosis after catheter ablation of atrial fibrillation. *Circulation* 1998; 98:1769–75.
103. Haissaguerre M, Shah DC, Jais P, et al. Electrophysiological breakthroughs from the left atrium to the pulmonary veins. *Circulation* 2000; 102:2463–5.
104. Nilsson B, Chen X, Pehrson S, Kober L, Hilden J, Svendsen JH. Recurrence of pulmonary vein conduction and atrial fibrillation after pulmonary vein isolation for atrial fibrillation: a randomized trial of the ostial versus the extraostial ablation strategy. *Am Heart J* 2006; 152(3):537.e1–8.
105. Oral H, Scharf C, Chugh A, et al. Catheter ablation for paroxysmal atrial fibrillation: segmental pulmonary vein ostial ablation versus left atrial ablation. *Circulation* 2003; 108:2355–60.
106. Katritsis DG, Ellenbogen KA, Panagiotakos DB, et al. Ablation of superior pulmonary veins compared to ablation of all four pulmonary veins. *J Cardiovasc Electrophysiol* 2004; 15:641–5.
107. Gerstenfeld EP, Callans DJ, Dixit S, Zado E, Marchlinski FE. Incidence and location of focal atrial fibrillation triggers in patients undergoing repeat pulmonary vein isolation: implications for ablation strategies. *J Cardiovasc Electrophysiol* 2003; 14:685–90.
108. Pappone C, Oreto G, Rosanio S, et al. Atrial electroanatomic remodeling after circumferential radiofrequency pulmonary vein ablation: efficacy of an anatomic approach in a large cohort of patients with atrial fibrillation. *Circulation* 2001; 104:2539–44.
109. Pappone C, Rosanio S, Oreto G, et al. Circumferential radiofrequency ablation of pulmonary vein ostia: A new anatomic approach for curing atrial fibrillation. *Circulation* 2000; 102:2619–28.
110. Oral H, Pappone C, Chugh A, et al. Circumferential pulmonary-vein ablation for chronic atrial fibrillation. *N Engl J Med* 2006; 354:934–41.
111. Natale A, Raviele A, Arentz T, et al. Venice Chart international consensus document on atrial fibrillation ablation. *J Cardiovasc Electrophysiol* 2007; 18:560–80.
112. Callahan TD 4th, Natale A. Catheter ablation of atrial fibrillation. *Med Clin North Am* 2008; 92:179–201, xii.
113. Kanj M, Wazni O, Natale A. Pulmonary vein antrum isolation. *Heart Rhythm* 2007; 4:S73–9.
114. Verma A, Marrouche NF, Natale A. Pulmonary vein antrum isolation: intracardiac echocardiography-guided technique. *J Cardiovasc Electrophysiol* 2004; 15:1335–40.
115. Hocini M, Jais P, Sanders P, et al. Techniques, evaluation, and consequences of linear block at the left atrial roof in paroxysmal atrial fibrillation: a prospective randomized study. *Circulation* 2005; 112:3688–96.
116. Jais P, Hocini M, Hsu LF, et al. Technique and results of linear ablation at the mitral isthmus. *Circulation* 2004; 110:2996–3002.
117. Fassini G, Riva S, Chiodelli R, et al. Left mitral isthmus ablation associated with PV Isolation: long-term results of a prospective randomized study. *J Cardiovasc Electrophysiol* 2005; 16:1150–6.
118. Kottkamp H, Tanner H, Kobza R, et al. Time courses and quantitative analysis of atrial fibrillation episode number and duration after circular plus linear left atrial lesions: trigger elimination or substrate modification: early or delayed cure? *J Am Coll Cardiol* 2004; 44:869–77.
119. Willems S, Klemm H, Rostock T, et al. Substrate modification combined with pulmonary vein isolation improves outcome of catheter ablation in patients with persistent atrial fibrillation: a prospective randomized comparison. *Eur Heart J* 2006; 27:2871–8.
120. Knecht S, Hocini M, Wright M, et al. Left atrial linear lesions are required for successful treatment of persistent atrial fibrillation. *Eur Heart J* 2008; 29(19):2359–66.
121. Todd DM, Skanes AC, Guiraudon G, et al. Role of the posterior left atrium and pulmonary veins in human lone atrial fibrillation: electrophysiological and pathological data from patients undergoing atrial fibrillation surgery. *Circulation* 2003; 108:3108–14.
122. Roberts-Thomson KC, Stevenson IH, Kistler PM, et al. Anatomically determined functional conduction delay in the posterior left atrium relationship to structural heart disease. *J Am Coll Cardiol* 2008; 51:856–62.
123. Kumagai K, Muraoka S, Mitsutake C, Takashima H, Nakashima H. A new approach for complete isolation of the posterior left atrium including pulmonary veins for atrial fibrillation. *J Cardiovasc Electrophysiol* 2007; 18:1047–52.
124. Nademanee K, McKenzie J, Kosar E, et al. A new approach for catheter ablation of atrial fibrillation: mapping of the electrophysiologic substrate. *J Am Coll Cardiol* 2004; 43:2044–53.
125. Konings KT, Kirchhof CJ, Smeets JR, Wellens HJ, Penn OC, Allessie MA. High-density mapping of electrically induced atrial fibrillation in humans. *Circulation* 1994; 89:1665–80.
126. Oral H, Chugh A, Good E, et al. Radiofrequency catheter ablation of chronic atrial fibrillation guided by complex electrograms. *Circulation* 2007; 115:2606–12.
127. Liu J, Scherlag BJ, Zhou J, et al. Autonomic mechanism to explain complex fractionated atrial electrograms (CFAE). *J Cardiovasc Electrophysiol* 2007; 18:1197–205.
128. Scherlag BJ, Yamanashi W, Patel U, Lazzara R, Jackman WM. Autonomically induced conversion of pulmonary vein focal firing into atrial fibrillation. *J Am Coll Cardiol* 2005; 45:1878–86.
129. Pappone C, Santinelli V, Manguso F, et al. Pulmonary vein denervation enhances long-term benefit after circumferential ablation for paroxysmal atrial fibrillation. *Circulation* 2004; 109:327–34.

130. Wright M, Haissaguerre M, Knecht S, et al. State of the art: catheter ablation of atrial fibrillation. *J Cardiovasc Electrophysiol* 2008; 19:583–92.
131. Oral H, Knight BP, Tada H, et al. Pulmonary vein isolation for paroxysmal and persistent atrial fibrillation. *Circulation* 2002; 105:1077–81.
132. O'Neill MD, Jais P, Takahashi Y, et al. The stepwise ablation approach for chronic atrial fibrillation--evidence for a cumulative effect. *J Interv Card Electrophysiol* 2006; 16:153–67.
133. Haissaguerre M, Hocini M, Sanders P, et al. Catheter ablation of long-lasting persistent atrial fibrillation: clinical outcome and mechanisms of subsequent arrhythmias. *J Cardiovasc Electrophysiol* 2005; 16:1138–47.
134. Haissaguerre M, Sanders P, Hocini M, et al. Catheter ablation of long-lasting persistent atrial fibrillation: critical structures for termination. *J Cardiovasc Electrophysiol* 2005; 16:1125–37.
135. Ouyang F, Ernst S, Chun J, et al. Electrophysiological findings during ablation of persistent atrial fibrillation with electroanatomic mapping and double Lasso catheter technique. *Circulation* 2005; 112:3038–48.
136. Kobza R, Hindricks G, Tanner H, et al. Late recurrent arrhythmias after ablation of atrial fibrillation: incidence, mechanisms, and treatment. *Heart Rhythm* 2004; 1:676–83.
137. Skanes AC, Klein G, Krahn A, Yee R. Cryoablation: potentials and pitfalls. *J Cardiovasc Electrophysiol* 2004; 15:S28–34.
138. Tse HF, Reek S, Timmermans C, et al. Pulmonary vein isolation using transvenous catheter cryoablation for treatment of atrial fibrillation without risk of pulmonary vein stenosis. *J Am Coll Cardiol* 2003; 42:752–8.
139. Khairy P, Chauvet P, Lehmann J, et al. Lower incidence of thrombus formation with cryoenergy versus radiofrequency catheter ablation. *Circulation* 2003; 107:2045–50.
140. Tse HF, Kwong YL, Lau CP. Transvenous cryoablation reduces platelet activation during pulmonary vein ablation compared with radiofrequency energy in patients with atrial fibrillation. *J Cardiovasc Electrophysiol* 2005; 16:1064–70.
141. Moreira W, Manusama R, Timmermans C, et al. Long-term follow-up after cryothermic ostial pulmonary vein isolation in paroxysmal atrial fibrillation. *J Am Coll Cardiol* 2008; 51:850–5.
142. Schwartzman D, Kuck KH. Anatomy-guided linear atrial lesions for radiofrequency catheter ablation of atrial fibrillation. *Pacing Clin Electrophysiol* 1998; 21:1959–78.
143. Novak PG, Guerra PG, Thibault B, Macle L. Utility of a nonfluoroscopic navigation system for pulmonary vein isolation. *J Cardiovasc Electrophysiol* 2004; 15:967.
144. Kato R, Lickfett L, Meininger G, et al. Pulmonary vein anatomy in patients undergoing catheter ablation of atrial fibrillation: lessons learned by use of magnetic resonance imaging. *Circulation* 2003; 107:2004–10.
145. Oral H, Knight BP, Ozaydin M, et al. Clinical significance of early recurrences of atrial fibrillation after pulmonary vein isolation. *J Am Coll Cardiol* 2002; 40:100–4.
146. Neumann T, Erdogan A, Dill T, et al. Asymptomatic recurrences of atrial fibrillation after pulmonary vein isolation. *Europace* 2006; 8:495–8.
147. Senatore G, Stabile G, Bertaglia E, et al. Role of transtelephonic electrocardiographic monitoring in detecting short-term arrhythmia recurrences after radiofrequency ablation in patients with atrial fibrillation. *J Am Coll Cardiol* 2005; 45:873–6.
148. Steven D, Rostock T, Lutomsky B, et al. What is the real atrial fibrillation burden after catheter ablation of atrial fibrillation? A prospective rhythm analysis in pacemaker patients with continuous atrial monitoring. *Eur Heart J* 2008; 29:1037–42.
149. Wazni OM, Marrouche NF, Martin DO, et al. Radiofrequency ablation vs antiarrhythmic drugs as first-line treatment of symptomatic atrial fibrillation: a randomized trial. *JAMA* 2005; 293:2634–40.
150. Pappone C, Augello G, Sala S, et al. A randomized trial of circumferential pulmonary vein ablation versus antiarrhythmic drug therapy in paroxysmal atrial fibrillation: the APAF Study. *J Am Coll Cardiol* 2006; 48:2340–7.
151. Jais P, Cauchemez B, Macle L, et al. Catheter ablation versus antiarrhythmic drugs for atrial fibrillation: the A4 study. *Circulation* 2008; 118:2498–505.
152. Stabile G, Bertaglia E, Senatore G, et al. Catheter ablation treatment in patients with drug-refractory atrial fibrillation: a prospective, multi-centre, randomized, controlled study (Catheter Ablation For The Cure Of Atrial Fibrillation Study). *Eur Heart J* 2006; 27:216–21.
153. Noheria A, Kumar A, Wylie JV Jr, Josephson ME. Catheter ablation vs antiarrhythmic drug therapy for atrial fibrillation: a systematic review. *Arch Intern Med* 2008; 168:581–6.
154. Tsao HM, Wu MH, Huang BH, et al. Morphologic remodeling of pulmonary veins and left atrium after catheter ablation of atrial fibrillation: insight from long-term follow-up of three-dimensional magnetic resonance imaging. *J Cardiovasc Electrophysiol* 2005; 16:7–12.
155. Jayam VK, Dong J, Vasamreddy CR, et al. Atrial volume reduction following catheter ablation of atrial fibrillation and relation to reduction in pulmonary vein size: an evaluation using magnetic resonance angiography. *J Interv Card Electrophysiol* 2005; 13:107–14.
156. Scharf C, Sneider M, Case I, et al. Anatomy of the pulmonary veins in patients with atrial fibrillation and effects of segmental ostial ablation analyzed by computed tomography. *J Cardiovasc Electrophysiol* 2003; 14:150–5.
157. Lemola K, Desjardins B, Sneider M, et al. Effect of left atrial circumferential ablation for atrial fibrillation on left atrial transport function. *Heart Rhythm* 2005; 2:923–8.
158. Verma A, Kilicaslan F, Adams JR, et al. Extensive ablation during pulmonary vein antrum isolation has no adverse impact on left atrial function: an echocardiography and cine computed tomography analysis. *J Cardiovasc Electrophysiol* 2006; 17:741–6.
159. Pappone C, Rosanio S, Augello G, et al. Mortality, morbidity, and quality of life after circumferential pulmonary vein ablation for atrial fibrillation: outcomes from a controlled nonrandomized long-term study. *J Am Coll Cardiol* 2003; 42:185–97.
160. Roy D, Talajic M, Nattel S, et al. Rhythm control versus rate control for atrial fibrillation and heart failure. *N Engl J Med* 2008; 358:2667–77.
161. Tondo C, Mantica M, Russo G, et al. Pulmonary vein vestibule ablation for the control of atrial fibrillation in patients with impaired left ventricular function. *Pacing Clin Electrophysiol* 2006; 29:962–70.

162. Khan MN, Jais P, Cummings J, et al. Pulmonary-vein isolation for atrial fibrillation in patients with heart failure. *N Engl J Med* 2008; 359:1778–85.
163. Balasubramaniam R, Kistler PM. AF and Heart failure: the chicken or the egg? *Heart* 2009; 95(7):535–9.
164. Cappato R, Calkins H, Chen SA, et al. Worldwide survey on the methods, efficacy, and safety of catheter ablation for human atrial fibrillation. *Circulation* 2005; 111:1100–5.
165. Oral H, Chugh A, Ozaydin M, et al. Risk of thromboembolic events after percutaneous left atrial radiofrequency ablation of atrial fibrillation. *Circulation* 2006; 114:759–65.
166. Patel A, Au E, Donegan K, et al. Multidetector row computed tomography for identification of left atrial appendage filling defects in patients undergoing pulmonary vein isolation for treatment of atrial fibrillation: comparison with transesophageal echocardiography. *Heart Rhythm* 2008; 5:253–60.
167. Di Biase L, Fahmy TS, Wazni OM, et al. Pulmonary vein total occlusion following catheter ablation for atrial fibrillation: clinical implications after long-term follow-up. *J Am Coll Cardiol* 2006; 48:2493–9.
168. Ghia KK, Chugh A, Good E, et al. A nationwide survey on the prevalence of atrioesophageal fistula after left atrial radiofrequency catheter ablation. *J Interv Card Electrophysiol* 2009; 24:33–6.
169. Lemola K, Sneider M, Desjardins B, et al. Computed tomographic analysis of the anatomy of the left atrium and the esophagus: implications for left atrial catheter ablation. *Circulation* 2004; 110:3655–60.
170. Bunch TJ, Ellenbogen KA, Packer DL, Asirvatham SJ. Vagus nerve injury after posterior atrial radiofrequency ablation. *Heart Rhythm* 2008; 5:1327–30.
171. Chugh A, Oral H, Lemola K, et al. Prevalence, mechanisms, and clinical significance of macroreentrant atrial tachycardia during and following left atrial ablation for atrial fibrillation. *Heart Rhythm* 2005; 2:464–71.
172. Mesas CE, Pappone C, Lang CC, et al. Left atrial tachycardia after circumferential pulmonary vein ablation for atrial fibrillation: electroanatomic characterization and treatment. *J Am Coll Cardiol* 2004; 44:1071–9.
173. Gerstenfeld EP, Marchlinski FE. Mapping and ablation of left atrial tachycardias occurring after atrial fibrillation ablation. *Heart Rhythm* 2007; 4:S65–72.
174. Satomi K, Bansch D, Tilz R, et al. Left atrial and pulmonary vein macroreentrant tachycardia associated with double conduction gaps: a novel type of man-made tachycardia after circumferential pulmonary vein isolation. *Heart Rhythm* 2008; 5:43–51.
175. Gerstenfeld EP, Callans DJ, Sauer W, Jacobson J, Marchlinski FE. Reentrant and nonreentrant focal left atrial tachycardias occur after pulmonary vein isolation. *Heart Rhythm* 2005; 2:1195–202.
176. Sanders P, Hocini M, Jais P, et al. Characterization of focal atrial tachycardia using high-density mapping. *J Am Coll Cardiol* 2005; 46:2088–99.
177. Lickfett L, Mahesh M, Vasamreddy C, et al. Radiation exposure during catheter ablation of atrial fibrillation. *Circulation* 2004; 110:3003–10.
178. Gerber TC, Carr JJ, Arai AE, et al. Ionizing Radiation in Cardiac Imaging. A Science Advisory From the American Heart Association Committee on Cardiac Imaging of the Council on Clinical Cardiology and Committee on Cardiovascular Imaging and Intervention of the Council on Cardiovascular Radiology and Intervention. *Circulation* 2009; 119(7):1056–65.
179. Boersma LV, Wijffels MC, Oral H, et al. Pulmonary vein isolation by duty-cycled bipolar and unipolar radiofrequency energy with a multielectrode ablation catheter. *Heart Rhythm* 2008; 5:1635–42.
180. Mansour M, Forleo GB, Pappalardo A, et al. Initial experience with the Mesh catheter for pulmonary vein isolation in patients with paroxysmal atrial fibrillation. *Heart Rhythm* 2008; 5:1510–16.
181. Chun KR, Schmidt B, Metzner A, et al. The 'single big cryoballoon' technique for acute pulmonary vein isolation in patients with paroxysmal atrial fibrillation: a prospective observational single centre study. *Eur Heart J* 2008; 30(6):699–709.
182. Markowitz SM. Ablation of atrial fibrillation: patient selection, technique, and outcome. *Curr Cardiol Rep* 2008; 10:360–6.
183. Moe GK. On the multiple wavelet hypothesis of atrial fibrillation. *Arch Int Pharmacodyn Ther* 1962;1409:183–188.

7

Percutaneous Treatment of Valvular Heart Disease

S. CHIU WONG
ERIC AU
SUZANNE ZENTKO

OUTLINE

Population-based echocardiographic studies in the United States estimate that about 2.5% of the population have moderate to severe valvular dysfunction (1). Of the cardiac valvular disease categories reported, mitral regurgitation was found to be the most prevalent (1.7%), followed by aortic regurgitation and stenosis (0.5% and 0.4% respectively), while mitral stenosis was the least common (0.1%). The incidence of heart disease increased with age (0.7% between age 18 and 44 and 13.3% in subjects 75 years or older). There was a 1.36-fold increase in overall adjusted mortality in patients with valvular dysfunction compared to those without (1).

Much research has been conducted on the etiology of valvular dysfunction and the optimal timing for treatment. Pharmacologic treatment of valvular diseases with beta-blockers, ACE inhibitors, angiotensin receptor blockers and HMG-CoA reductase inhibitors can improve symptoms but has not been shown to effectively prolong survival. Thus, the treatment of choice for significant valvular disease has traditionally been open surgical repair or replacement. Surgical treatment of valvular diseases has made steady progress over the last few decades, resulting in substantial improvements in clinical outcomes following these procedures. However, with the need for general anesthesia and cardiopulmonary bypass, perioperative morbidity and mortality for open surgical valve operations remain problematic. In addition, recovery time can be prolonged and inpatient cardiac rehabilitation is often required.

With the aging of the population and improved survival of patients with both cardiac and noncardiac diseases, the prevalence of valvular diseases will continue to increase (1). In the coming years, this patient population will likely have more frequent comorbid conditions that place them at a even higher risk for periprocedural complications following any of the currently available open surgical treatment approaches. In fact, a significant portion of patients who would otherwise meet criteria to undergo surgical valve repair or replacement are not offered such options due to both higher surgical risk and patient preference (2).

Against this backdrop, research into less invasive approaches to treat valvular disease has been intensified. In the surgical realm, minimally invasive techniques, with its attendant patient and procedural related limitations, have been tried with some success but traditional valvular operations still remain the norm. At the same time, great strides have been made in percutaneous approaches to treatment of valvular disease. Two valvular disease states in which percutaneous balloon valvuloplasty have had great success are in the treatment of pulmonic stenosis and mitral stenosis.

The first use of percutaneous balloon valvuloplasty was described in 1982 for patients with pulmonic stenosis (3). By the late 1980s, this treatment modality had become the procedure of choice for this condition, first in children and later in adolescents and adults. For example, one seminal study published in 1996 showed that percutaneous balloon valvuloplasty could be performed for pulmonic stenosis in adolescents and adults with low rates of complications and excellent immediate and long-term outcomes (4). Current guidelines recommend percutaneous valvuloplasty as the procedure of choice for adolescents and adults with severe pulmonic stenosis requiring treatment (5).

With the success in treatment of pulmonic stenosis, percutaneous balloon valvuloplasty has been applied in the treatment of mitral stenosis since 1984. Clinical studies reveal that procedural outcomes are related to mitral valve anatomy; better results have been shown in patients with lower Echo Scores, a grading system that takes into account leaflet mobility, thickening, calcification and subvalvular thickening (6). Excellent immediate and long-term outcomes have been demonstrated by numerous studies, including head-to-head comparisons of balloon valvuloplasty with open surgical commissurotomy (7,8). Current AHA/ACC guidelines recommend percutaneous valvuloplasty as the procedure of choice for patients with severe mitral stenosis and suitable anatomy (5).

While percutaneous balloon valvuloplasty for pulmonic and mitral stenosis quickly became the treatment standard in selected patients with suitable valvular anatomy, this technique has met with less success when applied to aortic stenosis. The concept of a percutaneous treatment of aortic stenosis was first put into clinical use by Cribier in 1985, when he successfully performed an aortic balloon valvuloplasty by partially dilating the stenotic valve using repetitive balloon dilations (9). Subsequent data showed that postprocedure valve area rarely exceeded 1 cm^2. Despite acceptable rates of "procedural success" with moderate reduction in the transvalvular pressure gradient that translated into symptomatic relief, the beneficial effects rarely lasted more than 6 to 12 months due to a high rate of valve restenosis. Patients who underwent a repeat procedure had 36% 1-year mortality with only temporary benefit (10,11). Since the long-term clinical outcomes following balloon valvuloplasty in patients with severe aortic stenosis were similar to those left untreated, the procedure was largely abandoned, and it is now reserved for palliative or bridging therapy (12).

The limited clinical efficacy of balloon valvuloplasty alone in the treatment of aortic stenosis and other valvular heart diseases has prompted further research and development of novel technologies in the past decade. The era of percutaneous valve repair or replacement was first introduced by Dr. Bonhoffer in 2000 when a bovine jugular stent valve was first implanted successfully in a 12-year-old boy with combined pulmonic stenosis and regurgitation eight years following a Carpentier-Edwards conduit connecting the right ventricle and pulmonary artery (13). Subsequently, the more refined Melody® Transcatheter Pulmonary Valve and Ensemble® Transcatheter Delivery System (Medtronic B.V., The Netherlands) received (CE) mark on October 4, 2006, for percutaneous pulmonic valve replacement. Recently, Lurz et al. reproduced Dr. Bonhoeffer's experience in 155 patients who underwent percutaneous pulmonic valve implantation for treatment of pulmonic stenosis and/or regurgitation. The median follow up was 28.4 (ranged from 0 to 83.7) months. Freedom from reoperation was 70% and freedom from repeat transcather intervention was 73% at 70 months with 96.9% survival noted at 83 months (14). This procedure has no doubt transformed the landscape of interventional cardiology for pediatric and young adult patients with congenital heart disease with a marked reduction in the number of repeat procedures often necessary following pulmonic conduit surgery. The extension of this novel technology to treatment of other valvular disease states seems natural. Exciting research and development is currently underway for percutaneous treatment of mitral regurgitation and percutaneous valve replacement for aortic stenosis.

■ PERCUTANEOUS VALVE REPAIR AND REPLACEMENT FOR MITRAL REGURGITATION

Background

Normal mitral valve function requires intact leaflet structure, preserved subvalvular apparatus (i.e., chordae tendinae and papillary muscles), and a nondilated mitral annulus. Disruption of any one of these elements can lead to regurgitation of blood into the left atrium under the high pressure of left ventricular systole.

The most common cause of primary mitral regurgitation in the developed world is mitral valve prolapse due to degenerative disease, while the most common causes of secondary or functional mitral regurgitation are left ventricular systolic dysfunction and ischemic heart disease. Other etiologies of mitral regurgitation include rheumatic heart disease, infective endocarditis, inflammatory rheumatologic conditions, trauma and drug toxicity.

The clinical consequences of significant mitral regurgitation are numerous and include impaired quality of life (particularly with dyspnea and fatigue on exertion), left ventricular enlargement and dysfunction, arrhythmias such as atrial fibrillation, secondary pulmonary hypertension and sudden cardiac death. Concomitant mitral regurgitation can be particularly deleterious in patients with either congestive heart failure or ischemic heart disease (15,16).

Medical treatment of mitral regurgitation with afterload reduction and diuresis can effectively alleviate symptoms, but has not been shown to prolong survival. The currently recommended treatments for severe mitral regurgitation are surgical mitral valve repair or replacement. Mitral valve replacement with either a bioprosthetic or mechanical valve has the inherent drawbacks of a potential increase in periprocedural complications, compromise of left ventricular function, need for reoperation and lifelong anticoagulation. Therefore, whenever possible, mitral valve repair is the preferred technique and can involve surgically reshaping the leaflets, annuloplasty, and repositioning or replacing chordae (5). However, due to the complexity of the procedure, coupled with often difficult valve anatomy, less than half of the patients with mitral valve surgery underwent mitral valve repair both in the United States and Europe (17). Importantly, a significant portion of patients who would otherwise undergo surgical mitral valve repair or replacement do not undergo such surgeries due to both high surgical risk and patient preference (18). Thus, the advent of less invasive interventional approaches to treat mitral regurgitation is appealing, particularly for the growing number of elderly patients with frequent comorbidities. Currently there are multiple devices in either preclinical or clinical phase designed for percutaneous treatment of mitral regurgitation. They can be categorized into five different approaches (Table 7.1): (a) leaflet apposition, (b) coronary sinus annuloplasty, (c) direct subvalvular annuloplasty, (d) direct chamber and annular reshaping, and (e) mitral valve replacement.

Table 7.1 Percutaneous transcatheter mitral valve repair/replacement technologies

Mechanism Device	Company (State)	Development Stage
Leaflet apposition		
Mitral clip	Evalve (CA)	CE Mark Approved, U.S. phase 2 randomized trial completed
Mobius	Edwards LifeSciences (CA)	On hold
Coronary sinus annuloplasty		
MONARC system	Edwards LifeSciences (CA)	Clinical outside U.S.
Shape-changing rods	Viacor (MA)	Clinical outside U.S.
CARILLON system	Cardiac Dimensions (WA)	CE mark approved
Direct annuloplasty		
Sturure-based plication	Mitralign Inc. (NH)	Early clinical
Anchor-Cinch plication	Guided Delivery System (CA)	Early clinical
RF annulus remodeling	QuantumCor (CA)	Clinical outside U.S.
Direct chamber and annular reshaping		
PS3 system	Ample Medical (CA)	Early clinical
iCoapsys	Myocor (MN)	Early clinical
Valve replacement		
EndoValve	EndoVavle Inc. (NJ)	Preclinical

Percutaneous Mitral Valve Repair

Of the myriad percutaneous approaches currently proposed for the treatment of mitral regurgitation, the MitraClip™ (E-valve®, Menlo Park, CA) and CARILLON™ Mitral Contour System™ (Cardiac Dimension®, Kirkland, WA) have recently received CE Mark approval in Europe but none by the U.S. FDA.

The percutaneous method used to address mitral regurgitation that is furthest along in development and clinical trials to date is the MitraClip. This novel percutaneous approach is based on the open surgical "edge-to-edge" technique first described by Dr. Ottavio Alfieri in Italy, whereby central mitral regurgitation is repaired by the placement of sutures connecting the edges of the central portions of the anterior and posterior (A2 and P2 segments) mitral leaflets (Figure 7.1). This approach creates a double orifice, allowing blood to flow freely from the left atrium to the left ventricle during diastole, while aiding in coaptation of the leaflets during ventricular systole (Figure 7.2) (19). Follow-up in patients undergoing the open edge-to-edge technique showed a substantial decrease in mitral regurgitation without evidence of significant mitral stenosis (20).

The MitraClip is designed to produce a similar edge-to-edge result via a percutaneous approach performed on the beating heart without the need for cardiopulmonary bypass. A steerable 24 French guide catheter is inserted into the femoral vein and brought across the interatrial septum using a trans-septal approach to allow access to the left atrium and mitral valve. The MitraClip device (Figure 7.3), composed of cobalt chromium contrast with polyester covering, is then positioned so that the two arms capture the edges of the central portions of the anterior and posterior mitral valve leaflets. Real-time fluoroscopic and transesophageal echocardiographic image modalities are used to optimize clip placement. If the position of the MitraClip is not ideal, the device can be reopened and repositioned for optimal reduction in mitral regurgitation, or a second MitraClip device can be deployed in the same patient if necessary. Once optimal positioning has been achieved, the device is locked and then detached from the clip delivery system. After clip placement, patients are generally treated with aspirin for at least six months and with clopidogrel for at least one month.

Following encouraging studies in animals, the MitraClip was tested in humans in a nonrandomized phase 1 safety and feasibility trial, named the Endovascular Valve Edge-to-Edge Repair Study (EVEREST)

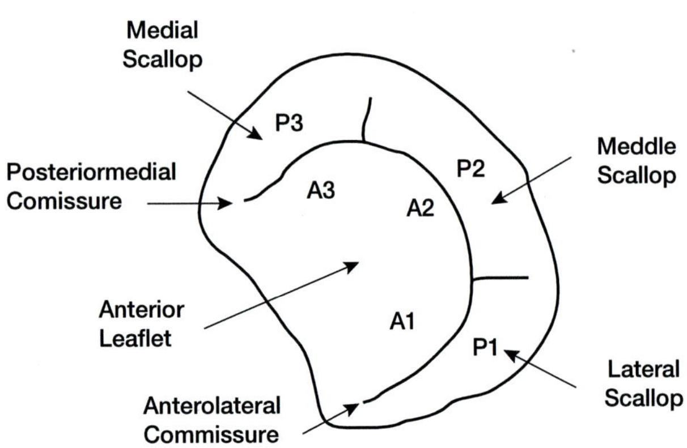

FIGURE 7.1 Mitral valve leaflet structure.

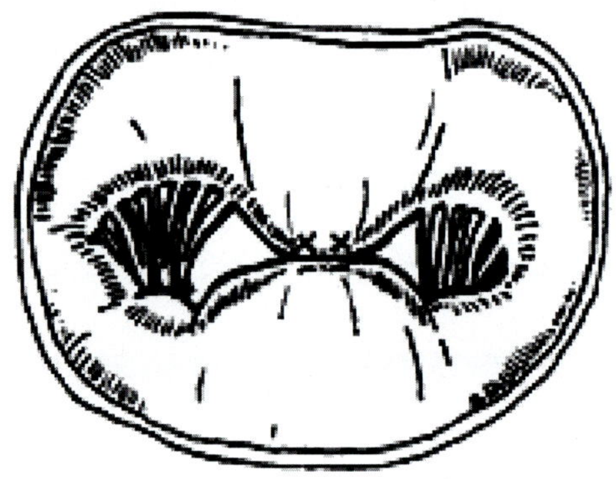

FIGURE 7.2 Double orifice created by the surgical edge-to-edge technique.

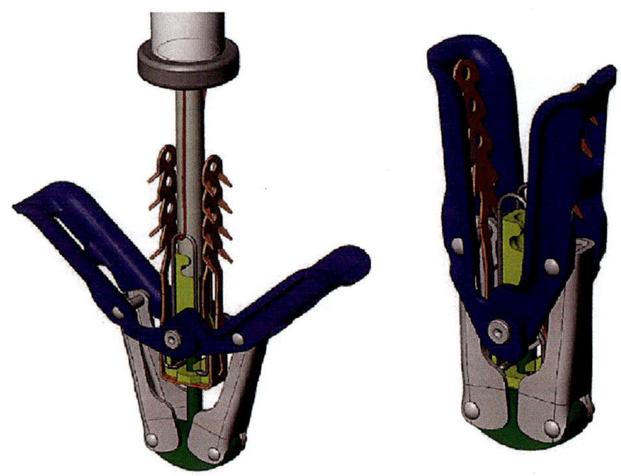

FIGURE 7.3 The MitraClip device. (Evalve Corporation; From Ref. 21, with permission.)

(21). In this study, the initial results of which were published in 2005, 27 patients with moderate-to-severe or severe mitral regurgitation involving the central portions of the leaflets and reduced left ventricular function (either ejection fraction less than 60% or left ventricular end-systolic dimension >45 mm) underwent the percutaneous procedure for MitraClip placement under general anesthesia. The etiology of the mitral regurgitation was degenerative in 93% of patients and ischemic in 7% of patients. The MitraClip was successfully deployed in 24 of 27 patients (89%). At 30 days, 85% were free from major adverse events, which was the primary study endpoint. The authors reported that one patient sustained a nonembolic stroke associated with postprocedure hypotension. Clip detachment from one of the mitral leaflets was noted in three patients. Importantly, there were no cases of clip embolization for the entire cohort. Although reduction in the degree of mitral regurgitation was not the primary endpoint of this study, 64% of the 22 patients who were discharged with a MitraClip in place had ≤2+ mitral regurgitation at one month follow-up. Overall, the EVEREST trial demonstrated placement of the MitraClip to be safe and feasible, with significant improvements in mitral regurgitation.

Since the publication of the initial findings of EVEREST in 2005, additional follow-up analyses of the MitraClip have been either published or reported at national conferences. Serial echocardiographic monitoring of study participants in whom MitraClip devices were successfully deployed demonstrated no significant mitral stenosis after one year of follow-up (22).

At a national conference in October 2007, researchers presented data on 107 patients from the nonrandomized registry of EVEREST (a larger registry that continued to enroll patients following the initial EVEREST results mentioned earlier). They reported that 74% of patients had reduction in their mitral regurgitation to ≤2+ following implantation of MitraClip devices. In addition, 82% of patients who had undergone successful MitraClip placement remained free from surgery three years after the procedure. Finally, these investigators found that at one year following successful MitraClip implantation, there was echocardiographic evidence of reverse remodeling of the left ventricle (decreased left ventricular end diastolic and end systolic dimensions and volumes) and 94% of patients had improved or stable New York Heart Association (NYHA) class heart failure symptoms (23).

At a national conference in April 2008, investigators reported that 83% of the 23 patients who received the MitraClip demonstrated a reduction in the severity of functional mitral regurgitation and 89% of those had sustained improvement at two years of follow-up (24). They also noted that the mean length of stay following the MitraClip procedure was three days.

To further evaluate this device, the EVEREST II trial is an ongoing randomized phase 2 trial comparing the safety and efficacy of the MitraClip versus open mitral valve surgery. Enrollment in this trial was completed in September 2008 but final results are not currently available. The primary efficacy endpoint of EVEREST II is freedom from surgery for valve dysfunction, death, and moderate-to-severe or severe mitral regurgitation at one year. The primary safety endpoint is freedom from major adverse events at one month. A high-risk registry arm of the EVEREST II trial completed enrollment in January 2008 and evaluates the safety and efficacy of the MitraClip device in patients who are considered to be high risk for surgery.

Overall, the MitraClip device is an exciting novel percutaneous approach to an increasingly common valvular condition. As of September 2008, the device had been implanted in over 350 patients. Results thus far have been very encouraging for the treatment of degenerative and functional mitral regurgitation, in terms of both safety and efficacy. Importantly, investigators have noted that the MitraClip device has not been shown to preclude future surgical options for mitral regurgitation, including mitral valve repair surgery. The results of the EVEREST II trial comparing the safety and efficacy of MitraClip placement with open mitral valve surgery will certainly be anxiously awaited. In the interim, the FDA has approved the REALISM (Real World ExpAnded MuLtIcenter Study of the MitraClip® System) study, a prospective multicenter continued access registry of the EVEREST II study. The registry will enroll up to 120 U.S. patients in two arms: a high-risk and a nonhigh-risk cohort that will undergo 30-day, 6-, and 12-month clinical follow-up.

A second leaflet apposition technology, the Mobius™ (Edwards Lifesciences, Irvine, CA), shares a similar conceptual approach to the MitraClip in connecting the central portion of the anterior and posterior segments of the mitral leaflets together. Instead of covered metal clips, polypropylene suture material is used for the edge to edge apposition (25). However, further clinical evaluation has been put on hold due to technical as well as technological issues associated with the current device design.

Percutaneous Mitral Annuloplasty

Mitral annular support devices are frequently implanted to treat mitral regurgitation during open mitral valve repair surgery; in fact, over 50% of mitral valve repair surgeries consist solely of simple annuloplasty (26). The aim of such mitral annular rings is to decrease the annular diameter in order to improve leaflet coaptation and thus reduce functional mitral regurgitation related to left ventricular dilation. The morbidity and mortality inherent to open surgery and cardiopulmonary bypass limit the use of annular support devices to patients who are good surgical candidates. The availability of percutaneous methods to improve the mitral annular diameter would be potentially applicable for both patients who are at higher surgical risk (especially patients with ischemic cardiomyopathy) and for patients who do not have another indication for open cardiac surgery (e.g., coronary artery disease requiring coronary artery bypass surgery).

Numerous companies have developed devices and techniques to treat mitral annular dilatation percutaneously. Most of these devices take advantage of the close anatomic proximity of the coronary sinus to the posterior aspect of the mitral valve annulus, and involve the placement of a prosthetic device in the coronary sinus to decrease the anterior–posterior diameter of the mitral valve annulus, thereby improving mitral leaflet coaptation. Other techniques involve percutaneous direct plication of the mitral annulus with sutures or the use of a bridge to connect a coronary sinus anchor and a septal anchor.

Several animal studies have demonstrated the ability of percutaneous devices placed in the coronary sinus to reduce mitral antero-posterior diameter, improve mitral leaflet coaptation, and reduce mitral regurgitation (27–29). The first experiences with such devices in humans have been reported over the last few years. A 2006 case series reported results with the Edwards Viking annuloplasty device (Figure 7.4), which involved the implantation of a nitinol implant consisting of proximal and distal self-expanding anchors attached by a bridge (30). Device implantation was successful in four of five patients with chronic, ischemic mitral regurgitation, and the degree of mitral regurgitation was reduced at hospital discharge in three of these

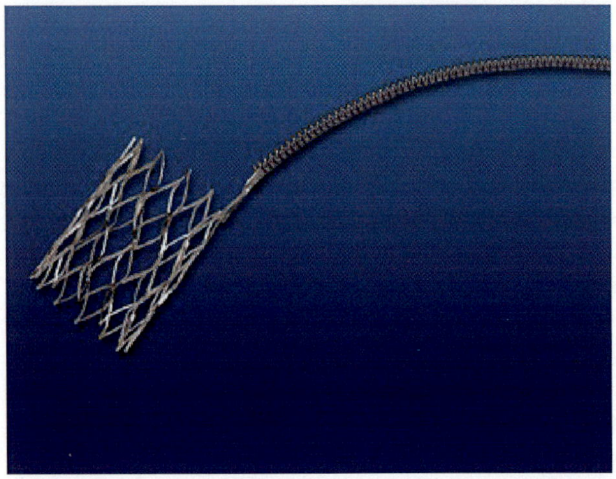

FIGURE 7.4 Percutaneous mitral annuloplasty device (MONARC System Edwards Lifesciences, Inc., with permission.)

four patients. Unfortunately, separation of the nitinol bridge was observed in three of the four patients in routine follow-up chest x-rays, prompting reconfiguration of the nitinol bridge and overall device design by the company.

The second generation coronary sinus annuloplasty Edwards MONARC™ System is a 9 French device delivered through a 12 French guide catheter via a jugular approach. It consists of a larger nitinol proximal coronary sinus anchor, a redesigned flexible shortening bridge segment and a smaller distal great cardiac vein anchor. The connecting bridge contains a biodegradable element which degrades over a 6-week period resulting in shortening of the spring bridge. This increases the tension around the mitral valve and gradually pushes the posterior mitral annulus and its associated structures forward, resulting in decreased mitral regurgitation which ideally results in more favorable left ventricular remodeling over a three to six-month period. EVOLUTION is an international multicenter registry using the MONARC system for treatment of functional mitral regurgitation. Of the 72 enrolled patients, the average left ventricular ejection fraction was 38 ± 11%, 61% had 2+, and 34% had 3–4+ mitral regurgitation at baseline, as documented by echocardiography by a corelab. Of the 59 devices implanted, 55 (93%) were delivered at the target location within the coronary sinus. There was no in-hospital mortality associated with the procedure, and the event-free survival was 91% at 30 days, 83% at six months, 81% at one year and 70% at two years. There were 15 major events reported: 10 deaths, three myocardial infarctions, and two cardiac tamponades. Along with the gradual tightening of the connecting bridge segment and left ventricular remodeling over time, ≥1 grade improvement in the severity of mitral regurgitation was observed in 41.2% of patients with 1+, 57.7% of patient with 2+, and 88.9% of patients with 3+ mitral regurgitation at 6 months follow-up (31).

The first experience in humans with another percutaneous mitral annuloplasty device (Viacor Inc.) was reported in 2007 (32). This device consists of a seven French multilumen delivery catheter and nitinol rods with nontraumatic silicone distal tips placed into the anterior interventricular vein. They are available in a variety of lengths (70, 90, 110, 120, 130, 140 mm), two stiffness levels (1000 and 200 g/cm of pressure), and three tapers (quarter, half, and full) to allow for adjustment during implantation until mitral regurgitation is minimized (Figure 7.5). The rigid rods exert outward forces at their proximal and distal ends, resulting in forward displacement of the mid segment of the coronary sinus and the associated annulus. This, in turn, reduces the antero-posterior distance of the mitral annulus. In this case series evaluating safety and feasibility, temporary implantation of the device was attempted in four patients (in the operating room immediately prior to mitral valve surgery for three patients and in the catheterization laboratory for the fourth patient) with ischemic mitral regurgitation via either the right internal jugular vein or the left subclavian vein. Device implantation was unsuccessful in one patient due to the angulation of the coronary sinus. The remaining three patients tolerated temporary device implantation without complications. The device appeared efficacious, with a decrease in both anterior–posterior diameter (from 40.75 ± 4.3 to 35.2 ± 1.6 mm) and mitral regurgitant volume (from 45.5 ± 24.4 to 13.3 ± 7.3 mL).

The CARRILLON Mitral Contour System is the second percutaneous device that received CE Mark approval in February 2009. The device consists of a nitinol-based distal (great cardiac vein) anchor and a proximal (coronary sinus) "crimp" with a connecting bridge that is manually tensioned to cinch the septal-lateral mitral annulus prior to deployment (Figure 7.6) (33). Temporary implantation via the right internal jugular vein under light sedation was successful in four of five patients, all of whom had a dilated cardiomyopathy (left ventricular ejection fraction 30–45%), grade 2 to 4 mitral regurgitation, and NYHA class II or III heart failure. The authors state that device implantation in one patient was not successful because the great cardiac vein was too small for

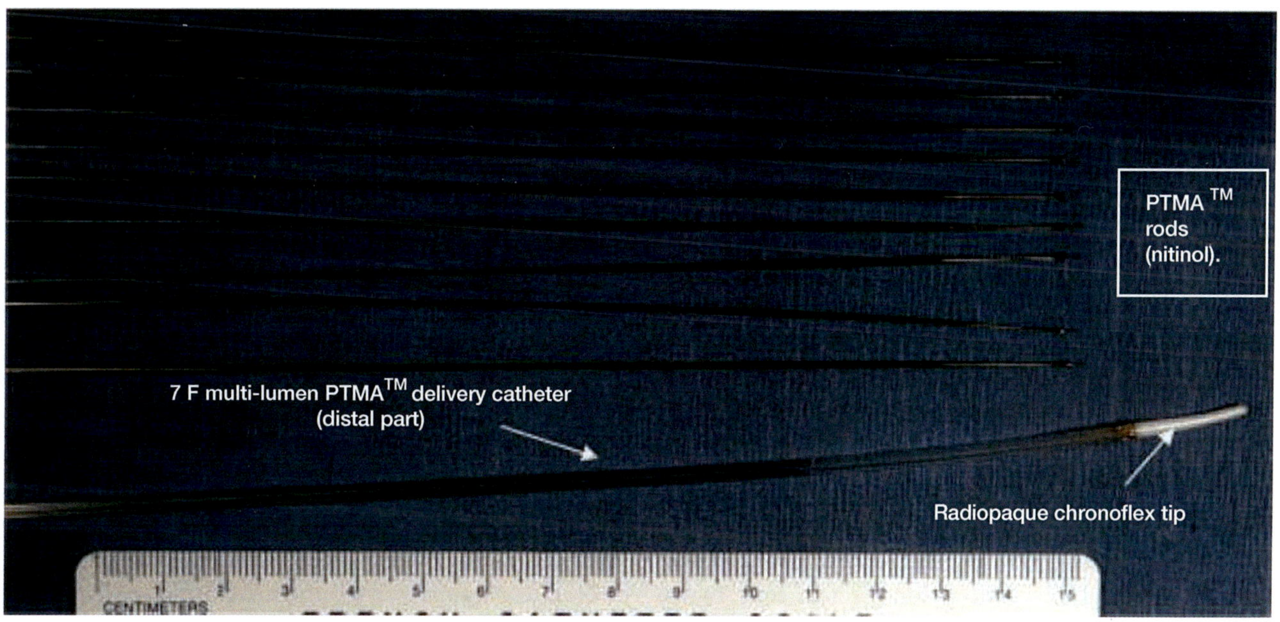

FIGURE 7.5 Percutaneous mitral annuloplasty device. (Viacor Inc.; From Ref. 32, with permission.)

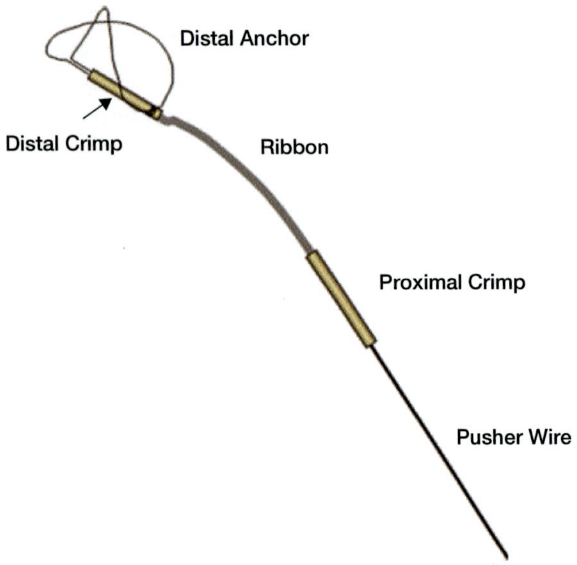

FIGURE 7.6 Percutaneous mitral annuloplasty device. (Cardiac Dimensions Inc.; From Ref. 33, with permission.)

the distal anchor device. Temporary deployment of the device (for less than one hour, on average) resulted in a decrease in the septal-lateral mitral annular dimension (from 35.5 ± 4.7 to 32.2 ± 4.6 mm, $P = 0.02$), a reduction in mitral regurgitation color Doppler area (from 98.3 ± 43.6 to 83.3 ± 35.1 mm^2, $P = 0.09$), and a reduction in mitral regurgitation jet as a percentage of left atrial area (from 36 ± 18% to 30 ± 14%, $P = 0.11$). No adverse events occurred during or after temporary placement of the device. This case series demonstrated the safety and feasibility of this device and approach.

The AMADEUS registry is a prospective multicenter European registry to evaluate the safety and efficacy of the CARILLON Mitral Contour System™ in patients with function mitral regurgitation. Joachim Schofer recently presented 6-month clinical outcomes of 48 patients (34). Among the 30 patients with successful device placement, cardiac perforation was noted in three patients at one month and there were two deaths (6.9%) and three myocardial infarctions reported at six months. The regurgitant volume was reduced from 35 ± 16 mL at baseline to 24 ± 12 at six months (P <0.001) and six-minute walk test increased from a mean of 307 meters to 403 meters (P <0.001).

These reports of early clinical experience in humans have shown that the concept of percutaneous mitral annuloplasty may be feasible for many patients with ischemic or functional mitral regurgitation. However, some potential limitations have been identified. Most notably, variability in coronary sinus anatomy, including the degree of ostial angulation in the right atrium, overall vessel size, lateral extent, relationship to the mitral annulus, and proximity of the left circumflex artery could make coronary sinus device approaches impossible or unhelpful in some patients.

Despite these limitations, CARILLON Mitral Contour System™ has recently received CE Mark approval. More clinical experience is clearly warranted to further assess the role of percutaneous annuloplasty via coronary sinus remodeling in the treatment of mitral regurgitation.

Direct Annulus Plication

Placement of an annuloplasty ring is a common surgical approach for treatment of mitral regurgitation. There are currently a number of novel devices designed to simulate suture mitral annuloplasty surgery percutaneously. All are currently in preclinical and early pilot clinical phase of development.

Both the Mitralign device (Mitralign Inc., Tewksbury, MA) and the AccuCinch System (Guided Delivery Systems, Inc., Santa Clara, CA) are designed to place a delivery catheter retrograde across the aortic valve that directs posteriorly to facilitate insertion of stitches along the posterior annulus to enable direct annular "cinching," thus changing the geometry of the mitral valve apparatus with the goal of reducing the amount of mitral regurgitation. The Mitralign clinical investigation began in November 2008 with the first two implants performed by Drs. Eberhard Grube and Lutz Buellesfeld in Siegburg, Germany.

Another device, the QuantumCor technology (Q-Care, Lake Forest, CA) reduces mitral annulus circumference by applying radiofrequency energy directly to the mitral annulus, heating and thus contracting the collagen fibers over time.

Direct Chamber and Annular Reshaping

One of the major pathophysiologic mechanisms leading to functional mitral regurgitation is ventricular dilatation resulting in malapposition of the mitral valve leaflets. To that end, there are currently several devices designed to remodel the ventricle for the treatment of mitral regurgitation. Following initial encouraging animal studies, the first human use of a percutaneous septal-to-lateral cinching device, the PS3 system (Ample

Medical Inc, Foster City, CA) to reduce mitral annular diameter was reported in 2007 (35,36). This cinching device consists of a coronary sinus anchor and a septal anchor, attached by a bridge (Figure 7.7). Implantation is achieved with the use of two magnetically-linked catheters placed in the coronary sinus and the left atrium via a trans-septal puncture. Tension applied on this bridge decreases the septal-lateral mitral annular distance. In this report, two patients underwent device implantation immediately prior to surgical mitral valve repair. There were no complications following device implantation and mitral regurgitation grade was decreased in both patients.

The iCoapsys™ device (Myocar® Inc., Maple Grove, NM) is currently under early clinical development. It consists of two pads connected by a flexible cord that are positioned on the outside of the heart. A specially designed needle is used to gain access to the pericardial space. Subsequently, anchoring devices are placed on the outer left ventricular surfaces in an anterior–posterior orientation connected by a tethering suture that passes horizontally through the left ventricle. By increasing tension to the anchoring suture, a change in ventricular shape along with position of the mitral annulus may facilitate proper mitral leaflet coaptation. The Valvular and Ventricular Improvement Via iCoapsys Delivery (VIVID) study is a four-site U.S. registry of 30 patients approved by the FDA on November 3, 2007, to assess the safety and feasibility of iCoapsys™ for the treatment of functional mitral regurgitation.

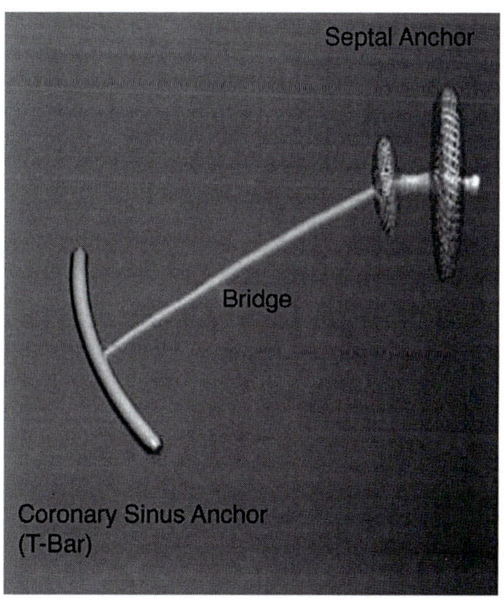

FIGURE 7.7 Percutaneous mitral annuloplasty device. (From Ref. 36, with permission.)

Direct Valve Replacement

The idea of percutaneous mitral valve replacement may be more challenging than mitral valve repair techniques due to the unique shape and location of the mitral valve and associated apparatus. The Endovalve-Hermann mitral valve replacement system (Endovalve Inc., Princeton, NJ) is a bioprosthetic foldable redeployable valve that allows antegrade trans-septal placement via a 24 French sheath. An early animal study in four sheep has been reported by Hermann at TCT 2007 (Figure 7.8).

In addition, a recent publication described the feasibility of placing a transcatheter bioprosthetic valve at the site of a surgical mitral valve replacement in a bovine model (37). This type of approach may eventually be used in lieu of repeat open surgical replacement for patients with a failing mitral valve bioprosthesis.

■ PERCUTANEOUS AORTIC VALVE REPLACEMENT

Background

In adult patients with single native left-sided history of valvular heart disease, aortic stenosis was the most frequently reported valve lesion in the 2001 Euro Heart

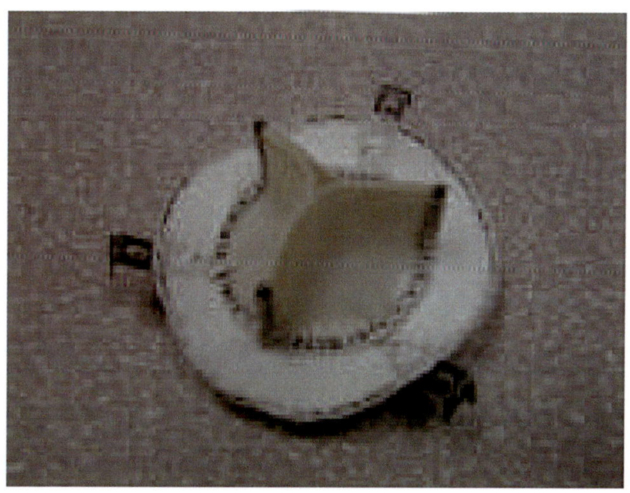

FIGURE 7.8 Endovalve.

Survey and its incidence continues to increase along with the growth of elderly population in Western societies (2). Aortic stenosis mostly occurs due to calcific degeneration of a normal trileaflet and less frequently in the setting of a congenital bicuspid valve. While still common in some parts of the world, rheumatic valve disease is now a rare cause in developed countries.

The natural history of aortic stenosis generally involves a prolonged asymptomatic period with the onset of symptoms as stenosis worsens. Although individual courses vary, longitudinal studies have shown that once stenosis develops, the mean transaortic gradient increases at an average rate of 7 mm Hg per year, with a corresponding decrease of about 0.1 cm^2 per year in valve area (38). A minimal gradient is present until the valve orifice is less than 50% normal and patients tend to be asymptomatic until the valve area is less than 1 cm^2. Once this occurs and patients present with the classic symptoms of angina, heart failure and syncope, clinical deterioration can be rapid and mortality dramatically increases.

The onset of clinical symptoms indicates hemodynamically significant disease and is a pivotal point for making management decisions since the average overall survival is two to three years, with a high risk of sudden death (39). To date, no pharmacological treatments have been proven to delay or prevent the progression of aortic stenosis. The hypothesis that lipid-lowering therapy may slow the disease course has been repudiated by two randomized controlled trials which failed to demonstrate any clinical benefit with atorvastatin, simvastatin and ezetimibe (40,41).

On the other hand, favorable perioperative and long-term outcomes with surgical aortic valve replacement have been shown in multiple longitudinal studies, estimating that after the initial perioperative period which carries <5% mortality in first time isolated aortic valve replacements (42) and about 9% mortality in older patients (43), the average long-term survival in older patients after surgery is similar to controls without aortic stenosis. Hence, surgical correction has remained the mainstay of therapy for aortic stenosis because it dramatically improves both survival and quality of life, earning the procedure a class I indication for symptomatic severe aortic stenosis (5).

However, a number of prior studies had showed that 30% to 60% of patients who have an indication for aortic valve replacement do not undergo surgery due to advanced age, poor left ventricular function, prior surgery and comorbid conditions such as renal, pulmonary, and neurologic diseases that render them too high risk for surgery (2,44,45). Since the prevalence of aortic stenosis increases with age, as the elderly population gets larger, it can be inferred that the number of patients unsuitable for surgery will increase as well. Given that the mortality for uncorrected symptomatic severe aortic stenosis is 44% at one year (46) and up to 70% in the high-risk population (47), the need for alternative, less invasive strategies for valvular disease is clearly warranted.

Two percutaneous aortic valves have recently received CE Mark approval (CoreValve in May 2007 and Edwards-Sapien in September 2007) and several other valved stent designs are in development with first-in-man reports or in preclinical testing. Only the Edwards-Sapien valve is currently undergoing evaluation in a randomized multicenter clinical trial against surgery in the United States.

The Edwards-Sapien Valve

Dr. Alain Cribier reported the first human implantation of percutaneous aortic heart valve in 2002 and changed the landscape in the treatment of aortic valvular heart disease (48). The initial prototype, developed by Percutaneous Valve Technologies, Inc. (Fort Lee, NJ), consisted of three bovine pericardial leaflets mounted on a balloon-expandable stainless steel stent designed to have an effective diameter range of 21 to 23 mm following deployment. The implantation was performed using a transvenous, or antegrade approach, where the femoral vessels are exposed via surgical cut down and the femoral vein is cannulated with a 24 French sheath for access. The delivery catheter is advanced through the right atrium into the left atrium using trans-septal puncture, then across the mitral valve into the left ventricle, and finally into the left ventricular outflow tract to be positioned between the diseased leaflets, thus approaching the valve in an antegrade direction (Figure 7.9).

The prototypic percutaneous aortic valve was implanted in a 57-year-old male with calcified critical aortic stenosis who failed previous balloon valvuloplasty and was in cardiogenic shock as well as leg ischemia at the time of procedure. Following the procedure, the aortic pressure rose from a 70 mmHg systolic to 120 mm Hg with the aortic valve gradient decreased from 30 to 6 mm Hg. The calculated valve

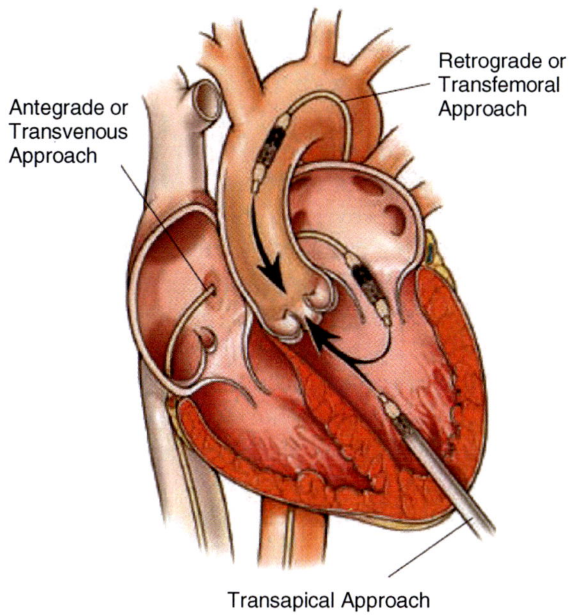

FIGURE 7.9 Schematic of percutaneous valve implantation techniques. (From Ref. 62, with permission.)

area increased from 0.6 to 1.9 cm². Unfortunately, the patient died 17 weeks after the procedure due to a myriad of comorbidities (48).

In December 2003, Edwards LifeSciences (Irvine, CA) acquired Percutaneous Valve Technologies. The ongoing single-center phase 1 pilot the Initial Registry of EndoVascular Implantation of Valves in Europe (I-REVIVE) study had already been initiated in August of the same year. Minor changes were then added to the protocol and the study was continued as Registry of Endovascular Critical Aortic Stenosis Treatment (RECAST) trial. The Cribier-Edwards valve was redesigned into a sutureless balloon-expandable trileaflet valve consisting of equine pericardial tissue sewn into a 14 mm long stainless steel frame with an external diameter of 22 to 26 mm on implantation. The stent was partly covered with fabric on the ventricular side in order to form a seal against the aortic annulus and mounted on a delivery balloon catheter.

Despite the advantages of using the femoral vein, which can readily accommodate larger sheaths, provide greater ease of crossing severely stenotic valves and generally has lower bleeding complications with venous compared to arterial access, there is a significant risk of mitral valve injury potentially resulting in severe mitral regurgitation with the antegrade approach. The procedure itself is also often very complex and difficult to reproduce. With refinements of the sheath and delivery systems and accumulation of clinical experience, the transarterial retrograde approach has become the preferred technique. In the retrograde method, arterial access is gained either through a surgical cutdown or with percutaneous arterial puncture. Once access is established, the prosthetic stent compressed within a delivery catheter is advanced in a retrograde fashion into the stenotic valve (Figure 7.9). After stent deployment and catheter removal, open surgical closure or a percutaneous vascular closure device is used to achieve hemostasis.

While technically easier and generally faster than the antegrade method, the retrograde approach can be complicated by injury to the femoral artery or an inability to cross severely stenotic valves. In addition, it is not feasible in patients with severe aortoiliac peripheral vascular disease due to small caliber vessels and a high stroke risk. These limitations prompted the introduction of the transapical approach which was first described in a porcine model by Walther et al. from Leipzig, Germany (49). The transapical approach provides more direct access to the aortic annulus which obviates the need for large-bore access sites in diseased vessels and has been used with good results as well as fewer vascular complications. This technique is ideal for patients with small-diameter vessels, severe atherosclerotic disease or porcelain aortas. After a small anterolateral thoracotomy incision is made in the fifth or sixth intercostal space, the left ventricular apex is punctured with a needle. A sheath is inserted into the apex, which allows a delivery catheter with the mounted stent to reach the stenotic valve in an antegrade fashion (Figure 7.9). After valve deployment, the delivery catheter is withdrawn, and the apical puncture site is closed with purse string sutures. A major procedural consideration is stroke risk. Of the three approaches, the incidence of periprocedural stroke was demonstrated to be lowest with the transapical approach at rates of 0% to 5% versus the reported 4% to 10% with the transfemoral route. This observation is likely due to the minimal aortic manipulation offered with transapical access (47). The disadvantages of this technique stem from the need for general anesthesia, thoracotomy, apical repair and chest tube placement. Procedural complications include left ventricular aneurysm or pseudoaneurysm and pneumothorax. Despite these difficulties, outcomes data for this approach is favorable and comparable to the transfemoral technique. Procedural success has been reported to be between 88% and 97%, with a 30-day mortality ranging from 10% to 17% (47,50–54).

In all three approaches, the actual delivery of the valve is similar. Once the native valve is crossed and a guidewire is in place, a balloon valvuloplasty is initially performed to open the stenosed native valve. Positioning of the prosthesis is then guided by fluoroscopy, angiography and transesophageal echocardiography. The ideal stent position is with the mid-portion of the prosthetic valve abutting the native valve, making sure that the superior edge of the prosthesis does not occlude the coronary ostia and the inferior edge does not impinge on the motion of the mitral valve leaflets. Once proper positioning is ensured using the aforementioned modalities, the prosthesis is deployed using maximum inflation and rapid deflation of the delivery balloon (Figure 7.10). Both the valvuloplasty and the valve deployment are carried out with simultaneous rapid right ventricular pacing at rates between 180 and 220 bpm to reduce stroke volume, minimize forward flow, and ultimately decrease the risk of valve displacement during deployment. In cases of significant paravalvular leaks after valve insertion, a postballoon dilation with a larger balloon is frequently performed. In general, the selected valve size is slightly larger than the patient's native annular diameter in order to decrease the risk of paravalvular leaks; for example, a 23 mm valve would be used in a patient with an annular diameter of no more than 21 mm and a 26 mm valve is often implanted in patients with annulus diameter greater than 21 mm.

In clinical practice, the overall procedural success was reported between 70% in the earlier trials and 97% in later reports, with an average increase in aortic valvular area from 0.6 to 1.7 cm^2 and a decrease in transvalvular gradient from 42 to 10 mm Hg. The reduction in afterload translated into symptomatic relief, with an improvement of at least one NYHA functional class reported in most studies. In addition, a significant increase in ejection fraction was observed, most notably in patients with a preoperative ejection fraction of <45%. All improvements were sustained for the duration of follow-up, currently out to two years for some patients. The 30-day mortality was 10% to 22%, highest in the earlier experiences, with a six-month mortality estimated at an average of 77% (50,53–56). The decrease in procedural and clinical adverse events with time suggests that there is a learning curve with this procedure. This was highlighted when Webb et al. reported his experience on the first 25 patients with a procedural success of 76% and a 30-day mortality of 16%, while the numbers were 96% and 8%, respectively, in the subsequent 25 patients (50). Importantly, the reported survival rate at a median of 359 days was 81% for this cohort of patients which is much higher than expected with either balloon valvuloplasty or medical management alone.

The current generation of the Cribier-Edwards valve has been renamed the Edwards-Sapien valve (Figure 7.11). Instead of equine tissue, this iteration incorporates bovine pericardium within a similar stainless-steel frame, and the surrounding fabric now extends further to improve coaptation with the annulus

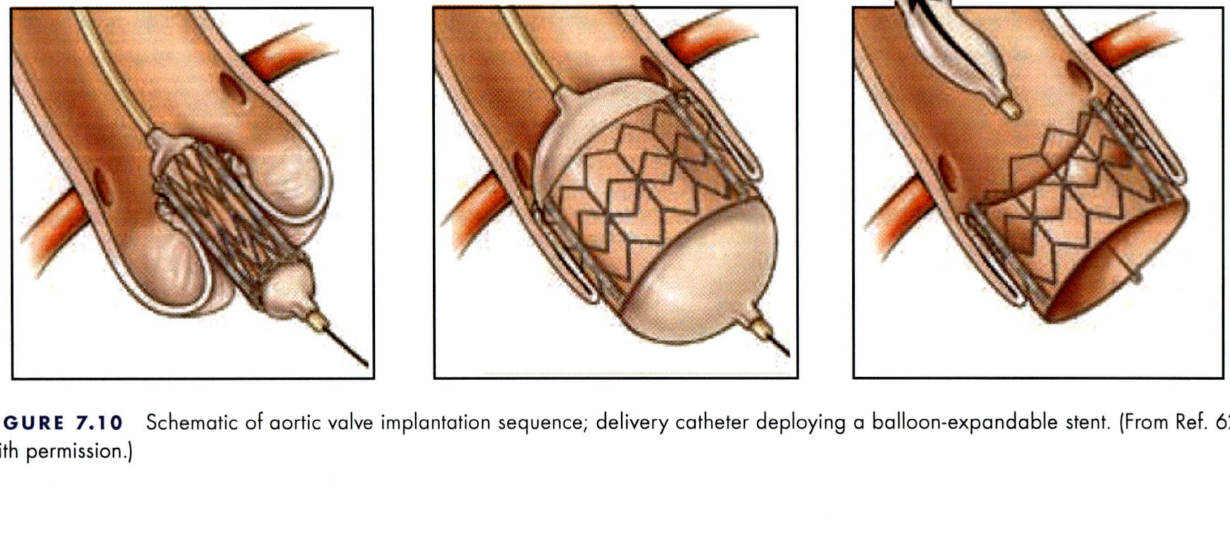

FIGURE 7.10 Schematic of aortic valve implantation sequence; delivery catheter deploying a balloon-expandable stent. (From Ref. 62, with permission.)

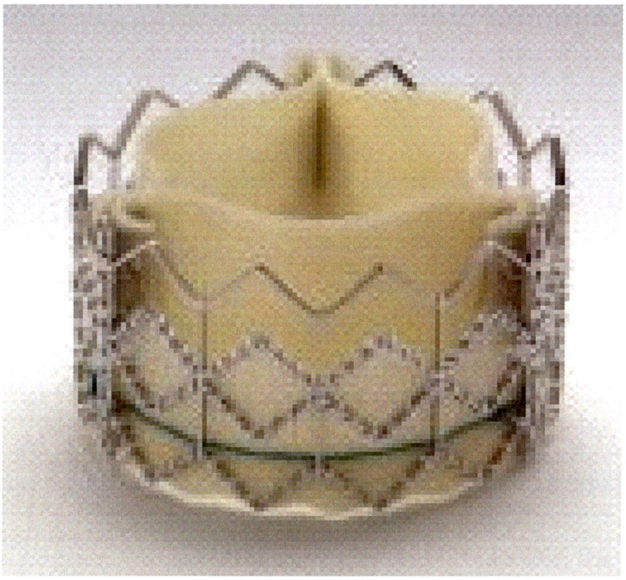

FIGURE 7.11 The Edwards-Sapien valve. (Edwards Lifesciences, Inc., with permission.)

and reduce paravalvular leaks. The current device is available in two expandable diameters: 23 and 26 mm, requiring 22F and 24F (previously 26F) sheaths, respectively. This second generation Edwards valve has been implanted via the retrograde and transapical approaches in clinical trials. The trans-septal approach has largely been abandoned due to technical difficulties and high procedural complications.

Investigations with the Edwards-Sapien valve have yielded good outcomes similar to those with its predecessor, documenting procedural success rates of 88% to 91% with 8% to 17% 30-day mortality. Survival at six months was 60% to 78% and Walther et al. (51) noted a 71% one-year survival. Measurable success is evidenced by an increase in valve area from 0.6 to 1.6 cm^2, and a decrease in mean aortic gradient from 38 to 8 mm Hg, on average. Significant improvements in both heart failure class (one on average) and ejection fraction were also reported (47,51,52,57). All hemodynamic measurements remained stable throughout the 6-month follow-up (47,57).

The Edwards-Sapien valve is currently in a phase 3 clinical trial in the United States, the ongoing Placement of AoRTic traNscathetER valve (PARTNER) trial is a prospective randomized multicenter study to assess the safety and efficacy of the Edwards-Sapien valve in the treatment of severe aortic stenosis in high-risk patients. Participants of the study are randomized within two separate arms of the trial. Cohort A is a surgical arm comparing the percutaneous technique with conventional surgery with the objective of demonstrating noninferiority of the catheter-based procedure in 690 patients. Cohort B involves 350 patients not eligible for surgery with at least a 50% estimated surgical morbidity and mortality. These patients will be randomized to be treated either medically with or without balloon valvuloplasty versus percutaneous replacement via femoral approach with the intention of showing superiority of the Edwards-Sapien valve placement over medically treated patients. As of January 31, 2009, 700 patients had been enrolled into the PARTNER trial.

The CoreValveRevalving System

In contrast to the balloon-expandable Edwards-Sapien valve, the CoreValve^{tm} (CoreValve Inc, Irvine CA) is a sutureless self-expanding valve designed to assume a predetermined hourglass shape once released from its constraining sheath (Figure 7.12). The first-generation valve used bovine pericardial leaflets, whereas the subsequent second- and third-generation devices have porcine tissue valves and sealing cuff. The 50-mm nitinol frame with a flared superior portion ensures adequate fixation along the ascending aorta. The frame is also designed to fully expand against the walls of the left ventricular outflow tract and the aortic root with minimal recoil, obliterating space between the prosthesis and the adjacent walls in order to minimize the risk of paravalvular leaks. Although the superior portion of the stent spans both coronary ostia, the large openings within the framework allow blood to flow freely into the coronaries. A unique advantage with this valve is the added capacity for the device to be retrieved and repositioned after partial implantation in order to minimize stent valve misplacement. The internal diameter of the stent is designed to expand between 21 and 22 mm and the device is deployed via a 24F (first generation), 21F (second generation), or more recently an 18F (third generation) delivery system (58).

The first-generation CoreValve prosthesis was evaluated in 2006 by Grube et al. (59), who reported an 84% procedural success with a 20% 30-day mortality, a reduction in transvalvular gradient (44–12 mm Hg) and a significantly higher functional class at a 30-day follow-up. Subsequently, Grube et al. (58) and Marcheix et al. (60) assessed the second and third-generation devices and reported procedural success at 74% and 100%, with a 30-day mortality of 12% and 20%,

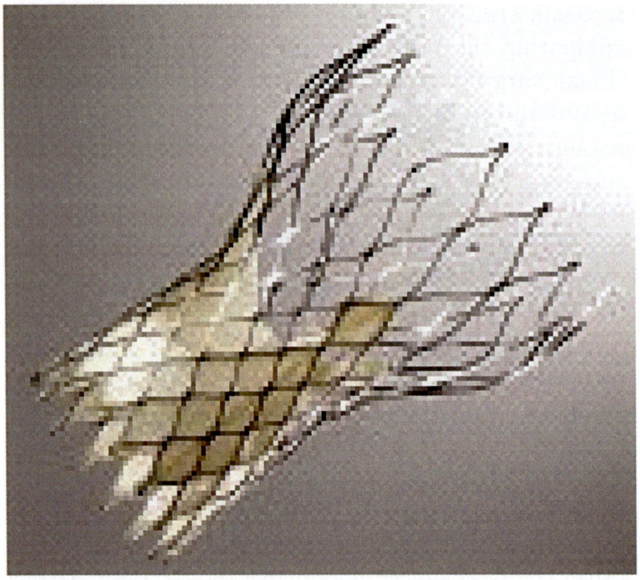

FIGURE 7.12 The CoreValve. (Medtronic, Inc., with permission.)

respectively. Both studies showed a significant improvement in hemodynamic aortic valve parameters (aortic orifice area increased from 0.6 to 1.2 mm Hg; gradient decreased from 47 to 9 mm Hg) as well as an average increase of at least one NYHA functional class.

Currently, the CoreValve still awaits FDA approval for an investigational device exemption (IDE) to initiate a clinical trial in the United States. In the meantime, Medtronic, Inc. (Minneapolis, MN) announced acquisition of CoreValve on February 23, 2009. Given Medtronic's longstanding involvement in the prosthetic valve technology, this transaction will certainly further help facilitate future clinical program developments of the CoreValve Revalving system in the coming years.

Procedural Complications

Several procedural complications are uniquely associated with percutaneous aortic valve procedures. Not unexpectedly, one of the most common complications is aortic regurgitation due to incomplete apposition of the valved stent to the aortic annulus and surrounding walls. In addition to adverse hemodynamic effects, the shear stress on red blood cells resulting from paravalvular leaks can result in low-grade hemolysis and other hematologic complications. Fortunately, postprocedure paravalvular insufficiency was generally mild and stable during subsequent follow-up (50). The risk of this complication can be minimized by oversizing the valve in reference to the target annular diameter.

Migration or embolization of the prosthesis is another major concern. Although infrequently encountered, such an event generally requires open retrieval of the device, although cases have been reported where the embolized stent lodged in the thoracic aorta without any resulting complications and was not retrieved. Meticulous imaging during device deployment to insure proper placement and the use of larger caliber valves has been associated with a lower rate of prosthesis migration and embolization.

While rarely observed, coronary obstruction can be a catastrophic complication. The prosthetic valves themselves can obstruct the coronary ostia. The CoreValve frame generally reaches above the level of the aortic root, but the large openings within the CoreValve stent strut generally do not obstruct blood flow and even allow catheter insertion into the coronary ostia. The Edwards-Sapien valve usually does not extend to the coronary origins. However, the possibility of the implanted stent displacing a fibrotic and thickened native aortic leaflet over a coronary ostium resulting in obstruction has been reported. To minimize this risk, operators currently use preprocedural CT measurement and intraprocedural echocardiographic doppler assessment during balloon valvuloplasty prior to actual valve placement to identify potential patients with bulky obstructive native leaflets which constitutes an anatomical exclusion for the procedure.

Stroke in this setting is generally due to an embolization of either friable native valve material or an atheroembolism from a plaque on the ascending aorta associated with catheter manipulation. It is a relatively common complication, occurring in up to 10% of cases. However, this number may be lower in the current practices since most patients with severe peripheral vascular disease, who are inherently at a higher risk for stroke, are more likely to undergo valve placement using the transapical technique as reported by Rodes-Cabau et al. (57).

Although no study observed structural valve deterioration during the short time of follow-up reported thus far (maximum two years), the lifespan of the valve remains to be determined. The Cribier-Edwards valve has a 2% failure rate at 12 years and 4% at 20 years (47). It remains to be seen whether the Edwards-Sapien and CoreValve implants will be as durable. The question of therapeutic options in the event of device failure also remains to be answered, although there have been multiple reports of successful valve-in-valve restenting with a second prosthesis placed within the first for severe aortic regurgitation or valve dysfunction (47,58).

Other Novel Percutaneous Aortic Valves

A major drawback of all of the current percutaneous valve designs is that once fully deployed, they cannot be repositioned. Given the necessity for optimal valve placement, an ideal device should be flexible and collapsible to allow for repeated retrieval and repositioning. To that end, Schofer et al. (61) recently published a first-in-man feasibility study using a novel nonmetallic prosthesis (Direct Flow Medical Inc, Santa Rosa, CA). The trileaflet valve is made of bovine pericardial tissue encased in a conformable fabric with two independently inflatable balloon rings attached to its superior and inferior borders. The device is 16 and 17 mm in length, with a 23 or 25 mm internal diameter, corresponding to an external diameter of 27 and 29 mm, and is delivered via a 22F sheath. After initial balloon valvuloplasty of the stenosed aortic valve, both stent valve rings are inflated with a contrast-containing saline mixture to expand the valve across the native annulus and subsequently deflated. They are then inflated individually and the apparatus is sequentially shifted within the outflow tract until it is in the desired location. Once satisfactory position and function are confirmed, the contrast solution within the rings is replaced by a polymer which solidifies within 24 hours to permanently fix the implant in place.

Using the retrograde technique, the authors reported an 80% procedural success rate, with a 6.7% 30-day mortality and a similar frequency of stroke. The average aortic valve area increased from 0.8 to 1.64 cm^2, with a concomitant decrease in gradient from ≥35 to 14 mm Hg and at least one NYHA functional class improvement. Although the mortality numbers for the percutaneous procedure may seem relatively high, the results have to be interpreted in light of the fact that all patients entering these trials are high risk, nonoperable candidates with multiple comorbidities and advanced age, with an average 30-day operative mortality in the range of 20% to 30%, as estimated by the EuroScore risk assessment.

Percutaneous aortic valve replacement is clearly in its early stages of development. Currently, there are a plethora of companies with various percutaneous aortic valve designs (Table 7.2) that promise to address

Table 7.2 Percutaneous aortic valve replacement technologies

Company (Location)	Name of Device	Development Stage
Edwards LifeSciences (CA, U.S.)	Edwards-Sapien	U.S. randomized CE mark
Medtronic (MN, U.S.)	CoreValve Revalving System	Outside U.S. CE mark
Direct Flow Medical (CA, U.S.)	Direct Flow	Outside U.S.
Endoluminal Technology Research (FL, U.S.)	Paniagua	Early clinical
ATS Medical (MN, U.S.)	3f Entrata	Preclinical
Hansen Medical (CA, U.S.)	AorTx	Preclinical
Sadra Medical (CA, U.S.)	Lotus Valve System	Early clinical
VenaValve Technology (Muenchen, Germany)	JenaValve	Preclinical
Sorin Group (Saluggia, Italy)	Perceval S	Outside U.S.
Heart Leaflet Technologies (MN, U.S.)	Heart Leaflet	Outside U.S.
Medtronic (MN U.S.)	Ventor Embracer	Outside U.S.

various limitations associated with the current CE Mark approved stent valves. The enhanced attributes of these more novel designs include a lower profile for safer and easier delivery as well as the capacity to reposition and retrieve devices to optimize valve placement. Down the road, tissue engineering, nanotechnology and novel biomaterials may produce valve surfaces that are more flexible and collapsible for delivery, more biocompatible and, at the same time, more durable than the current surgical bioprosthetic or mechanical valves.

FUTURE DIRECTIONS

The introduction of percutaneous heart valve technology has certainly changed the landscape in the treatment of patients with valvular heart disease. Although this field is in its early stages of development, it is an exciting and burgeoning area of clinical research. Preliminary clinical results have been encouraging for the MitraClip, mitral annular devices, as well as aortic stent valve prostheses. Importantly, they have also highlighted some of the limitations of these emerging technologies. For example, the current mitral valve leaflet apposition technology is limited by its applicability only to appose A_2P_2 segments. In addition, anatomical variability of the coronary sinus with respect to the mitral annulus has rendered coronary sinus based technologies less generalizable and their clinical efficacy less predictable. For aortic valve replacement, the current large profile of both the Edwards-Sapien and the CoreValve Revalving Systems presents significant barriers in applying these devices in patients with peripheral vascular disease including aortic arch disease. Whether the transapical approach is a safer alternative remains to be determined. Furthermore, long-term durability of treatment with these techniques is currently unknown. Further evaluation and integration of advanced imaging techniques (e.g., 3D echocardiography, cardiac CT, and cardiac MRI) to delineate aortic and mitral leaflets, mitral apparatus, and coronary sinus anatomy may help tailor specific treatment approaches and optimize placements of these novel devices.

Although early clinical outcomes with the current percutaneous valve technologies indeed offer considerable promise to those high-risk patients who are not deemed to be operative candidates, conventional open heart surgery should still be the method of choice for the majority of patients with valvular heart disease. The future role of percutaneous valve technology can only be evaluated through systematic analysis of clinical outcomes based on head-to-head randomized comparisons of these novel devices against standard surgical results with long-term follow-up as exemplified by the PARTNER and EVEREST II trials. Further technical improvements, cumulative operator experience and longer term clinical follow-up are clearly warranted before this novel therapeutic option can be extended to a broader spectrum of patients with valvular heart dysfunction.

Finally, this important field of percutaneous valve treatments can only be developed expeditiously and to its fullest extent through collaborative efforts from interventional cardiologists, cardiac surgeons, and imaging experts as well as the device industry. Through these coordinated efforts and concerted collaborations, one can certainly envision that some day percutaneous heart valve techniques will offer safer and less invasive treatment options for a broad spectrum of patients with valvular heart disease.

REFERENCES

1. Nkomo VT, Gardin JM, Skelton TN, et al. Burden of valvular heart diseases: a population-based study. *Lancet* 2006; 368:1005–11.
2. Iung B, Baron G, Butchart EG, et al. A prospective survey of patients with valvular heart disease in Europe: the Euro Heart Survey on valvular disease. *Eur Heart J* 2003; 24:1231–43.
3. Kan JS, White RI Jr, Mitchell SE, et al. Percutaneous balloon valvuloplasty: a new method for treating congenital pulmonary-valve stenosis. *N Eng J Med* 1982; 307:540.
4. Chen CR, Cheng TO, Huang T, et al. Percutaneous balloon valvuloplasty for pulmonic stenosis in adolescents and adults. *N Eng J Med* 1996; 335:21–5.
5. Bonow RO, Carabello BA, Chatterjee K, et al. Focused update incorporated into the ACC/AHA 2006 guidelines for the management of patients with valvular heart disease: a report of the American College of Cardiology/American Heart Association task force of practice guidelines. *Circulation* 2008; 118:e523–661.
6. Wilkens GT, Weyman AE, Abascal VM, et al. Percutaneous balloon dilatation of the mitral valve: an analysis of echocardiographic variables related to outcome and the mechanism of dilatation. *Br Heart J* 1988; 60:299–308.
7. Reyes VP, Raju BS, Wynne J, et al. Percutaneous balloon valvuloplasty compared with open surgical commissurotomy for mitral stenosis. *NEJM* 1994; 331:961–7.
8. Palacios IF, Sanchez PL, Harrell LC, et al. Which patients benefit from percutaneous mitral balloon valvuloplasty. *Circulation* 2002; 105:1465–71.

9. Cribier A, Savin T, Saoudi N, et al. Percutaneous transluminal valvuloplasty of acquired aortic stenosis in elderly patients: an alternative to valve replacement? *Lancet* 1986; 1:63–7.
10. American Heart Assn. Percutaneous balloon aortic valvuloplasty. Acute and 30-day follow-up results in 674 patients from the NHLBI Balloon Valvuloplasty Registry. *Circulation* 1991 Dec; 84(6): 2383–97.
11. Agarwal A, Kini AS, Attanti S, et al. Results of repeat balloon valvuloplasty for treatment of aortic stenosis in patients aged 59 to 104 years. *Am J Cardiol* 2005 Jan 1; 95(1):43–7.
12. Lieberman EB, Bashore TM, Hermiller JB, et al. Balloon aortic valvuloplasty in adults: failure of procedure to improve long-term survival. *J Am Coll Cardiol* 1995 Nov 15; 26(6): 1522–8.
13. Bonhoeffer P, Boudjemline Y, Saliba Z, et al. Percutaneous replacement of pulmonary valve in a right-ventricle to pulmonary-artery prosthetic conduit with valve dysfunction. *Lancet* 2000; 356:1403–5.
14. Lurz P, Coats L, Khambadkone S, et al. Percutaneous pulmonary valve implantation. Impact of evolving technology and learning curve on clinical outcome. *Circulation* 2008; 117:1964–72.
15. Blondheim DS, Jacobs LE, Kotler MN, et al. Dilated cardiomyopathy with mitral regurgitation: decreased survival despite a low frequency of left ventricular thrombus. *Am Heart J* 1991; 122(3 Pt 1):763–71.
16. Grigioni F, Enriquez-Sarano M, Zehr KJ, et al. Ischemic mitral regurgitation: long-term outcome and prognostic implications with quantitative Doppler assessment. *Circulation* 2001; 103(13):1759–64.
17. Fedak PW, McCarthy PM, Bonow RO. Evolving concepts and technologies in mitral valve repair. *Circulation* 2008; 117:963–74.
18. Mirabel M, Iung B, Baron G, et al. What are the characteristics of patients with severe, symptomatic mitral regurgitation who are denied surgery? *Eur Heart J* 2007; 28:1358–65.
19. Alfieri O, Maisano F, De Bonis M, et al. The double-orifice technique in mitral valve repair: a simple solution for complex problems. *J Thorac Cardiovasc Surg* 2001; 122:674–81.
20. Bhudia SK, McCarthy PM, Smedira NG, et al. Edge-to-edge (Alfieri) mitral repair: results in diverse clinical settings. *Ann Thorac Surg* 2004; 77:1598–606.
21. Feldman T, Wasserman HS, Herrmann HC, et al. Percutaneous mitral valve repair using the edge-to-edge technique: six-month results of the EVEREST phase I clinical trial. *J Am Coll Cardiol* 2005; 46:2134–40.
22. Herrmann HC, Rohatgi S, Wassermann HS, et al. Mitral valve hemodynamic effects of percutaneous edge-to-edge repair with the MitraClip device for mitral regurgitation. *Catheter Cardiovasc Interv* 2006; 68:821–8.
23. Evalve press release of presentations at the Transcatheter Cardiovascular Therapeutics symposium. October 24, 2007. Washington D.C.
24. Evalve press release of presentations at The Society for Cardiovascular Angiography and Interventions-American College of Cardiology i2 Summit(SCAI-ACCi2). April 1, 2008. Chicago, IL.
25. Naqvi TZ, Buchbinder M, Zarbatany D, et al. Beating-heart percutaneous mitral valve using a transcatheter endovascular suturing device in an animal model. *Catheter Cardiovasc Interv* 2007; 69:525–31.
26. Savage EB, Ferguson TB Jr, DiSesa VJ, et al. Use of mitral valve repair: analysis of contemporary United States experience reported to the Society of Thoracic Surgeons National Cardiac Database. *Ann Thorac Surg* 2003; 75:820–5.
27. Kaye DM, Byrne M, Alferness C, et al. Feasibility and short-term efficacy of percutaneous mitral annular reduction for the therapy of heart failure-induced mitral regurgitation. *Circulation* 2003; 108:1795–7.
28. Byrne MJ, Kaye DM, Mathis M, et al. Percutaneous mitral annular reduction provides continued benefit in an ovine model of dilated cardiomyopathy. *Circulation* 2004; 110:3088–92.
29. Daimon M, Shiota T, Gillinov AM, et al. Percutaneous mitral valve repair for chronic ischemic mitral regurgitation: a real-time three-dimensional echocardiographic study in an ovine model. *Circulation* 2005; 111:2183–9.
30. Webb JG, Harnek J, Munt BI, et al. Percutaneous transvenous mitral annuloplasty: initial human experience with device implantation in the coronary sinus. *Circulation* 2006; 113:851–5.
31. Alec Vahanian. 12–Month interim results of the percutaneous MONARC™ system for the treatment of functional mitral regurgitation. The Evolution Study. Presented at TCT 2008.
32. Dubreuil O, Basmadjian A, Ducharme A, et al. Percutaneous mitral valve annuloplasty for ischemic mitral regurgitation: first in human experience with a temporary implant. *Catheter Cardiovasc Interv* 2007; 69:1053–61.
33. Duffy SJ, Federman J, Farrington C, et al. Feasibility and short-term efficacry of percutaneous mitral annular reduction for the therapy of functional mitral regurgitation in patients with heart failure. *Catheter Cardiovasc Interv* 2006; 68: 205–10.
34. Schofer J. The Carillon mital annuloplasty device European Union Study (AMADEUS): 6-Month outcomes. Presented at ESC 2008.
35. Rogers JH, Macoviak JA, Rahdert DA, et al. Percutaneous septal sinus shortening: a novel procedure for the treatment of functional mitral regurgitation. *Circulation* 2006; 113:2329–34.
36. Palacios IF, Condado JA, Brandi S, et al. Safety and efficacy of acute percutaneous septal sinus shortening: first in human experience. *Catheter Cardiovasc Interv* 2007; 69:513–18.
37. Kempfert J, Blumenstein JM, Borger MA, et al. Minimally invasive off-pump valve-in-a-valve implantation: the atrial transcatheter approach for re-operative mitral valve replacement. *Eur Heart J* 2008; 29:2382–7.
38. Otto CM, Burwash IG, Legget ME, et al. Prospective study of asymptomatic valvular aortic stenosis. Clinical, echocardiographic and exercise predictors of outcome. *Circulation* 1997; 95:2262–70.
39. Livanainen AM, Lindroos M, Tilvis R, et al. Natural history of aortic valve stenosis of varying severity in the elderly. *Am J Cardiol* 1996; 78:97–101.
40. Cowell SJ, Newby DE, Prescott RJ, et al. A randomized trial of intensive lipid-lowering therapy in calcific aortic stenosis. *N Engl J Med* 2005; 352:2389–97.
41. Rossebo AB, Pedersen TR, Boman K, et al. Intensive lipid low ering with simvastatin and ezetimibe in aortic stenosis. *N Engl J Med* 2008 Sep 25; 359(13):1343–56.
42. Astor BC, Kaczmarek RG, Hefflin B, et al. Mortality after aortic valve replacement: results from a nationally representative database. *Ann Thorac Surg* 2000 Dec; 70(6):1939–45.

43. Goodney PP, O'Connor GT, Wennberg DE, et al. Do hospitals with low mortality rates in coronary artery bypass also perform well in valve replacement? *Ann Thorac Surg* 2003; 76:1131–7.
44. Varadarajan P, Kapoor N, Bansal RC, et al. Clinical profile and natural history of 453 nonsurgically managed patients with severe aortic stenosis. *Ann Thorac Surg* 2006 Dec; 82(6):2111–15.
45. Pai RG, Kapoor N, Bansal RC, et al. Malignant natural history of asymptomatic severe aortic stenosis: benefit of aortic valve replacement. *Ann Thorac Surg* 2006 Dec; 82(6):2116–22.
46. Pellika PA, Sarano ME, Nishimura RA, et al. Outcome of 622 adults with asymptomatic, hemodynamically significant aortic stenosis during prolonged follow-up. *Circulation* 2005; 111(24):3290–5.
47. Svensson LG, Dewey T, Kapadia S, et al. United States feasibility study of transcatheter insertion of a stented aortic valve by the left ventricular apex. *Ann Thorac Surg* 2008 Jul; 86(1):46–54.
48. Cribier A, Eltchaninoff H, Bash A, et al. Percutaneous transcatheter implantation of an aortic valve prosthesis for calcific aortic stenosis: first human case description. *Circulation* 2002 Dec 10; 106(24):3006–3008.
49. Walther T, Dewey T, Wimmer-Greinecker G, et al. Transapical approach for sutureless stent-fixed aortic valve implantation: experimental results. *Eur J Cardio-thoracic Surg* 2006; 29:703–8.
50. Webb JG, Pasupati S, Humphries K, et al. Percutaneous transarterial aortic valve replacement in selected high-risk patients with aortic stenosis. *Circulation* 2007 Aug 14; 116(7):755–63.
51. Walther T, Falk V, Kempfert J, et al. Transapical minimally invasive aortic valve implantation; the initial 50 patients. *Eur J Cardiothorac Surg* 2008 Jun; 33(6):983–8.
52. Walther T, Simon P, Dewey T, et al. Transapical minimally invasive aortic valve implantation: multicenter experience. *Circulation* 2007 Sep 11; 116(11 Suppl):I240–5.
53. Walther T, Falk V, Borger MA, et al. Minimally invasive transapical beating heart aortic valve implantation—proof of concept. *Eur J Cardiothorac Surg* 2007 Jan; 31(1):9–15.
54. Lichtenstein SV, Cheung A, Ye J, et al. Transapical transcatheter aortic valve implantation in humans: initial clinical experience. *Circulation* 2006 Aug 8; 114(6):591–6.
55. Cribier A, Eltchaninoff H, Tron C, et al. Treatment of calcific aortic stenosis with the percutaneous heart valve: mid-term follow-up from the initial feasibility studies: the French experience. *J Am Coll Cardiol* 2006 Mar 21; 47(6):1214–23.
56. Ye J, Cheung A, Lichtenstein SV, et al. Six-month outcome of transapical transcatheter aortic valve implantation in the initial seven patients. *Eur J Cardiothorac Surg* 2007 Jan; 31(1):16–21.
57. Rodés-Cabau J, Dumont E, De La Rochellière R, et al. Feasibility and initial results of percutaneous aortic valve implantation including selection of the transfemoral or transapical approach in patients with severe aortic stenosis. *Am J Cardiol* 2008 Nov 1; 102(9):1240–6.
58. Grube E, Schuler G, Buellesfeld L, et al. Percutaneous aortic valve replacement for severe aortic stenosis in high-risk patients using the second- and current third-generation self-expanding CoreValve prosthesis: device success and 30-day clinical outcome. *J Am Coll Cardiol* 2007;50:69–76.
59. Grube E, Laborde JC, Gerckens U, et al. Percutaneous implantation of the CoreValve self-expanding valve prosthesis in high-risk patients with aortic valve disease: the Siegburg first-in-man study. *Circulation* 2006 Oct 10; 114(15):1616–24.
60. Marcheix B, Lamarche Y, Berry C, et al. Surgical aspects of endovascular retrograde implantation of the aortic CoreValve bioprosthesis in high-risk older patients with severe symptomatic aortic stenosis. *J Thorac Cardiovasc Surg* 2007 Nov; 134(5):1150–6.
61. Schofer J, Schlüter M, Treede H, et al. Retrograde Transarterial implantation of a nonmetallic aortic valve prosthesis in high-surgical-risk patients with severe aortic stenosis: a first-in-man feasibility and safety study. *Circ Cardiovasc Intervent* 2008; 1:126–33.
62. Singh IM, Tuzcu EM, Sishehbor MH, et al. Percutaneous treatment of aortic value stenosis. *Cleve Clin J med.* 2008;75(11): 805–812.

8 Advances in Pulmonary Hypertension

IRINA SOBOL
EVELYN M. HORN

OUTLINE

Pulmonary arterial hypertension (PAH) is an organ-specific vasculopathy characterized by endothelial and smooth muscle (SM) cell proliferation, which leads to occlusion of the medium-sized vessels and in situ thrombosis. This may lead to destruction of some vessels, abnormal growth of other vessels, and the evolution of an "apoptotic resistant" state. This obliterative vasculopathy leads to the progressive increase in pulmonary vascular resistance and ensuing right ventricular (RV) failure. Much progress in this field has occurred due to the availability of new therapeutic agents, the discovery of molecular mechanisms—including the genetics of the subgroup of patients with familial pulmonary hypertension (FPAH) (1)—and the delineation of some of the pathways through which newer agents work. Nevertheless, for many, this disease has an ominous prognosis (2).

Although the prostacyclin analogues, endothelin receptor antagonists (ERA), and phosphodiesterase-5 (PDE-5) inhibitors all have been clinically beneficial and have been associated with modest gains, it is less evident that long-term prognosis has been seriously effected (3). Furthermore, the availability of these medications has promoted consideration of this therapy in nonapproved patient populations in the hope of ameliorating secondary pulmonary hypertension, which now is sometimes the "treatable" part of these other diseases. Yet the newer therapies have been approved only for the limited World Health Organization (WHO) group I patients (Table 8.1). There is a need to differentiate the disease for which the newer expensive approved drugs are useful and those for whom there is either no data or negative data. Lastly, a better understanding of the phenotype of pulmonary hypertension and its complex pathophysiological mechanisms may provide insight into the disease process, and ultimately lead to successful interventions in the more encompassing group of pulmonary hypertension patients with more specific targeted therapies.

CLASSIFICATION

Classification of PAH has evolved over the years with the 1998 WHO classification, the 2003 revised WHO classification (4), and most recently updated at Dana Point, California in 2008 (Table 8.1) (5). Group I PAH includes patients with a unifying pathologic appearance and similar response to treatments, although aspects of the pathophysiological mechanisms may be quite distinct. It includes patients with idiopathic (IPAH), previously known as primary pulmonary hypertension

Table 8.1 Updated clinical classification of pulmonary hypertension

1. Pulmonary arterial hypertension (PAH)
    - 1.1 Idiopathic PAH
    - 1.2 Heritable
        - 1.2.1 BMPR2
        - 1.2.2 ALK1, endoglin (with or without hereditary hemorrhagic telangiectasia)
        - 1.2.3 Unknown
    - 1.3 Drug- and toxin-induced
    - 1.4 Associated with
        - 1.4.1 Connective tissue diseases
        - 1.4.2 HIV infection
        - 1.4.3 Portal hypertension
        - 1.4.4 Congenital heart diseases
        - 1.4.5 Schistosomiasis
        - 1.4.6 Chronic hemolytic anemia
    - 1.5 Persistent pulmonary hypertension of the newborn

1′. Pulmonary veno-occlusive disease and/or pulmonary capillary hemangiomatosis

2. Pulmonary hypertension owing to left heart disease
    - 2.1 Systolic dysfunction
    - 2.2 Diastolic dysfunction
    - 2.3 Valvular disease
3. Pulmonary hypertension owing to lung diseases and/or hypoxia
    - 3.1 Chronic obstructive pulmonary disease
    - 3.2 Interstitial lung disease
    - 3.3 Other pulmonary diseases with mixed restrictive and obstructive pattern
    - 3.4 Sleep-disordered breathing
    - 3.5 Alveolar hypoventilation disorders
    - 3.6 Chronic exposure to high altitude
    - 3.7 Developmental abnormalities
4. Chronic thromboembolic pulmonary hypertension
5. Pulmonary hypertension with unclear multifactorial mechanisms
    - 5.1 Hematologic disorders: myeloproliferative disorders, splenectomy
    - 5.2 Systemic disorders: sarcoidosis, pulmonary Langerhans cell histiocytosis: lymphangioleiomyomatosis, neurofibromatosis, vasculitis
    - 5.3 Metabolic disorders: glycogen storage disease, Gaucher disease, thyroid disorders
    - 5.4 Others: tumoral obstruction, fibrosing mediastinitis, chronic renal failure on dialysis

Source: From Ref. 4, with permission.

(PPH), heritable pulmonary hypertension, drug- and toxin-induced pulmonary hypertension, "associated with known disease" (APAH), persistent pulmonary hypertension of the newborn, and pulmonary veno-occlusive disease (PVOD) and/or pulmonary capillary hemangiomatosis (PCH).

The prevalence of IPAH is one to two cases per million. The NIH cohort survival rates in untreated patients are poor, with a one-year survival rate of 68%, three-year survival rate of 48% and five-year survival rate of 34%. Survival is related to baseline functional status at the time of diagnosis, such that patients who present as functional

New York Heart Association (NYHA) class III or IV or six-minute walk tests less than 332 meters do poorly (6). Of note, the prognosis of patients treated in the modern era with intravenous epoprostenol is improved. Although survival data is limited, comparisons are made to outdated historical controls of the 1991 NIH study, and most randomized clinical data are limited to industry-sponsored studies of 12- to 16-week duration with extension phases. This disease has a female predominance, with a mean age of diagnosis of 36.4 years.

Heritable forms of PAH (previously familiar or FPAH) remains a rare occurrence, includes approximately 300 families, and has been linked to BMPR-2, endoglin and TGF-β receptor mutations (7). The discovery of the BMPR-2 abnormality led to the focus on the TGF-β and SMAD pathways (8). Drug and toxin induced pulmonary hypertension is now a separate subcategory.

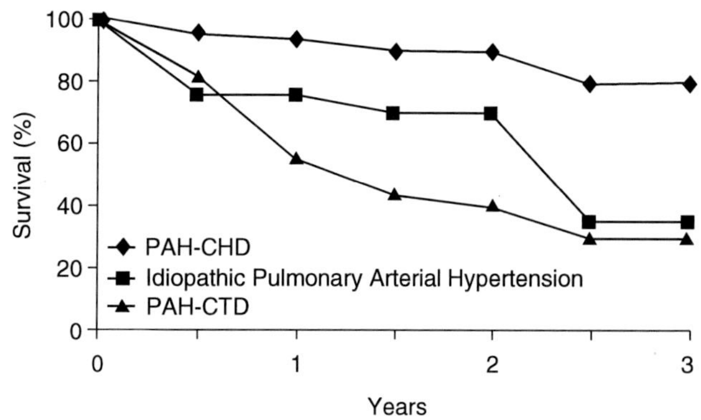

FIGURE 8.1 Comparisons of survival in primary pulmonary hypertension, congenital heart defects, and collagen vascular disease (unpublished data). (CHD, congenital heart disease; CTD, connective tissue disease.) (From Ref. 4.)

APAH is a group with multiple associated diseases, including but not limited to connective tissue diseases (CTD), congenital shunts, portal hypertension, HIV, schistosmiasis and chronic hemolytic anemia. Notably, most clinical studies have included CTD, nonhypoxic CHD, and patients with history of anorexigen use, but excluded HIV (except for a small number of studies and subsequent tracking of patients), portopulmonary hypertension (PPHTN), and hemoglobinopathies. Importantly, although these associated diseases are grouped together, there are significant distinctions in their pathophysiology. Scleroderma spectrum of disease (SSD) is characterized by lung fibrosis causing elevated pulmonary vascular resistance, whereas lupus and mixed connective tissue diseases may have a reversible inflammatory vascular component and HIV may also have a significant inflammatory component. Baseline survival for these distinct populations prior to treatment also varies significantly (Figure 8.1). Also included in WHO group I are patients with pulmonary veno-occlusive disease and pulmonary capillary hemangiomatosis who prior to 2003 were considered as distinct entities; importantly, these individuals may develop pulmonary edema in response to pulmonary vasodilators. Lastly, a small yet distinct subset is persistent pulmonary hypertension of the newborn.

WHO group II patients with pulmonary venous hypertension include patients with systolic heart failure, preserved ejection fraction heart failure (PEFHF), valvular heart disease, and hypertrophic, restrictive, or infiltrative cardiomyopathies. Particular care should be exercised to correctly diagnose and differentiate these patients since targeted pulmonary vasodilator therapy may actually worsen their symptoms, presumably due to increased flow to the left side with an increase in left atrial pressure leading to pulmonary edema. Unfortunately, multiple trials (Table 8.2) have yielded negative results, including use of intravenous (IV) epoprostenol in patients awaiting heart transplant with secondary pulmonary hypertension where treatment was associated with a worse survival (9); treatment with bosentan in chronic stable left ventricular dysfunction (10) and sildenafil (16) also had negative results. An exception is a few promising studies of sildenafil in stable New York Heart Association Class III patients on maximal heart failure therapy using hemodynamic, exercise and quality of life (QOL) parameters (11,12,17,18).

Differentiating diastolic heart failure with secondary pulmonary hypertension from pulmonary hypertension with secondary left ventricular diastolic abnormities is not always a straightforward assessment and is a commonly occurring diagnostic dilemma in light of the increasing prevalence of diastolic heart failure in the aging population. Any patient who is being evaluated for pulmonary hypertension and in whom the measurement of the pulmonary capillary wedge pressure (PCWP) is at all questionable should have a direct assessment of the left ventricular end diastolic pressure. An erroneously elevated wedge pressure may be encountered in patients with severe pulmonary hypertension due to bowing of the septum into the left ventricle.

Table 8.2 Major trials with pulmonary vasodilators in patients with heart failure

Study (Ref.)	Agent	Condition	*N* patients randomized	Clinical Improvement	Hemodynamic Improvement
FIRST(9)	Epoprostenol	Advanced HF	471	Worse than placebo	Yes
REACH-1 (10)	Bosentan	Severe HF	377	Worse than placebo, then similar	n/a
Long-term use of Sildenafil in HF (11)	Sildenafil	Stable HF	46	Yes	Yes (aerobic efficiency)
Sildenafil improved exercise capacity in HF (12)	Sildenafil	HF and secondary pulmonary HTN	34	Yes	Yes
RITZ-5 (13)	Tezosentan	Pulmonary edema	84	Yes	n/a
VERITAS (14)	Tezosentan	ADHF	1300	Similar to placebo	
ENABLE (15)	Bosentan	Severe HF	1613	Probable worse than placebo	n/a
FDHF01	Sitaxsentan	PEFHF	Target 150	Results pending	n/a
RELAX	Sildenafil	PEFHF	Target 190	Results pending	Results pending

HF, heart failure; HTN, hypertension; ADHF, acute decompensated heart failure; PEFHF, preserved ejection fraction; HF, heart failure.

Treatment strategies for progressive pulmonary venous hypertension should focus on treatment of the underlying disease. For patients with advanced decompensated systolic heart failure and secondary pulmonary hypertension, it is essential to reduce the pulmonary vascular resistance prior to heart transplantation to prevent acute RV failure of the donor heart. The use of continuous milrinone, occasionally nesiritide, and earlier intervention with mechanical circulatory device support (19) as a bridge to cardiac transplantation is considered a standard approach for this group of patients. Earlier intervention with valve repair or replacement for patients with mitral valve disease and aortic valve disease with associated pulmonary hypertension is recommended.

The most difficult patient population to address is that which includes patients with diastolic heart failure and PEFHF with secondary pulmonary venous hypertension, given the lack of effective treatment strategies for this large and growing group of patients. The comorbidities of obesity, sleep apnea, hypertension, diabetes, older age, anemia, and chronic renal failure are all associated with PEFHF and secondary pulmonary hypertension. A pilot study using the selective endothelin receptor antagonist sitaxsentan (not approved in the United States) has been completed; early reports are promising and warrant further investigation. The ongoing RELAX study using PDE-5 inhibitors to improve clinical status and exercise capacity in diastolic heart failure in this patient population is ongoing and will also be of interest. It remains speculative as to why some patients with the same degree of left atrial hypertension develop progressive and irreversible PAH and others do not. Perhaps here too a genetic predisposition for such exists, and the exogenous trigger leads to the manifestation of the pulmonary hypertension phenotype similar to the "two-hit hypothesis" of FPAH.

WHO group III is comprised of patients with lung diseases and hypoxemia. Hypoxic vasoconstriction is specific to the lung vasculature and not to the systemic vasculature. This initially adaptive response to hypoxemia—to decrease ventilation/perfusion (V/Q) mismatch—may become maladaptive and promote pathological hypoxic pulmonary vasoconstriction, with progressive elevation of pulmonary pressures and ensuing RV failure. Ultimately, this may result in increased intimal and adventitia thickness, causing increased pulmonary vascular resistance and a decrease in the number of blood vessels in the hypoxic lung (20).

The initial sensors and subsequent signal transduction systems of hypoxic vasoconstriction (HPV) remain an area of intense investigation (21,22). At the cellular level, pulmonary artery smooth muscle (PASM) contraction depends on an increase in cytosolic calcium from the extracellular space as well as release from intracellular stores, and membrane depolarization due to closure of K^+ channels. Many argue that the mitochondria is a primary oxygen sensor such that electron transport chain inhibitors can specifically inhibit HPV and/or prevent the hypoxia-specific response. Reactive oxygen species are also implicated in HPV. Two different models are proposed: one describes an increase in mitochondrial ROS mediated via increased intracellular calcium release, and the second describes a decrease in mitochondrial ROS mediated via inhibition of the Kv channel (Figure 8.2).

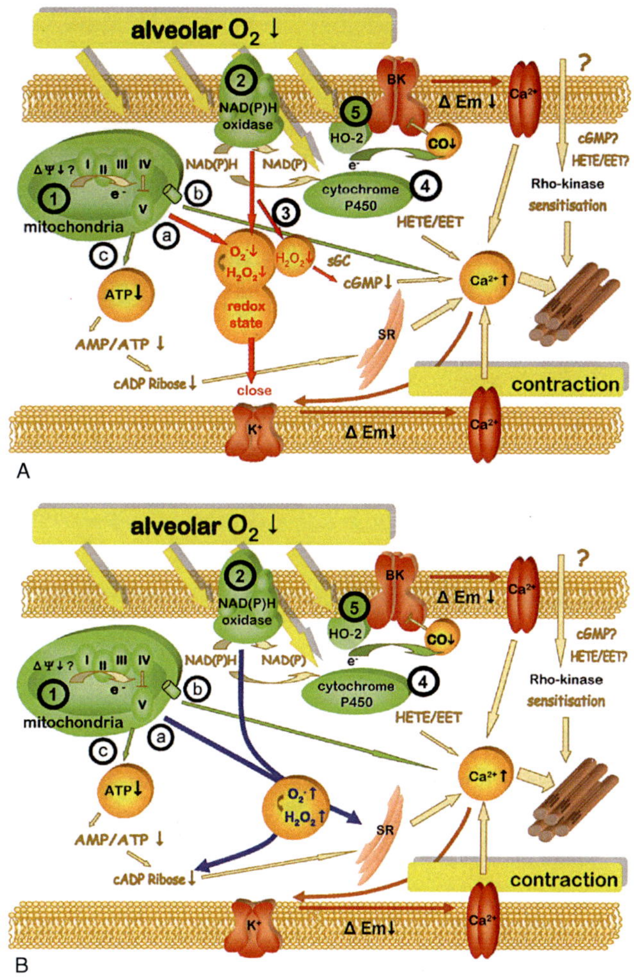

FIGURE 8.2 Current concepts of the oxygen sensing in hypoxic pulmonary vasoconstriction (HPV). There is a controversy regarding levels of reactive oxygen species (ROS) that mediate HPV. Panel A describes concepts that comprise a decrease in ROS. Panel B describes concepts that comprise an increase in ROS. This figure highlights the complexity of proposed mechanisms for HPV that include mitochondria-dependent model, NAD(P)H-oxidase dependent model, and cytochrome *P450* and heme oxygenase-2 as possible oxygen sensors of HPV. (From Ref. 16, with permission.)

There are a variety of hypoxic lung diseases that may be associated with secondary pulmonary hypertension which have different pathophysiological mechanisms and ultimately need to be addressed independently. ILD associated with SSD and CTD is one area with some published data (addressed in the Special Population section of this chapter). Thus far, evidence is lacking that targeted pulmonary vasodilator therapy is useful in patients with nonspecific interstitial pneumonitis; however, due to the limited options for the primary disease, patients are often referred for treatment of the "treatable" ancillary component of the disease, a hypothesis that needs to be studied (limited ongoing studies). Experimentally, pneumonectomy and hypoxemia are models used to study pulmonary hypertension (23), and evidence of pathological changes has been established in a study of hypoxic lung disease—including an increase in intimal and adventitia thickness and a decrease in the number of blood vessels (23). Thus, ILD, COPD, obesity and hypoventilation, prior pneumonectomy, and regional hypoxemia all may lead to pulmonary hypertension in the susceptible, perhaps genetically predisposed patient.

WHO group IV includes patients with chronic thrombotic and embolic disease. For those with chronic thromboembolic disease, diagnosis and well-timed surgery may be curative if performed at a center proficient in performing pulmonary thromboendarterectomies. However, even with successful thromboendarterectomy some patients develop progressive pulmonary hypertension. Here, the pathology may also be reactive prethrombotic occlusion, postocclusion with remodeling, or reactive vasoconstriction in unaffected areas of the lung (Figure 8.3).

Finally, WHO group V includes diagnoses not fitting into any of the above categories, such as sarcoidosis, pulmonary histiocytosis, extrinsic compression of pulmonary artery, etc. Sarcoidosis may involve chronic lung disease, an active vasculitis, extrinsic compression, or cardiac disease.

■ SYMPTOMS

Symptoms of pulmonary hypertension include dyspnea on exertion, chest pain, palpitations, syncope, ascites and lower extremity edema. Anginal symptoms may occur and are thought to be due to increased RV oxygen demand, decreased right coronary artery perfusion due to decreased pressure difference between aorta and RV end diastolic pressure, and rare instances of compression of the left main coronary artery by the dilated pulmonary trunk. Right ventricular hypertrophy (RVH) correlates with EKG findings including RV strain pattern with precordial T-wave inversions; severity of RVH is more likely to be associated with symptoms although EKG evidence of RVH cannot be used as a screening test. Pericardial and pleural effusions may also contribute to sensations of chest discomfort, heaviness or dyspnea. Accumulation of fluid is due to abnormal drainage of lymphatics and pericardial and pleural venous return into the right atrium. Palpitations may be due to sinus tachycardia, atrial tachycardia, or atrial fibrillation, atrial flutter, and AV nodal reentrant tachycardia (25). Syncope is a worrisome presentation in this disease, and may be exertional, cough mediated or vasodepressor in nature (26). The mechanism of syncope in PAH may be due to the failure to adequately augment cardiac output—the right-sided equivalent to aortic stenosis—or due to a Bezold-Jarisch vasodepressor reflex. Exertional syncope despite targeted pulmonary vasodilator therapy is one of the indications for atrial septostomy in patients with advanced PAH (27).

Different patient populations may be more prone to certain associated manifestations. In particular, pericardial effusions are found more commonly in patients with CTD; tachyarrhythmias are more common in patients with SSD, CHD, and non-WHO group I disease, and less common in IPAH patients.

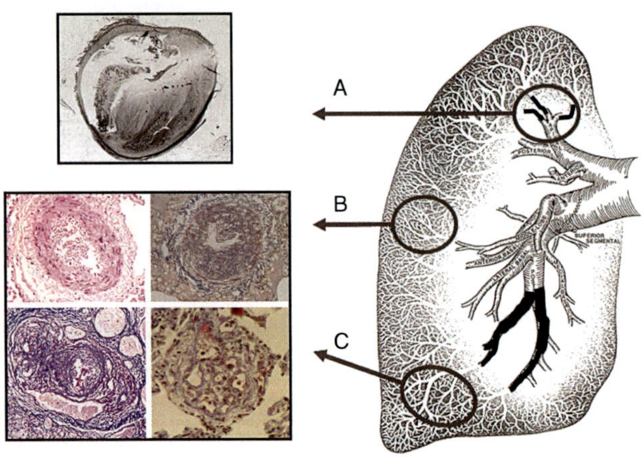

FIGURE 8.3 Schematic representation of three mechanisms of small-vessel disease in CTEPH. (A) Obstruction of small, elastic, subsegmental arteries not amenable to surgical treatment. (B) Pulmonary arteriopathy in small muscular arteries and arterioles distal to nonobstructed elastic vessels (medial thickening, intimal proliferation, and plexiform and colander lesions are shown). (C) Pulmonary arteriopathy in small muscular arteries and arterioles distal to obstructed large elastic vessels (virtually identical changes as in B). (From Ref. 24, with permission.)

■ EVALUATION

Hemodynamics

Pulmonary hypertension is defined hemodynamically as a mean pulmonary artery pressure (mPAP) ≥25 mm Hg concomitant with pulmonary capillary wedge pressure measurement ≤15 mm Hg and pulmonary vascular resistance of <3 Wood units (28) using right heart catheterization (RHC). These criteria were used for enrolling patients into the NIH registry, which was originally assembled to provide definitions and classification of this disease, subsequently used for litigation in the anorexigen cases, and ultimately used by the regulatory agencies in industry-sponsored clinical trials for new drug approvals. This initial NIH database enrolled patients from 1981 until 1985. Of note, the patient population eventually assessed had a mPAP ≥42 mm Hg with normal or decreased cardiac index.

A comprehensive hemodynamic assessment can provide diagnosis and rationale for outpatient treatment. During the course of the evaluation, hypoxia should be treated with 100% oxygen to assess the role of hypoxic pulmonary vasoconstriction and the degree of its reversibility. An elevated pulmonary capillary wedge pressure which signifies pulmonary venous hypertension—that is, left heart failure—should be assessed with systemic vasodilators or inodilators like nitroprusside, nitroglycerine, milrinone, or nesiritide to assess the degree to which pulmonary vascular resistance can be reversed with unloading of the left ventricle or improving cardiac output. Sometimes, the addition of superimposed targeted pulmonary artery vasodilators to systemic vasodilators or inodilators is indicated. In some patients, this may be the appropriate assessment for cardiac interventions such as high-risk valve replacement, ventricular assist device, and cardiac transplant eligibility.

Finally, a comprehensive hemodynamic evaluation in IPAH patients should include assessment of pulmonary vasoreactivity with inhaled nitric oxide (10–40 ppm), inhaled iloprost, IV epoprostenol, or adenosine in patients with precapillary hypertension. If with these treatments mPAP decreases by 10 mm Hg to levels ≤40 mm Hg, IPAH patients are considered "responders." This denotes a small but very important population (<15% of IPAH patients) with significantly improved outcomes when treated with high doses of calcium channel blockers (29,30). For the select patients who are deemed "responders" and are subsequently treated with calcium antagonists, close follow-up to confirm a sustained hemodynamic improvement is essential.

For the growing number of patients with combined pulmonary hypertension and abnormal left ventricular hemodynamics, a careful hemodynamic study can help to delineate the subtleties of both diseases and response to therapies. Exercise catheterization is recommended in those patients with normal hemodynamics at rest, but with a pretest likelihood of PAH and/or other data suggesting exercise-induced symptoms, for instance, exercise echo or cardiopulmonary stress test. Unfortunately, to date there is no consensus as to the best exercise protocols for an appropriate hemodynamic assessment. Among those used include: upright bicycle with neck pulmonary arterial (PA) lines at 75% predicted maximum exercise, supine bicycle, supine arm exercise, and supine volume loading. In all cases, it is essential to carefully measure PCWP, cardiac outputs, and PA pressures at consistent parts of the respiratory cycle, and not merely PA pressures.

Imaging

Echocardiography is a noninvasive tool that can provide assessment of possible causes, shunts, left atrial hypertension, left ventricular dysfunction, valvular heart disease, and consequences of pulmonary hypertension. Measurements of RV systolic and diastolic pressures, and associated findings of paradoxical septal motion, diminished IVC collapse, RVH, right atrial (RA) or right ventricular (RV) enlargement, pericardial effusion, and decreased RV ejection time should all be included in the assessment of these patients. The measurement of PA pressures can be done with relative precision and varying degrees of correlation with invasive measures.

Although many studies report a high correlation between transthoracic echochardiography (TTE) and RHC measurements of pulmonary artery systolic pressure (PAPs) (31), Arcasoy et al. (32) demonstrated the inaccuracy of this correlation in patients with lung disease. Measurements of PAPs are dependent on age, sex, and BMI. Methods to determine right atrial pressures vary, with wide confidence intervals around each measurement creating a source of potentially large error in adding this pressure to the tricuspid velocity. Thus, some centers report "TR jet plus RA pressure" leaving it to the clinician to assess the RA pressure. Furthermore, although these measurements have been somewhat validated at rest they have not been validated with exercise or interventions. More importantly, there remains difficulty in the noninvasive measurement of left atrial pressure that is independent of the loading conditions. One of the proposed methods that is thought to be load-independent is the e/e' ratio assessment. It denotes a ratio between the velocity of the movement of the red blood cells across the mitral valve in early diastole and the velocity of the movement of the mitral annulus during the same time interval. Despite early reports to the contrary, there still appears to be a correlation between preload and the e/e' ratio (33).

Thus, echocardiography is recommended as a screening tool, but not as the definitive diagnostic tool in patients suspected of having pulmonary hypertension. For a particular patient, following the initial correlation of the echo estimate of PA pressure with direct catheterization measurement will allow subsequent patient specific correlations. Tricuspid annular plane systolic excursion (TAPSE) has been shown to correlate strongly with RV ejection fraction as assessed by radionuclide angiography (34). It has been used in both two- and three-dimensional evaluations, and as a means of serial follow-up studies of

RV function. Another technique to assess RV function is the measurements of isovolumic relaxation time (IVRT). Prolonged right ventricular IVRT in IPAH patients was found to be the strongest predictor of clinical status and survival (35). Another novel method of predicting outcomes in patients with IPAH is Doppler measurement of pulmonary vascular capacitance, which is calculated by utilization of the relationship between stroke volume and pulmonary pulse pressure. In multivariate analysis, echo-calculated pulmonary vascular capacitance correlated more strongly with outcomes than invasively measured mPAP, RA pressure, and pulmonary vascular resistance (PVR) (36).

Other new echocardiographic methods have been employed in evaluation of PAH. One of them is strain imaging, which measures deformation over time; it has been used in concert with TAPSE and RV Tei index (isovolumic contraction time and relaxation time/ejection time; [TVt – RVt]/RVt), and has been shown to be reduced in patients with acute pulmonary embolus and improved after stabilization (37). Using parameters of the eccentricity index, which highlight RV/LV interdependence, it was shown that an eccentricity index less than median was associated with improved survival and freedom from a composite endpoint (38). Lastly, the newer technique of vector velocity imaging applied to the right ventricle is promising as a quantitative assessment of RV function and reserve.

All of these data are at best correlative at rest but not with interventions. Exercise echocardiography for pulmonary hypertension has emerged as another screening technique which is not well validated, despite early studies of its use in patient populations at risk, relatives of BMPR-2 + FPAH (39), and more recently in the SSD patient population (40,41). Many of the previously described echocardiographic techniques have not been verified under volume or exercise challenges. Furthermore, data with respect to the normal exercise response of athletes may show increased flow and elevated left atrial and PA pressures (42), and highlight the need to correlate echocardiographic findings with true hemodynamics. Ultimately, three-dimensional echocardiography may emerge as a better means of evaluating the RV given its unusual geometry, but little data is available.

Magnetic Resonance Imaging (MRI)

One of the most important markers of survival in PAH patients is RV function, both its ability to withstand an increased afterload as well as favorable ventricular remodeling in response to effective treatments. MRI has evolved as the gold standard to evaluate RV structure and function. Due to the complex shape of the RV, which is thin walled, crescent shaped, and wrapped around the LV with a peristaltic nature of contraction, echocardiography has been limited to, at best, semi-quantitative assessments of the RV. MRI is uniquely suited for evaluation of RV morphology due to its high resolution and relative absence of confounders that affect echocardiographic image quality. It is independent of geometric assumptions and has superior reproducibility. Cardiac MRI has been successful in correlating RV dimensions, hypertrophy, mass, and LV septal-to-free wall curvature ratio with mPAP (43–45). Delayed contrast enhancement (DCE) is a tissue parameter derived from the contrast enhanced MRI images. It is thought to detect fibrosis in the areas of high mechanical stress. The presence and extent of DCE is inversely related to RV function and PA pressures (46,47); however, it has also been found in patients with dilated cardiomyopathies. Thus, the specificity of this finding has not been fully established; it may be related to hemodynamics, but additional correlative studies are needed (Figure 8.4). Some authors have used algorithms which combine morphologic measurements of the RV and the pulmonary artery with biophysical parameters, and they have found a strong correlation with mPAP by RHC (48). Others, however, have not reproduced these findings (49). One of the key roles of RHC has been to define acute responders to vasodilator therapy; that is, those who may benefit from high-dose calcium channel blockade. MRI assessment of pulmonary artery distensibility correlated highly with vasodilator response with 100% sensitivity and 56% specificity (50). With respect to the functional correlations of MRI findings, one study correlated the increase in the RV stroke volume and decrease in PVR with an increase in six-minute walk distance in IPAH patients treated with epoprostenol (51). In conclusion, MRI is evolving as the gold standard in quantitative RV imaging, may provide additional excellent data with respect to PVR, and ultimately may become a useful surrogate endpoint in clinical trials with respect to RV remodeling. However, this is not in lieu of RHC to evaluate patients with PAH (52).

High-resolution Computed Tomography (HRCT)

Computed tomography (CT) is being applied to the evaluation of patients with PAH. Among the feasible

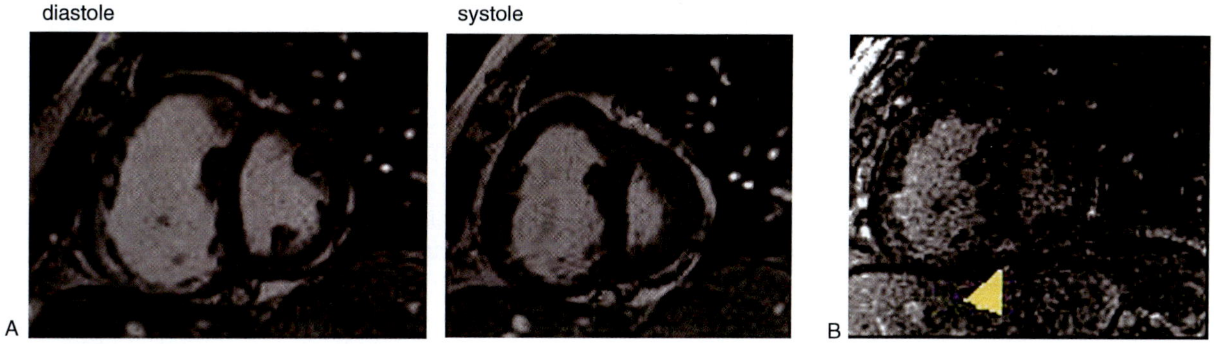

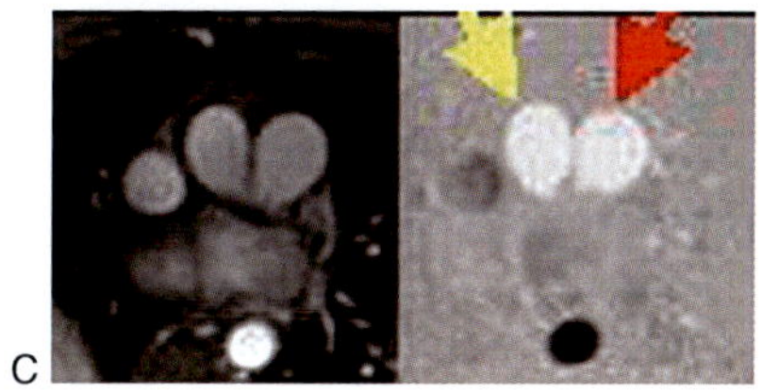

FIGURE 8.4 MRI of a representative patient with pulmonary arterial hypertension showing: (A) right ventriculation dilation, right ventricular hypertrophy, septal flattening; (B) mid-myocardial scar; (C) normal AO/PA flow without evidence of shunt.

findings are the determination of pulmonary artery diameter, presence of bronchial collaterals, and interventricular septal position, all of which have been shown to correlate with echocardiographic indices (53) and ultimately may be useful in directly imaging the complete pulmonary vascular tree. Spiral multidetector (MDCT) can allow for image reconstruction in any part of the cardiac cycle. Thus, end systolic and diastolic images can be produced to assess for volume and function. Various authors found the presence of pulmonary hypertension in patients in whom CT scans were performed for other indications; for example, during evaluation for lung transplantation for intrinsic lung disease (54). CT is particularly useful in the evaluation of patients with chronic thromboembolic pulmonary hypertension (CTEPH) and parenchymal lung disease. CT angiography is often used as an adjunctive tool in patients with suspected or diagnosed CTEPH and in defining a population that would benefit from thromboendarterectomy. Furthermore, HRCT scanning is crucial in the evaluation of patients with pulmonary hypertension in order to define the extent and severity of parenchymal lung disease.

The strongest predictor of mortality in pulmonary hypertension is RV function. The debate goes on as to the best modality to evaluate the RV function while prospectively following patients. Some of the options include various echo criteria, cardiac MRI, cardiac CT, hemodynamic assessments and likely a combination of the above.

Evaluation for Associated Diseases

The initial workup of patients for the presence of pulmonary hypertension should be guided by history, physical exam, pretest likelihood of disease, clinical suspicion, noninvasive evaluation, and ultimately RHC with a low threshold for obtaining complete LV hemodynamic measurements and response to interventions. This should be done in order to tease out pulmonary venous hypertension, hypoxic pulmonary vasoconstriction response, and assessment for the minority of "responsive" IPAH patients. No patient should be started on the newer therapies without a complete evaluation, or be erroneously labeled with the diagnosis of PAH. Transesophageal echo, cavitation echo, or MRI should be done to assess for subtle shunts in CHD, balanced shunt physiology, anomalous and partial anomalous venous return, and/or arterio-venous malformations. Care should be taken to address all possible etiologic and contributing factors, including: family history of pulmonary hypertension, use of anorexigen drugs, recreational substance abuse, symptoms or family history of CTD including SSD, lupus, rheumatoid arthritis, Sjogren's syndrome, HIV, portal hypertension, primary lung disease, left sided cardiac disease, autoimmune substrate, hypogammaglobulinemia, POEMs, hemoglobinopathies, thrombophilia, or embolic disease.

Evaluation for Chronic Thromboembolic Pulmonary Hypertension

Another necessary part of the evaluation should consist of tests to exclude potentially treatable causes. It is essential to exclude chronic thromboembolic disease, as it is the only potentially reversible form of pulmonary hypertension. Current recommendations to screen patients with V/Q lung scan were addressed in a recent study comparing sensitivity and specificity of V/Q scan versus HRCT scan in patients with angiographically proven diagnosis of CTEPH. The sensitivity of V/Q scan as opposed to CT angiogram were 96% to 97% versus 51%, and the specificity of 90% to 95% versus 99% (55). Combined V/Q and CTA are sufficient to exclude CTEPH. Surgical treatment of this disease has evolved where surgical mortality in an experienced center is less than 5%. Following thromboendarterectomy, approximately 90% of patients experience normalization of the PVR, which is maintained for months to years with most patients experiencing at least some degree of hemodynamic benefit from this surgery (56).

FUNCTIONAL TESTS

Pulmonary Function Tests

Pulmonary function tests are obtained to assess for intrinsic lung disease as well as to provide prognostic information. Although in the majority of young IPAH patients these parameters may be quite normal, there is prognostic significance of the diffusing capacity of the lung (DLCO) in patients with SSD with mild ILD. Specifically, a decreased DLCO correlates with poor outcomes in these patients (51). DLCO—which is reduced out of proportion to forced vital capacity (FVC) in these patients—is also highly suggestive of primary associated vasculopathy. A ratio of FVC/DLCO greater than 1.6 carries important diagnostic and predictive significance (41).

Six-Minute Walk

One of the most important and frequently used outcomes in PAH studies is the six-minute walk test. It strongly correlates with both invasive and noninvasive hemodynamic parameters and is an independent predictor of mortality. One study showed that patients walking less than 332 meters have a 20% three-year survival, compared with a 92% survival in those walking farther (6). Furthermore, arterial oxygen desaturation greater than 10% measured during a six-minute walk test is associated with a 2.9-fold increased risk of mortality over a median follow-up of 26 months. The six-minute walk test has been used as the primary outcome in most industry sponsored studies evaluating the efficacy of a new treatment. However, there are limitations to this assessment given the lack of correlation between changes in six-minute walk and mortality. Certainly, when one considers interventions in the non-WHO group 1 patients, endpoint assessments will need to be more robust than modest improvements in six-minute walk distance. Nevertheless, utilizing the Borg dyspnea score with the six-minute walk test has been a useful marker both for evaluation of new therapies for an "orphan disease" as well as to clinically follow patients. In this patient population it often serves as a surrogate for a near maximal stress test. There are major discussions ongoing as to whether this is truly the appropriate primary endpoint to be followed in future studies.

Cardiopulmonary Stress Testing

The gold standard of assessing exercise tolerance is cardiopulmonary exercise testing (CPET). Exertional dyspnea, which remains the primary symptom of PAH, results from physiological abnormalities that are easily assessed by the CPET. The basis of the test lies in our ability to measure O2 and CO2 concentrations using breath-by-breath analysis during bicycle or treadmill exercise. In particular, one can measure the ability to augment O2 transport to tissues with exercise, which is measured by the peak oxygen consumption (VO2), a marker of cardiac output. Anaerobic threshold (AT) is a measure of the highest VO2 that can be sustained without developing lactic acidosis. In PAH, there is a decrease in maximal VO2 and AT compared to normals and is similar to that seen in heart failure patients. Whereas in normal patients the ventilatory response to exercise is tightly linked to CO2 output, in pulmonary hypertension patients the ventilation of underperfused alveoli causes an increase in dead space ventilation. Physiologically this is manifested by a hyperbolic increase in the ventilatory equivalent (VE) relative to CO2 production and a decrease in end tidal CO2. Thus, VE/VCO2 at AT is significantly elevated in PAH patients in contrast to those with LV dysfunction. These parameters closely correlate with NYHA class and survival (58) although use of the CPET in multicenter studies was fraught with limitations due to significant center-to-center variability and each center's learning curve for the procedure (59). The presence of even a functional shunt is characterized by an abrupt decrease in O2 saturation with increasing exercise, due to shunting across a patent foramen ovale when RA pressure increases in response to the increased PA pressures.

Other testing for possible etiologies of pulmonary hypertension should be guided by clinical suspicion and any associated risk factors. For example, patients with HIV have 1:200 risk of developing pulmonary hypertension and their mortality is predicated on the PAH, with poor clinical outcomes when compared to patients with CTD, PPHTN, or IPAH (60), although recent reports are more optimistic about their response to first-line PAH therapy. PAH associated with SSD (see next section) defines a unique subset of patients whose outcomes are significantly worse than other forms of PAH. Furthermore, pulmonary complications are now the leading cause of death in this patient population. Of note, these patients may have lower PA pressures at presentation and yet be more symptomatic, related to abnormal RV to PA coupling. Their systemic disease can also affect both ventricles independently, thus adding a layer of complexity to their presentation and treatment. (61).

Clearly, a complete evaluation for the presence of lung disease and pulmonary hypertension should be done so that appropriate therapy can be initiated early in the course of disease. Other rheumatologic conditions that may predispose to development of PAH are rheumatoid arthritis and systemic lupus erythematosus, especially in patients with Raynauds phenomenon. For patients in whom there is a reason to suspect acute inflammation or vasculitis, response to immunomodulation therapy may at least partially treat pulmonary hypertension (62). This may be particularly relevant in the lupus or mixed-connective tissue patient population. In particular, pulmonary hypertension also markedly improved in a series of patients who were responders to cyclophosphamide therapy. In the appropriate lupus patient who does not have fulminant systemic disease, one may have to consider lung biopsy to assess for inflammation and vasculitis.

Portopulmonary hypertension (PPHTN) is essential to diagnose and treat, particularly in patients who require liver transplantation. Reports of the prevalence of PAH in patients with portal hypertension vary, but range between 0.7% and 2% (63,64). In patients undergoing liver transplantation, the prevalence is higher: between 3.5% and 16.1% (65). Outcomes of liver transplantation are worse in patients with systolic PA pressures greater than 60 mm Hg or mPAP >35 mm Hg and are associated with high perioperative risk. Recent studies have shown that genetic variation in estrogen signalling and cell growth regulators is associated with the risk of PPHTN in patients with liver disease. These biologic pathways may elucidate the mechanism for the development of PPHTN in patients with severe liver disease (66). A finding of high PA pressures in liver transplant patients often warrants treatment, with repeat hemodynamic assessment to demonstrate improvement in PA pressures. The data for treatment of PPHTN with advanced therapies is limited to small observational studies and case reports. An improvement in hemodynamics and NYHA class was reported in 14 patients treated with epoprostenol for one year (67,68). Some case reports exist of treatment with treprostinil, iloprost, sildenafil, bosentan, and ambrisentan.

■ SPECIAL POPULATIONS

An important subset of PAH is SSD. Scleroderma is a complex disorder that may affect primarily skin, or have wide-spread systemic involvement of almost any organ system. Pulmonary disease complicates up to 80% of all cases and is now the leading cause of death in this population. Given the potential for cardiac and pulmonary involvement, SSD also presents the complexities of differentiating the multiple etiologies of pulmonary hypertension which may include PEFHF, microvascular cardiac disease, progressive calcific valvular disease, primary pulmonary vascular disease, or pulmonary vascular disease associated with more significant ILD. More commonly than in IPAH, there is the associated finding of a pericardial effusion, which may be due to right heart failure or the underlying systemic disease. Thus, the two important subtypes of PAH associated with SSD are: one group characterized predominantly by a primary vascular disease with pathology similar to IPAH, albeit more fibrosis and intimal hyperplasia; and a second group with more significant ILD. These two pathologies can co-exist in the same patient, which sometimes may complicate treatment algorithms. ILD is a process associated with myofibroblast proliferation of the interstitial compartment (which is found between endothelial and epithelial basement membranes) and infiltration by inflammatory cells causing varying degrees of fibrosis. ILD is diagnosed by a constellation of serologic markers, pulmonary function testing, and appearance on HRCT. Most studies involving APAH and SSD excluded those patients with more significant ILD, although many patients had mild basilar fibrosis consistent with some degree of the myofibroblastic proliferation. Patients with SSD and pulmonary hypertension associated with ILD have the worst prognosis (69).

Patients with APAH associated with systemic lupus should also be differentiated as a distinct cohort, inasmuch as patients who respond to immunosuppressive therapy have a much better outcome (70). Overall, SSD APAH has a significantly worse prognosis than IPAH; this is true both with respect to the natural history of the disease as well as following treatment (Figure **8.1**).

SSD patients are more symptomatic with less severe hemodynamic parameters during first presentation (60). All of the approved drugs have a less impressive response in patients with SSD versus IPAH. In response to epoprostenol, exercise capacity, hemodynamics, and functional class all improved, but outcome and responses were less robust than the previous parallel PPH epoprostenol trial (71). A subgroup analysis of the BREATHE-1 bosentan trial in PAH patients showed a "decreased risk of worsening" in the treatment group (72); relative improvement in six-minute walk distance was predominantly due to the deterioration in the placebo group with a less impressive improvement in the active treatment group. However, bosentan may also be useful in the treatment of digital ulcers in this patient population (73). In the SUPER study (74) with sildenafil, some concern was raised that beyond the initial study period, at the 12-month mark, when there was a worsening status in the SSD APAH patient group. In contrast to this follow-up, Mathai et al. (75) have demonstrated improvement in myocardial parameters with PDE-5 inhibitors in this patient population.

In conclusion, SSD patients are sicker at the time of diagnosis and the magnitude of elevation of their PA pressures may under-represent the severity of their clinical status. Natural history and current medical interventions are less effective in this cohort of PAH patients. On the other hand, this patient population also represents the one cohort in whom one could ask the question: Can interventions limit the risk of development of disease? Thus, the most important question is how to predict or follow SSD patients for development of PAH to determine the onset of the disease process, which can be heralded by myofibroblast activation and a subclinical proinflammatory state. Among the suggestions for screening of the SSD patients for the development of PAH have been utilizing DLCO, a ratio of FVC:DLCO >1.6, exercise echo, and exercise catheterization (41) to risk-stratify scleroderma patients for clinical worsening, and utilizing MRI to assess RV function prior to overt progression.

Another unique group of patients are those with congenital systemic to pulmonary cardiac shunts, including atrial and ventricular septal defects (ASDs, VSDs), patent ductus arteriosus, and aorto-pulmonary window patients. Increased flow across the pulmonary vascular bed causes vascular remodeling in a susceptible group of patients. It is not known what makes some patients develop pulmonary hypertension or Eisenmenger physiology as opposed to others. The prevalence of pulmonary vascular disease varies among different populations; up to 50% of patients with large VSDs develop pulmonary hypertension as opposed to only 10% of those with ASDs (76). The two-hit hypothesis would explain this phenomenon with a genetic susceptibility present in those patients who develop PAH with smaller flow shunts. Supporting this theory is that some patients with very small shunts still develop the disease, and some children who develop Eisenmenger syndrome associated with small shunts have mothers with IPAH (77). Moreover, pathologic findings are similar between PAH associated with CHD and IPAH.

Fewer medications have been shown to be efficacious for treatment in this patient cohort. Outside of the standard management with digoxin, warfarin, oxygen, and diuretics, patients have been treated with both bosentan and epoprostenol. The BREATHE-5 study demonstrated improvement in pulmonary vascular resistance and exercise capacity in NYHA class III patients with the use of bosentan with a 16-week follow-up (78). Importantly, patients with Eisenmenger syndrome randomized to bosentan walked farther and did not increase their desaturation, the usual concern with these patients. A small study of IV epoprostenol in PAH associated with CHD showed efficacy in terms of NYHA class, hemodynamic response, and exercise capacity over one year (79), although there is the added concern of paradoxical embolus with a central venous line and shunt. Overall, the natural history of these patients is better compared to other subsets of PAH despite suprasystemic PA pressures given a compensated RV. We can expect growth of this patient population as the childhood survival of patients with cardiac shunts continues to improve.

Elevated PA pressures in non-WHO group IPAH, are a negative prognostic indicator for LV heart failure (80), COPD (81), sickle cell (82), and other diseases. Although PAH is a rare disease, these other diseases are widespread. Given effective treatments for PAH, there has been more aggressive screening and diagnosis as well as growing interest in treatment of pulmonary hypertension component of their disease. However, it is imperative to emphasize that there is very little data for efficacy of expensive targeted pulmonary vasodilator treatment in these patients, and in some the data is negative. Significant interest has been generated in pulmonary hypertension secondary to dilated or ischemic cardiomyopathy (WHO group II section), and in patients with hypoxemia and lung disease (WHO group III section). Studies are underway evaluating current PAH therapy in sickle cell disease and other hemoglobinopathies although initial enthusiasm has been dampened with early termination of a study of sildenafil in sickle cell patient population. The degree to which these diverse etiologies may all lead to a similar phenotype is an area of intense interest, both biologically and clinically. From a clinical perspective, in these nonorphan disease patient populations, future studies would need to utilize mortality or combined efficacy endpoint measurements, and not merely an improvement in six-minute walk distance. From a biological perspective, understanding the pathophysiology and the "downstream pathways" may open the door for other, more effective treatments in these patients.

■ PATHOPHYSIOLOGY

The advancement of specific therapies which target the known endothelin, prostacyclin, and nitric oxide pathways (Figure 8.5) has led to some of the successes in understanding the shortcomings of the vasodilator theory of pulmonary hypertension and in development of other therapies. The initial construct of vasoconstriction and subsequent triad of vascular proliferation, vasoconstriction and in situ thrombosis was the paradigm for pathophysiology of this disease. Therapies primarily targeted against vasoconstriction also happened to be beneficial with respect to vascular remodeling.

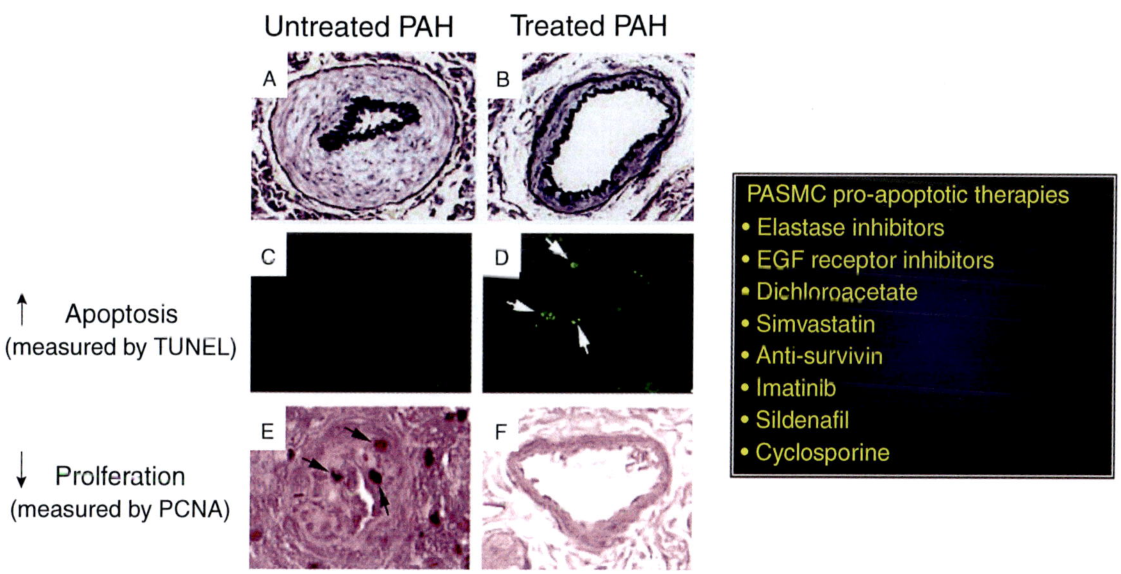

FIGURE 8.5 Proapoprotic experimental therapies in pulmonary arterial hypertension (PAH). A common denominator of these therapies is the induction of apoptosis as well as suppression of proliferation in the pulmonary artery wall. On the left are untreated rats with monocrotaline-induced PAH and on the right are rats treated with elastase inhibitors. Increased apoptosis of the intima-media is showed by TUNEL (terminal deoxynucleotidyl transferase biotin-dUTP nick end labeling), and decreased proliferation is imaged by staining for proliferation cell nuclear antigen (PCNA). The same pattern has been shown in the media of treated rats by all the therapies shown in the box. (From Ref. 116, with permission.)

The pathophysiology of PAH is thought to be due to unchecked cellular proliferation of the vascular wall, obliteration of the small and medium sized vessels, and in situ thrombosis with loss of the capillaries and small vessels. Endothelial dysfunction and vascular damage is accompanied by an imbalance of the proliferative vasoconstrictors (endothelin, thromboxane, serotonin) versus growth inhibitor vasodilators (prostacyclin, nitric oxide) with an increase in the pulmonary artery smooth muscle cells (PASMC) [Ca^{2+}] and the loss of the apoptotic response to unchecked growth.

The two-hit hypothesis implicates a preexisting genetic predisposition in addition to environmental insults. Some of the genetic factors that predispose to the development of pulmonary hypertension are the BMPR-2 mutations described in familial PAH, as well as some IPAH, and the ALK-1 and endoglin mutations found in some hereditary hemorrhagic telangiectasia patients (84). These genes encode for proteins in transforming growth factor (TGF)-beta super family. The BMPR-2 gene confers autosomal dominant inheritance with incomplete penetrance (only 20% of patients with this gene mutation acquire the disease), and female predominance with genetic anticipation (84). There is still not a clear link between genetics of this disease and its pathologic expression although the role of the TGF pathway is thought to be associated with the development of unchecked growth. One group in San Diego has also documented the acquisition of BMPR-1 via the TIE1-angiopoietin (85), although other labs have not been able to verify this finding.

Biopsy specimens of PAH include constrictive lesions and complex lesions. Constrictive lesions comprise medial hypertrophy and intimal thickening. Medial hypertrophy is defined as the increase in both number and cross-sectional area of the SM cells lining the walls of the pre- and intra-acinar pulmonary arteries; intimal thickening implies an increased number of fibroblasts in the thin layer between a SM cell and lamina propria of the blood vessel. These changes can be seen in both IPAH and pulmonary venous hypertension. In contrast, complex lesions are considered pathognomonic for PAH. The complex or plexiform lesion consists of focal proliferation of endothelial channels consisting of fibroblasts, SM cells, and connective tissue matrix. These lesions disrupt vascular vessel wall and serve as a nidus for in situ thrombosis.

A model proposed by Michelakis et al. (117) suggests a Venn Diagram of three disease characteristics of PAH which include the proliferative-antiapoptotic, degenerative, and inflammatory aspects of the disease. The "neoplasia model" of accelerated proliferation and suppressed apoptosis in the cell wall suggests a downregulation of distal apoptotic pathways including both the receptor mediated—BMPR-2 and Smad signaling—as well as the mitochondria-induced apoptosis. A state of "mitochondrial hyperpolarization" occurs with a switch to glycolytic pathways, effectively the Warburg effect of cancer cells. It is characterized by enhanced cellular glycolysis and suppression of mitochondrial cellular metabolism with upregulated glucose uptake and downregulation of the Kv channels. This inhibition of Kv channels leads to increased levels of intracellular K^+ and inhibition of caspases, which are directly implicated in promoting apoptosis with possible coordination by nuclear factor of activated T cells (NFAT). The degenerative disease model occurs due to the loss of microvascular endothelial cells distal to vascular obliteration and is mediated by excess cellular growth and loss of distal arterioles and capillaries. There is both a spatial and temporal gradient of vascular endothelial changes from the proximal PA to the distal PAs such that the distal vessels go through a reparative attempt to restore normal flow, although this repair process may inadvertently lead to the development of the plexogenic lesion. Earlier changes may be due to apoptosis of the small vessel pulmonary artery endothelial cells (PAEC) with the eventual development of apoptotic resistant PAECs and PASMCs later in the course of disease. There is data in animal models and a clinical association that suggest a role of inflammatory cells in IPAH (86,87). Severe PAH may occur in patients with systemic inflammatory disease and findings of autoantibodies such as antinuclear, antiendothelial, and antifibroblast antibodies. Furthermore, proinflammatory cytokines IL-1 and IL-6 may target endothelial cells and promote apoptosis and the development of PAH (88).

■ TREATMENT

The treatment paradigm for PAH includes "conventional" medications and "advanced" or disease-specific pulmonary vasodilator therapies that target three major pathways (Figure 8.5). The former group includes diuretics to maintain euvolemia, warfarin to prevent in situ thrombosis, digoxin, and supplemental oxygen to maintain systemic saturation of >92%. One study supporting the use of warfarin followed 64 patients with PPH treated with high-dose calcium channel blockers, of whom 55% were also treated with warfarin (89). Survival was better in both high dose calcium channel blocker responders and nonresponders receiving anticoagulation.

Prostacyclin, a product of arachidonic acid metabolism, is a pulmonary and systemic vasodilator, inhibitor of SM cell growth and platelet aggregation. Its biochemical effector is cyclic AMP (Figure 8.5). There are currently several alternative prostacyclin analogues approved for the treatment of PAH: 1) continuous IV infusion of epoprostenol; 2) continuous treprostinil which may either be continuous subcutaneous (SC) or IV delivery; 3) inhaled iloprost dosed six to nine times daily; and 4) most recently, an inhalation system for treprostinil dosed four times daily is also available. All three have been approved for WHO group I PAH patients with class III–IV symptoms; treprostinil is officially also approved for class II patients, although with the advent of oral drugs it is unlikely for a SC or IV delivery system to be used by patients who are less symptomatic.

Intravenous epoprostenol has been used since the 1980s and has been the gold standard in treating PAH. It has been shown that levels of prostacyclin are decreased in lungs of patients with severe pulmonary hypertension (90). The two randomized trials using epoprostenol introduced the randomized controlled studies for patients with this devastating disease. The first study followed 41 patients with NYHA class III PPH for 12 weeks. At the end of the follow-up period there were 8 total deaths, all of which were in the placebo arm (91). This remains the only short-term study ever to demonstrate a mortality improvement with therapy. The subsequent randomized study for patients with CTD and PAH showed efficacy but not a mortality benefit (71). In a long-term follow up study, 162 patients with PPH were followed for a median of 31 months with observed survival of 87.8%, 76.3%, and 62.8% at one, two, and three years, respectively. These results compared favorably with the natural history of PPH (now IPAH) patients enrolled in the NIH registry, with survival of 58.9%, 46.3%, and 35.4% at one, two, and three years, respectively (48). Epoprostenol has also been shown to improve six-minute walk distance, RV function, and hemodynamic parameters. Its therapeutic benefit is limited by the requirement for central venous access for continuous infusion; its short half-life, daily mixing, large pump, and need for ice packs; the concomitant complications of central line infection; and the fact that any abrupt cessation of infusion can result in severe rebound pulmonary hypertension and death.

Treprostinil is a synthetic analogue of prostacyclin with a longer half-life, and thus theoretically poses less danger of a severe adverse event in the setting of inadvertent discontinuation. It can be delivered via a subcutaneous infusion system utilizing a beeper-sized insulin delivery pump, but the local infusion may cause pain at the infusion site. Treprostinil may also be delivered intravenously either with a similar pump to epoprostenol or with a smaller pump (although not as small as the subcutaneous pump). Other side effects common to all prostanoids include nausea, flushing, jaw pain, diarrhea, and nervousness. Treprostinil has been shown to improve six-minute walk distance (92), functional class (93) and hemodynamics, and has been observed to improve survival compared to historic controls (94). Studies with inhaled treprostinil have recently led to approval by the regulatory agencies. Ongoing studies utilizing oral treprostinil are in progress.

Inhaled iloprost is administered via a special inhaler six to nine times daily and was initially approved as solo therapy based on the European data (95). It targets the pulmonary vascular bed and ultimately goes to the well-ventilated areas of the lung, thus effectively decreasing V/Q mismatch. It has also been shown to improve six-minute walk distance, hemodynamics, and functional class. The study is also one of the very few trials that looked at the composite clinical endpoint (96) and enrolled patients with CTEPH. A subsequent U.S. study added iloprost to bosentan therapy, and thus initiated the advent of inhaled therapy added to oral therapies as well as the growing trend of a polypharmacy drug approach (addressed later). Recently, inhaled treprostinil has been approved with a different delivery system and dosed four times daily which is likely to make it easier for patients and enhance compliance with an inhaled regimen.

Another target of pulmonary hypertension therapies is endothelin (Figure 8.5), which is elevated in this disease, correlates to disease severity, and is localized immunohistochemically to the plexogenic lesions. There are two endothelin receptors: ETa and ETb. ETa is found primarily on vascular SM cells, mediates the vasoconstrictive and mitogenic response, and is a direct target of both ETa-specific and nonspecific endothelin antagonists. ETb is located on the SMs where it mediates vasoconstriction, and is also found on endothelial cells where it mediates vasodilation; in experimental models it improves regional renal vasodilation (96). In disease states, specifically interstitial fibrosis, SM ETb receptors are upregulated and may become pathological (97).

The two FDA-approved ERA are bosentan and ambrisentan. Sitaxsentan is not approved in the United States although it has been approved in Europe, Canada, Australia, and Israel.

Bosentan is an oral nonselective endothelin receptor antagonist with multiple drug interactions due to P450 enzyme metabolism. Bosentan was the first oral therapy approved for pulmonary hypertension and markedly changed the treatment algorithms, which previously included only calcium antagonists for the small minority of responders and IV epoprostenol for others sick enough to warrant the cumbersome therapy. Patients with either IPAH or APAH associated with CTD enrolled in the studies showed improvements in six-minute walk distance, Borg dyspnea score, functional capacity, and increased time to clinical worsening (98). Long-term survival was assessed in a study following patients over 36 months and compared their outcome to the original cohort of patients in the NIH registry. The results showed significant improvement in the event-free survival, although this and all other similar comparisons are made to outdated historical controls (99). Bosentan has an approximate 11% incidence of transaminitis and thus requires monthly liver function test (LFT) monitoring and distribution by a specialty pharmacy. Long-term data regarding bosentan drug-drug interactions are available through the European TRAC database, which has shown the feasibility of its use in HIV patients who are concurrently on triple therapy. This database has also been useful in assessment of bosentan-sildenafil interactions. Despite in vivo drug-drug interactions, which increase bosentan levels and decrease sildenafil levels, there have been no reports of increased side effects when combining these medications that would require dose adjustments

Ambrisentan is a selective ETa receptor with a lower incidence of liver toxicity (closer to 3%), is a once-daily medication, and has fewer drug-drug interactions. It is the only treatment evaluated in all functional classes and it showed an improvement in exercise capacity and symptoms in patients with IPAH, CTD, anorexigen use and HIV infection (54). The pivotal ambrisentan trials, ARIES I & II, showed significant improvements in six-minute walk distance, dyspnea, functional capacity, decreased BNP as a biomarker, and increased time to clinical worsening (100). It remains unproven as to whether selectivity or nonselectivity is preferred. Peripheral edema may be a side effect of both drugs requiring diuretic adjustment similar to the introduction of beta-blockers in patients with congestive heart failure. Whether ambrisentan has a higher incidence of edema or may be related to its increased potency remains to be seen. Teratogenicity is a class effect as well. Thus, women of childbearing age require monthly pregnancy testing in addition to monthly liver function tests. It is yet to be determined whether ambrisentan—which has fewer drug-drug interactions—will ultimately be safer.

Sitaxsentan is approved outside of the United Sates, is a more selective ETa receptor antagonist, and is also a once daily drug. It has significant interactions with warfarin and is more similar to ambrisentan with respect to incidence of transaminitis. A nonblinded, nonrandomized extension study suggested a more favorable response to sitaxsentan than bosentan in the CTD patient population (101).

The final pathway for targeted therapy is enhancing the nitric oxide-cGMP mediated pathway (Figure 8.5). Nitric oxide (NO) is a free radical with a short half-life and has pleiotropic effects in the lungs, including vasorelaxation, bronchodilation, inhibition of platelet and leukocyte activation, and modulation of vascular SM proliferation. It is synthesized from L-arginine and oxygen by three NO synthases in the lung. Inhaled nitric oxide (iNO) is approved for treatment in term and near-term neonates with hypoxemia and PAH. It is used off-label acutely both in the evaluation of pulmonary hypertension in the cardiac catheterization lab and in the ICU settings, particularly in perioperative management of right heart failure and pulmonary hypertension (102,103). Although there are some cGMP independent effects, NO effectively stimulates guanylate cyclase, which activates cGMP, stimulates the cGMP-mediated protein kinases and promotes vascular relaxation. cGMP is limited by its breakdown by PDE inhibitors. Sildenafil selectively binds to PDE-5, which is abundantly expressed in the lung tissue and the net effect is to increase cGMP, promote SM relaxation and thereby enhance pulmonary vasodilation with minimal effects on systemic blood pressure.

There remains some debate as to whether there is enhanced RV inotropy with PDE-5 inhibitors. More recent work suggests that in the failing RV there is an inotropic effect of PDE-5 inhibitors not apparent in the normal RV and, most recently, LV (103). Placebo-controlled studies have shown an improvement in six-minute walk distance, functional capacity, hemodynamics, and QOL indices (73,104). Sildenafil 20, 40, and 80 mg three times daily were all associated with improvements in six-minute walk distance; therefore, the lowest dose was approved by the FDA for treatment. However, there also was a hemodynamic dose dependency such that higher doses of sildenafil were associated with a greater hemodynamic benefit. A unique side effect of this medication is change in color vision, blurred vision, or sensitivity to light, which has been reported in up to 11% of patients receiving greater than 100 mg of sildenafil per day which may be due to sildenafil's cross-reactivity of PDE-6 involved in the retinal phototransduction pathway.

Tadalafil has recently been approved with data showing efficacy at the 40 mg once daily dosing (two 20 mg tablets) (105).

A polypharmacy approach for treating pulmonary hypertension, which combines the targeting of the three different second messenger systems, has become more common with a combination of an endothelin receptor antagonist, a PDE-5 inhibitor and a prostanoid. However, there is a dearth of clinical data addressing this hypothetically attractive approach. One of the combination therapy trials evaluated a combination of bosentan and epoprostenol, and showed its safety and a tendency to hemodynamic improvement in patients with IPAH and CTD-related APAH (106). Addition of inhaled iloprost to bosentan showed a trend to improvement in six-minute walk distance, functional capacity, and time to clinical worsening (107). Sildenafil added to IV epoprostenol significantly delayed time to clinical worsening (108). In the 16 week Tadalafil study, approximately 53% of the patients were already on background Bosentan therapy and although their response to Tadalafil was not as robust (23 meter improvement, P = .05) as compared to the 44 meter improvement, P = .01 in treatment naive patients, (109) it clearly supports the concept of a polypharmacy approach

There are still many unanswered questions that remain in the evaluation and treatment paradigms for pulmonary hypertension. Because of the low prevalence of IPAH and only a more recently increased awareness of APAH, most of the trials looked at the surrogate outcomes. There is ample data to show correlation between baseline six-minute walk test, hemodynamic parameters, and mortality (110) in patients with pulmonary hypertension. However, concerns have been raised about the correlation of six-minute walk improvement with hard clinical outcomes, and about its ability to predict improvement after therapy. This issue was looked at in the meta-analysis combining all trials of pulmonary hypertension since 1985 and looking at the prevalence of clinical events in the treatment groups (3). Overall, treatment was associated with a nonsignificant reduction in all-cause mortality. In contrast, another recent meta-analysis review showed that active therapy was associated with a 43% reduction in mortality (111). Furthermore, in the Macchia et al. study (3), there was no relationship between the degree of end-of-study improvement in exercise capacity and the degree of reduction of death. While there is unambiguous improvement in the degree of dyspnea and exercise capacity in treated patients, questions remain as to the degree of mortality advantage offered to patients with all available newer therapies, given that all studies have been 12 to 16 weeks in duration.

The final consideration for advanced pulmonary hypertension should be given to surgical interventions. They include atrial septostomy and lung transplantation. Septostomy is done in the setting of progressive pulmonary hypertension despite maximal medical therapy to unload the RV, decompress a bowing right atrium, and to decrease syncope and sudden death in these patients. It is potentially a bridge to lung transplantation, a means of stabilizing RV function (112), and can be done in areas in the world where expensive pulmonary hypertension therapy is not an option. The rationale for the procedure is the observation that patients with Eisenmenger syndrome and congenital shunts have a better prognosis, and that the shunt physiology is "protective" compared with IPAH and no shunt or mechanism to decompress the right side. It has been shown that catheter-based atrial septostomy results in an increase in cardiac output due to increased LV filling; however, it comes at the cost of decreased oxygenation due to right to left shunting.

Finally, lung transplantation should be considered in severely symptomatic patients with pulmonary hypertension. While three-year survival of lung transplantation is approximately 50% (113), advanced IPAH carries an even worse prognosis. A careful risk-benefit assessment should be made regarding the timing and decision to proceed for lung transplantation. Guidelines for selection of patients for lung transplantation include NYHA IIIb or IV, mean RA pressure >10, mPAP >50, cardiac index <2.5, and rapidly progressive disease (114).

FUTURE DIRECTIONS

Future directions in the field of pulmonary hypertension are likely to be related to the delineation of the molecular mechanisms of endothelial injury; among them, the use of simvastatin in treatment of established pulmonary hypertension, which has been investigated in hypoxic PAH rats. There was a striking improvement in mPAP and medial thickening of PAs compared with controls (115). Another area is that of bone-marrow-derived endothelial-like progenitor cells. The hypothesis is that the progenitor cells would repair and regenerate blood vessels and subsequently improve pulmonary hemodynamics. In the rat model, this treatment has been shown to prevent pulmonary hypertension and, more importantly, reverse established pulmonary hypertension. A subgroup of these cells was transfected with human endothelial NO-synthase, which showed the best survival advantage over controls. A different model is used in an effort to treat PAH with gene therapy using a TIE2 receptor antagonist, which is used to inhibit angiopoietin-1 models. This treatment resulted in the prevention of pulmonary hypertension induced by hypoxia, angiopoietin stimulation, or monocrotaline administration (which is the most widely used rat model of pulmonary hypertension) and one in which most interventions show promise (116).

Newer targets for therapy challenge our understanding of "successful" strategies and emphasize the need to change our overall approach (Figure 8.6) to truly change the outcome of the disease (3). Furthermore, beyond the prostanoid infusions, hemodynamic responses with oral agents have been underwhelming. Thus, there is an emerging consensus that we should be focusing on vascular remodeling, perhaps with agents such as statins, rapamycin, cyclosporine, or elastase inhibitors. Moving beyond where we presently are requires shifting the emphasis to restore the ability for apoptosis; to that end, therapeutic possibilities include epidermal growth factor receptor inhibitors, platelet-derived growth factor (PDGF) inhibitors such as imatinib, survivin inhibitors, and metabolic modulators such as dichloroacetate to activate mitochondria-based apoptosis (117). Evidence of the link between inflammation and PAH exists in experimental models and certain clinical scenarios. Treatment strategies that aim at targeting specific inhibition of NFAT at the myocardial, SM, and endothelial cells are also promising.

CONCLUSION

Pulmonary hypertension is a disease of the pulmonary vasculature that progressively leads to an elevated PVR and RV failure. We have made significant progress in therapies for the WHO group I patient population, although response, QOL, hemodynamics, and NYHA class still remain much less than what we would like to see. The diagnosis of the disease needs to be established with RHC. Prognosis is predominantly determined by cardiac output and RV function. Thus, for both prognosis and follow-up, significant information is provided by close monitoring of the RV with various imaging modalities, including echocardiography, 3D echo, cardiac MRI, and cardiac CT. Functional evaluation should include QOL assessments, NYHA assessment, pulmonary function testing, six-minute walk test, and CPET. There is still an urgent need to further improve our understanding of this disease, develop useful animal models that more accurately mimic the pathology, change our paradigms of pathophysiology and treatment strategies, truly improve survival instead of merely improving six-minute walk distance, and thereby move beyond the current strategies of endothelin receptor antagonists, prostacyclin analogues, and NO-cGMP stimulation. Furthermore, differentiating the non-WHO group I patient population, in whom there is no data that our present therapies are useful, is essential. Nevertheless, acknowledging the increasing prevalence of secondary pulmonary hypertension, its association with a variety of diseases in which it is a marker of increased mortality, and understanding its mechanisms may ultimately provide insight into additional pathophysiology and the divergent pathways that lead to a similar organ-specific vasculopathy, the phenotype of which is pulmonary hypertension.

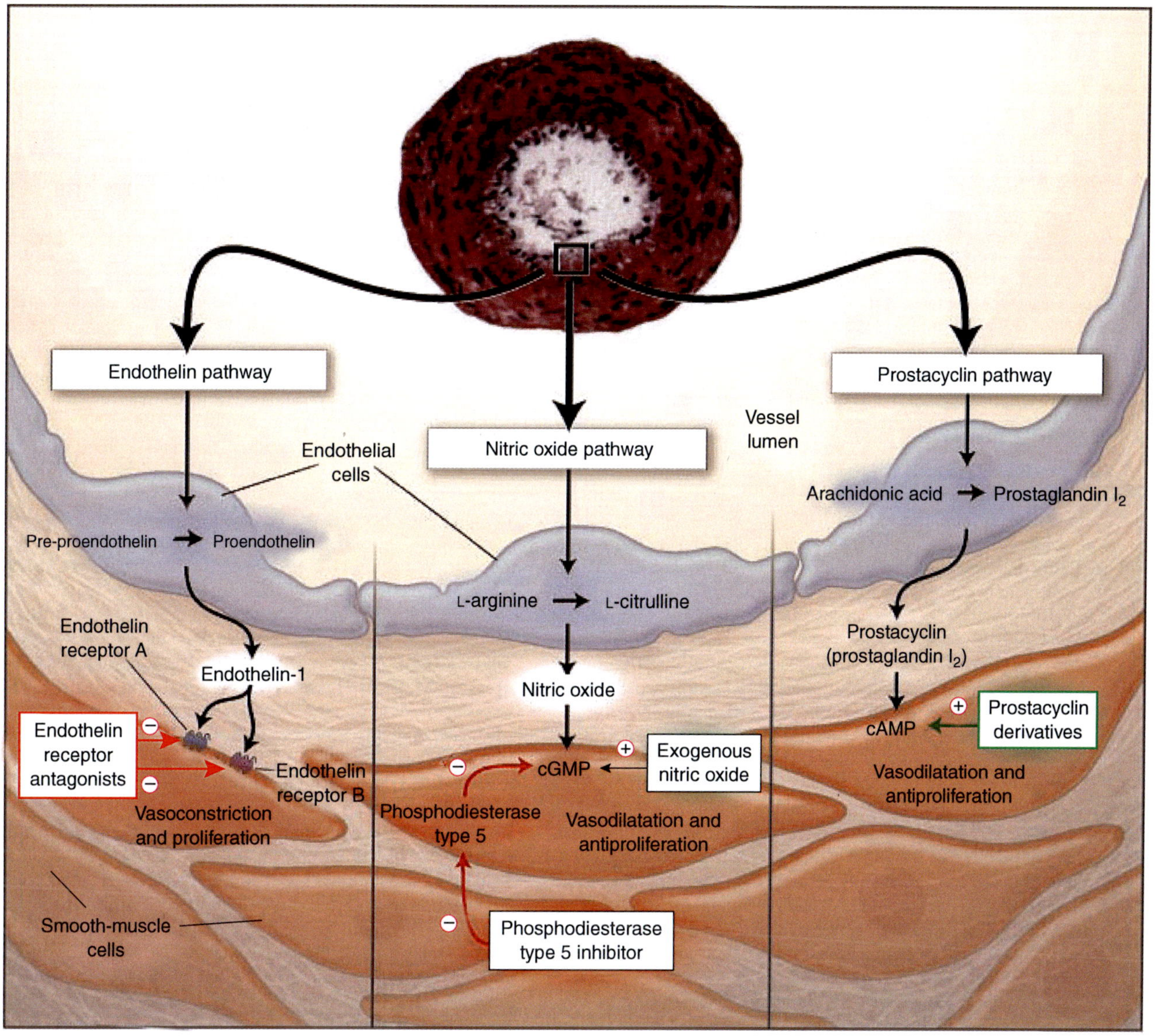

FIGURE 8.6 Targets for current therapies in pulmonary arterial hypertension (PAH) and their three major pathways: endothelin, nitric oxide, and prostacyclin. (From Ref. 83, with permission.)

REFERENCES

1. Austin ED, Loyd JE. Genetics and mediators in pulmonary arterial hypertension. *Clin Chest Med* 2007 Mar; 28(1):43–57,vii–viii.
2. D'Alonzo GE, Barst RJ, Ayres SM, et al. Survival in patients with primary pulmonary hypertension. Results from a national prospective registry. *Ann Intern Med* 1991; 115(5):343–9.
3. Macchia A, Marchioli R, Marfisi R, et al. A meta-analysis of trials of pulmonary hypertension: a clinical condition looking for drugs and research methodology. *Am Heart J* 2007; 153(6):1037–47.
4. Simonneau G, Galie N, Rubin LJ, et al. Clinical classification of pulmonary hypertension. *J Am Coll Cardiol*. 2004;43:5S–12S
5. Simonneau, G, Robbins IM, Beghetti M, et al. Updated clinical classification of pulmonary hypertension. *J Am Coll Cardiol* 2009; 54:S43-54.
6. Miyamoto S, Nagaya N, Satoh T, et al. Clinical correlates and prognostic significance of six-minute walk test in patients with primary pulmonary hypertension. *Am J Respir Crit Care Med* 2000; 161:487–92.

7. Newman JH, Trembath RC, Morse JA, et al. Genetic basis of pulmonary arterial hypertension: current understanding and future directions. *J Am Coll Cardiol* 2004 Jun 16; 43(12 Suppl S):33S–9S.
8. Yang X, Long L, Southwood M, et al. Dysfunctional Smad signaling contributes to abnormal smooth muscle cell proliferation in familial pulmonary arterial hypertension. *Circ Res* 2005; 96(10):1053–63.
9. Califf R, Adams KF, McKenna WJ, et al. A randomized controlled trial of epoprostenol therapy for severe congestive heart failure: The Flolan International Randomized Survival Trial (FIRST). *Am Heart J* 1997; 134:44–54.
10. Packer M, McMurray J, Massie BM, et al. Clinical effects of endothelin receptor antagonism with bosentan in patients with severe chronic heart failure: results of a pilot study. *J Cardiac Fail* 2005; 1:12–20.
11. Guazzi M, Samaja M, Arena R, et al. Long-term use of sildenafil in the therapeutic management of heart failure. *J Am Coll Cardiol* 2007; 50:2136–44.
12. Lewis GD, Lachmann J, Camuso J , et al. Sildenafil improves exercise hemodynamics and oxygen uptake in patients with systolic heart failure. *Circulation* 2007; 115(1):59–66.
13. Kaluspi E, Kobrin I, Zimlichman R, et al. RITZ-5: randomized intravenous tezosentan (an endothelin-A-B antagonist) for the treatment of pulmonary edema: a prospective, multicenter, double-blind, placebo-controlled study. *J Am Coll Cardiol* 2003;41:204–14.
14. McMurray JJV. Value of endothelin receptor inhibition with tezosentan in acute heart failure studies (VERITAS): Two multicenter, double blind, placebo-group trials assessing the efficacy, safety and tolerability of tezosentan in acute heart failure. Presented at the American College of Cardiology Meeting, March 2005.
15. Packer M. Effects of the endothelin antagonist bosentan on the morbidity and mortality in patients with chronic heart failure. Results of the ENABLE 1 and 2 trial program. Presented at the American College of Cardiology Meeting, March 2002.
16. Lepore JJ, Maroo A, Bigatello LM, et al. Hemodynamic effects of sildenafil in patients with congestive heart failure and pulmonary hypertension: combined administration with inhaled nitric oxide. *Chest* 2005; 127:1647–53.
17. Lewis GD, Shah R, Shahzad K , et al. Sildenafil improves exercise capacity and quality of life in patients with systolic heart failure and secondary pulmonary hypertension. *Circulation* 2007; 116:1555–62.
18. Behling A, Rohde LE, Colombo FC , et al. Effects of 5'-phosphodiesterase four-week long inhibition with sildenafil in patients with chronic heart failure: a double-blind, placebo-controlled clinical trial. *J Card Fail* 2008; 14:189–97.
19. Salzberg S, Lachat ML, von Harbou K , et al. Normalization of high pulmonary vascular resistance with LVAD support in heart transplantation candidates. *Eur J Cardiothorac Surg* 2005; 27:222–5.
20. Hopkins N, McLoughlin P. The structural basis of pulmonary hypertension in chronic lung disease: remodeling, rarefaction or angiogenesis? *J Anat* 2002; 201(4):335–48.
21. Weissmann N, Sommer N, Schermuly RT, et al. Oxygen sensors in hypoxic pulmonary vasoconstriction. *Cardiovasc Res* 2006; 71(4):620–9.
22. Weir EK, Olschewski A. Role of ion channels in acute and chronic responses of the pulmonary vasculature to hypoxia. *Cardiovasc Res* 2006; 71(4):630–41.
23. Rabinovitch MGW, Nadas AS, Miettinen OS, Reid L. Rat pulmonary circulation after chronic hypoxia: hemodynamic and structural features. *Am J Physiol* 1979; 236:H818–27.
24. Galiè N, Kim N. Pulmonary Microvascular Disease in Chronic Thromboembolic Pulmonary Hypertension. *Proc Am Thorac Soc* 2006; 3:571–6.
25. Tongers J, Schwerdtfeger B, Klein G, et al. Incidence and clinical relevance of supraventricular tachyarrhythmias in pulmonary hypertension. *Am Heart J* 2007; 153(1):127–32.
26. Rich S, Dantzker DR, Ayres SM, et al. Primary pulmonary hypertension. A national prospective study. *Ann Int Med* 1987; 107:216–223.
27. Kerstein D, Levy PS, Hsu DT, et al. Blade balloon atrial septostomy in patients with severe primary pulmonary hypertension. *Circulation* 1995; 91(7):2028–35.
28. Barst RJ, McGoon M, Torbicki A, et al. Diagnosis and differential assessment of pulmonary arterial hypertension. *J Am Coll Cardiol* 2004; 43(12 Suppl S):40S–7S.
29. Rich S, Kaufmann E, Levy PS. The effect of high doses of calcium channel blockers on survival in primary pulmonary hypertension. *N Engl J Med* 1992; 327(2):76–81.
30. Sitbon O, Humbert M, Jais L, et al. Long-term response to calcium channel blockers in idiopathic pulmonary hypertension. *Circulation* 2005; 111(23):3105–11.
31. Berger M, Haimowitz A, Van Tosh A, et al. Quantitative assessment of pulmonary hypertension in patients with tricuspid regurgitation using continuous wave Doppler ultrasound. *J Am Coll Cardiol* 1985; 6(2):359–65.
32. Arcasoy SM, Christie JD, Ferrari VA, et al. Echocardiographic assessment of pulmonary hypertension in patients with advanced lung disease. *Am J Respir Crit Care Med* 2003; 167(5):735–40.
33. Rivas-Gotz C, Manolios M, Thohan V, Nagueh SF. Impact of left ventricular ejection fraction on estimation of left ventricular filling pressures using tissue Doppler and flow propagation velocity. *Am J Cardiol* 2003; 91(6):780–4.
34. Kaul S, Tei C, Hopkins JM, et al. Assessment of right ventricular function using two-dimensional echocardiography. *Am Heart J* 1984; 107(3):526–31.
35. Tei C, Dujardin KS, Hodge DO, et al. Doppler echocardiographic index for assessment of global right ventricular function. *J Am Soc Echocardiogr* 1996; 9(6):838–46.
36. Mahapatra S, Nishimura RA, Oh JK, et al. The prognostic value of pulmonary vascular capacitance determined by Doppler echocardiography in patients with pulmonary arterial hypertension. *J Am Soc Echocardiogr* 2006; 19:1045–50.
37. Park JH, Park YS, Park SJ, et al. Midventricular peak systolic strain and Tei index of the right ventricle correlated with decreased right ventricular systolic function in patients with acute pulmonary thromboembolism. *International Journal of Cardiology* 2008; 125(3):319–24.
38. RaymondRJ,HinderliterAL,WillisPW,etal.Echocardiographic predictors of adverse outcomes in primary pulmonary hypertension. *J Am Coll Cardiol* 2002; 39(7):1214–19.
39. Grunig, E, Janssen, B, Mereles, D, et al. Abnormal pulmonary artery pressure response in asymptomatic carriers of primary pulmonary hypertension gene. *Circulation* 2000; 102:1145–50.
40. Pignone A, Mori F, Pieri F, et al. Exercise Doppler echocardiography identifies preclinic asymptomatic pulmonary hypertension in systemic sclerosis. *Ann N Y Acad Sci* 2007; 1108:291–304.

41. Steen V, Chou M, Shanmugam V, et al. Exercise-Induced Pulmonary Arterial Hypertension in Patients With Systemic Sclerosis. *Chest* 2008; 134:146–51.
42. Bossone E, Rubenfire M, Bach DS, et al. Range of tricuspid regurgitation velocity at rest and during exercise in normal adult men: implications for the diagnosis of pulmonary hypertension. *J Am Coll Cardiol* 1999; 33:1662–6.
43. Frank H, Globints S, Glogar D, et al. Detection and quantification of pulmonary artery hypertension with MR imaging: results in 23 patients. *Am J Roentgenol* 1993; 161:27–31.
44. Katz J, Whang J, Boxt LM, et al. Estimation of right ventricular mass in normal subjects and in patients with primary pulmonary hypertension by nuclear magnetic resonance imaging. *J Am Coll Cardiol* 1993; 21:1475–81.
45. Dellegrottaglie S, Sanx J, Poon M, et al. Pulmonary hypertension: accuracy of detection with left ventricular septal-to-free wall curvature ratio measured at cardiac MR. *Radiology* 2007; 243:63–9.
46. Blyth KG, Groenning BA, Martin TN, et al. Contrast enhanced-cardiovascular magnetic resonance imaging in patients with pulmonary hypertension. *Eur Heart J* 2005; 26:1993–9.
47. McCann GP, Van Dockum WG, Beek AM, et al. Extent of MRI delayed enhancement of myocardial mass is related to right ventricular dysfunction in pulmonary artery hypertension. *Am J Roentgenol* 2007; 188:349–55.
48. Laffon E, Allard M, Marthan R, et al. A computed method for noninvasive MRI assessment of pulmonary arterial hypertension. *J Appl Physiol* 2004; 96:463–8.
49. Roeleveld RJ, Marcus JT, Boonstra A, et al. A comparison of noninvasive MRI-based methods of estimating pulmonary artery pressure in pulmonary hypertension. *J Magn Reson Imaging* 2005; 22:67–72.
50. Jardim C, Rochitte CE, Humbert M, et al. Pulmonary artery distensibility in pulmonary arterial hypertension: a MRI pilot study. *Eur Respir J* 2006; 29:476–81.
51. Roeleveld RJ, Vonk-Noordegraaf A, Marcus JT, et al. Effects of epoprostenol on right ventricular hypertrophy and dilatation in pulmonary hypertension. *Chest* 2004; 125:572–9.
52. Benza R, Biederman R, Murali S, et al. Role of cardiac magnetic resonance imaging in the management of patients with pulmonary arterial hypertension. *J Am Coll Cardiol* 2008; 52:1683–92.
53. Grubstein A, Benjaminov O, Dayan DB, et al. Computed tomography angiography in pulmonary hypertension. *Israel Med Assoc J: Imaj* 2008; 10(2):117–20.
54. Perez-Enguix D, Morales P, Tomas JM, et al. Computed tomographic screening of pulmonary arterial hypertension in candidates for lung transplantation. *Transplantation Proc* 2007; 39:2405–8.
55. Tunariu N, Gibbs SJ, Win Z, et al. Ventilation-perfusion scintigraphy is more sensitive than multidetector CTPA in detecting chronic thromboembolic pulmonary disease as a treatable cause of pulmonary hypertension. *J Nucl Med* 2007; 48:680–4.
56. Auger W, Kim NH, Kerr KM, Test VJ, Fedullo PF. Chronic thromboembolic pulmonary hypertension. *Clin Chest Med* 2007;28:255–269.
57. Steen VD, Graham G, Conte C, et al. Isolated diffusing capacity reduction in systemic sclerosis. *Arthritis Rheum* 1992; 35(7):765–70.
58. Sun XG, Hansen JE, Oudiz RJ, et al. Exercise pathophysiology in patients with primary pulmonary hypertension. *Circulation* 2001; 104:429–35.
59. Hansen JE, Sun XG, Yasunobu Y, et al. Reproducibility of cardiopulmonary exercise measurements in patients with pulmonary arterial hypertension. *Chest* 2004; 126:816–24.
60. Speich R, Jenni R, Opravil M, et al. Primary pulmonary hypertension in HIV infection. *Chest* 1991; 100(5):1268–71.
61. Fisher MR, Mathai SC, Champion HC, et al. Clinical differences between idiopathic and scleroderma-related pulmonary hypertension. *Arthritis Rheum* 2006; 54:3043–50.
62. Sanchez O, Sitbon O, Jais X, et al. Immunosuppressive therapy in connective tissue diseases-associated pulmonary arterial hypertension. *Chest* 2006; 130(1):182–9.
63. McDonnell PJ, Toye PA, Hutchins GM, et al. Primary pulmonary hypertension and cirrhosis: are they related? *Am Rev Respir Dis* 1983; 127(4):437–41.
64. Hadengue A, Benhayoun MK, Lebrec D, et al. Pulmonary hypertension complicating portal hypertension: prevalence and relation to splanchnic hemodynamics. *Gastroenterology* 1991; 100(2):520–8.
65. Colle IO, Moreau R, Godinhho E, et al. Diagnosis of portopulmonary hypertension in candidates for liver transplantation: a prospective study. *Hepatology* 2003; 37(2):401–9.
66. Roberts KE, Fallon MB, Krowka MJ, et al. Serotonin transporter polymorphisms in patients with portopulmonary hypertension. *Chest* 2009; 135(6):1470–5.
67. McLaughlin VV, Genthner DE, Panella MM, et al. Compassionate use of continuous prostacyclin in the management of secondary pulmonary hypertension: a case series. *Ann Intern Med* 1999; 130(9):740–3.
68. Krowka MJ, Frantz RP, McGoon MD, et al. Improvement in pulmonary hemodynamics during intravenous epoprostenol (prostacyclin): A study of 15 patients with moderate to severe portopulmonary hypertension. *Hepatology* 1999; 30(3):641–8.
69. Mathai SC, Hummer LK, Champion HC, et al. Survival in pulmonary hypertension associated with the scleroderma spectrum of diseases: impact of interstitial lung disease. *Arthritis Rheum* 2009; 60:569–77.
70. Sanchez O, Sitbon O, Jais X, et al. Immunosuppressive therapy in connective tissue diseases-associated pulmonary arterial hypertension. *Chest* 2006; 130:182–9.
71. Badesch DB, Tapson VF, McGoon MD, et al. Continuous intravenous epoprostenol for pulmonary hypertension due to the scleroderma spectrum of disease. *Ann Intern Med* 2000; 132(3):425–34.
72. Ahmadi-Simab K, Lamprecht P, Hellmisch B, Gross WL. Treatment of pulmonary arterial hypertension (PAH) with oral endothelin-receptor antagonist bosentan in systemic sclerosis: BREATHE–1 trial and clinical experience. *Z Rheumatol* 2004; 63(6):495–7. [Article in German]
73. García de la Peña-Lefebvre P, Rodríguez Rubio S, Valero Expósito M, et al. Long-term experience of bosentan for treat ing ulcers and healed ulcers in systemic sclerosis patients. *Rheumatology (Oxford)* 2008; 47(4):464–6.
74. Badesch DB, Hill NS, Burgess G, et al. Sildenafil for pulmonary arterial hypertension associated with connective tissue disease. *J Rheumatol* 2007; 34(12):2417–22.
75. Mathai SC, Girgis RE, Fisher MR, et al. Addition of sildenafil to bosentan monotherapy in pulmonary arterial hypertension. *Eur Respir J* 2007; 29(3):469–75.
76. Vongpatanasin W, Brickner ME, Hillis LD, et al. The Eisenmenger syndrome in adults. *Ann Intern Med* 1998; 128(9):745–55.
77. Rich S, Rubin LJ, Abenhaim L, et al. Executive Summary from the World Symposium on Primary Pulmonary

Hypertension (Evian, France, September 6–10, 1998). The World Health Organization publication. http://web.archive.org/web/20020408173726/http://www.who.int/ncd/cvd/pph.html. Accessed Sept. 27, 2009.

78. Galiè N, Beghetti M, Gatzoulis MA, et al. Bosentan therapy in patients with Eisenmenger syndrome: a multicenter, double-blind, randomized, placebo controlled study. *Circulation* 2006; 114(1):48–54.
79. Rosenzweig EB, Kerstein D, Barst RJ, et al. Long-term prostacyclin for pulmonary hypertension with associated congenital heart defects. *Circulation* 1999; 99(14):1858–65.
80. Ghio S, Gavazzi A, Campana C, et al. Independent and additive prognostic value of right ventricular systolic function and pulmonary artery pressure in patients with chronic heart failure. *J Am Coll Cardiol* 2001; 37(1):183–8.
81. Kessler R, Faller M, Fourgaut G, et al. Predictive factors of hospitalization for acute exacerbation in a series of 64 patients with chronic obstructive pulmonary disease. *Am J Respir Crit Care Med* 1999; 159(1):158–64.
82. Gladwin MT, Sachdev V, Jison ML, et al. Pulmonary hypertension as a risk factor for death in patients with sickle cell disease. *N Engl J Med* 2004; 350(9):886–95.
83. Humbert M, Sitbon O, Simonneau, G. Treatment of Pulmonary Arterial Hypertension. *N Engl J Med* 2004; 351: 1425–1436.
84. Humbert M, Morrell NW, Archer SL, et al. Cellular and molecular pathobiology of pulmonary arterial hypertension. *J Am Coll Cardiol* 2004; 43(12 Suppl S):13S–24S.
85. Du L, Sullivan CC, Chu D, et al. Signaling molecules in nonfamilial pulmonary hypertension. *N Engl J Med* 2003; 348(6): 500–9.
86. Taraseviciene-Stewart L, Nicolls MR, Kraskauskas. Absence of T cells confers increased pulmonary arterial hypertension and vascular remodeling. *Am J Respir Crit Care Med* 2007; 175:1280–9.
87. Ulrich S, Nicolls MR, Taraseviciene L. Increased regulatory and decreased cd8+ cytotoxic T cells in the blood of patients with IPAH. *Respiration* 2008; 75:272–80.
88. Perros F, Cohen-Kaminsky S, Humbert M. Understanding the role of CD4+CD25(high) (so-called regulatory) T cells in idiopathic pulmonary arterial hypertension. *Respiration* 2008; 75(3):253–6.
89. Johnson SR, Mehta S, Granton JT, et al. Anticoagulation in pulmonary arterial hypertension: a qualitative systematic review. *Eur Respir J* 2006; 25(5):999–1004.
90. Tuder RM, Cool CD, Geraci MW, et al. Prostacyclin synthase expression is decreased in lungs from patients with severe pulmonary hypertension. *Am J Respir Crit Care Med* 1999; 159:1925–32.
91. Barst R, Rubin LJ, Long WA, et al. A comparison of continuous intravenous epoprostenol (Prostacyclin) with conventional therapy for primary pulmonary hypertension. *N Engl J Med* 1996; 334(5):296–301.
92. Tapson VF, Gomberg-Maitland M, McLaughlin VV, et al. Safety and efficacy of IV treprostinil for pulmonary arterial hypertension. A prospective, multicenter, open-label, 12-week trial. *Chest* 2006; 129:683–8.
93. Gomberg-Maitland M, Tapson VF, Benza RL, et al. Transition from intravenous epoprostenol to intravenous treprostinil in pulmonary hypertension. *Am J Respir Crit Care Med* 2005; 172:1586–9.
94. Barst RJ, Galiè N, Naeije R, et al. Long-term outcome in pulmonary arterial hypertension patients treated with subcutaneous treprostinil. *Eur Respir J* 2006; 28(6):1195–203.
95. Olschewski H, Simonneau G, Galiè N, et al. Inhaled iloprost for severe pulmonary hypertension. *N Engl J Med* 2002; 347(5):322–29.
96. Benigni A, Remuzzi G. Endothelin antagonists. *Lancet* 1999; 353(9147):133–8.
97. Fagan KA, McMurtry IF, Rodman DM. Role of endothelin-1 in lung disease. *Respir Res* 2001; 2(2):90–101.
98. Rubin LJ, Badesch DB, Barst RJ, et al. Bosentan therapy for pulmonary arterial hypertension. *N Engl J Med* 2002; 346:896–903.
99. McLaughlin VV, Sitbon O, Badesch DB, et al. Survival with first line bosentan in patients with primary pulmonary hypertension. *Eur Respir J* 2005; 25:244–9.
100. Galiè N, Olschewski H, Oudiz R, et al. Ambrisentan for the treatment of pulmonary arterial hypertension: results of the ambrisentan in pulmonary arterial hypertension. Randomized, double-blind, placebo-controlled, multicenter, efficacy (ARIES) study 1 and 2. *Circulation* 2008; 117(23):3010–19.
101. Barst RJ, Langleben D, Badesch D, et al; STRIDE-2 Study Group. Treatment of pulmonary arterial hypertension with the selective endothelin-A receptor antagonist sitaxsentan. *J Am Coll Cardiol* 2006; 47(10):2049–56.
102. Ricciardi MJ, Knight BP, Martinez FJ, Rubenfire M. Inhaled nitric oxide in primary pulmonary hypertension: a safe and effective agent for predicting response to nifedipine. *J Am Coll Cardiol* 1998; 32(4):1068–73.
103. Fattouch K, Sbraga F, Sampognaro R, et al. Treatment of pulmonary hypertension in patients undergoing cardiac surgery with cardiopulmonary bypass: a randomized, prospective, double-blind study. *J Cardiovasc Med (Hagerstown)* 2006; 7(2):119–23.
104. Ghofrani H, Widemann R, Rose F, et al. Sildenafil for treatment of lung fibrosis and pulmonary hypertension: a randomized controlled trial. *Lancet* 2000; 360:895–900.
105. Galiè N, Brundage BH, Ghofrani HA, et al. Pulmonary Arterial Hypertension and Response to Tandalafil (PHIRST) Study Group. Tadalafil therapy for pulmonary arterial hypertension. *Circulation* 2009; 119(22):2894–903.
106. Humbert M, Barst RJ, Robbins IM, et al. Combination of bosentan with epoprostenol in pulmonary arterial hypertension: BREATHE-2. *Eur Respir J* 2004; 24:353–9.
107. McLaughlin VV, Oudiz RJ, Frost A, et al. Randomized study of adding inhaled iloprost to existing bosentan in pulmonary arterial hypertension. *Am J Respir Crit Care Med* 2006; 174:1257–63.
108. Simonneau G, Rubin LJ, Galiè N, et al. Addition of sildenafil to long-term intravenous epoprostenol therapy in patients with pulmonary arterial hypertension: a randomized trial. *Ann Intern Med* 2008; 149(8):521-30.
109. Galiè N, Brundage BH, Ghofrani HA, et al. Tadalafil therapy for pulmonary arterial hypertension. *Circulation* 2009; 119(22):2894-903.
110. Miyamoto S, Nagaya N, Satoh T, et al. Clinical correlates and prognostic significance of six-minute walk test in patients with primary pulmonary hypertension. Comparison with cardiopulmonary exercise testing. *Am J Respir Crit Care Med* 1999; 161:487–92.

111. Galiè N, Manes A, Negro L, et al. A meta-analysis of randomized controlled trials in pulmonary arterial hypertension. *Eur Heart J* 2009; 30(4):394–403.
112. Kurzyna M, Dabrowski M, Bielecki D, et al. Atrial septostomy in treatment of end-stage right heart failure in patients with pulmonary hypertension. *Chest* 2007; 131(4):977–83.
113. Trulock EP, Christie JD, Edwards LB, et al. Registry of the International Society for Heart and Lung Transplantation: twenty-fourth official adult lung and heart-lung transplantation report—1007. *J Heart Lung Transplant* 2007; 26(8):782–95.
114. Orens JB, Estenne M, Arcasoy S, et al. International guidelines for the selection of lung transplant candidates: 2006 update-a consensus report from the Pulmonary Scientific Council of the International Society for the Heart and Lung Transplantation. *J Heart Lung Transplant* 2006; 25(7):745–55.
115. Girgis RE, Mozammel S, Champion HC, et al. Regression of chronic hypoxic pulmonary hypertension by simvastatin. *Am J Physiol Lung Cell Mol Physiol.* 2007; 292(5):L1105-10
116. Zhao YD, Courtman DW, Deng Y, et al. Rescue of monocrotaline-induced pulmonary arterial hypertension using bone marrow-derived endothelial-like progenitor cells: efficacy of combined cell and eNOS gene therapy in established disease. *Circ Res* 2005; 96:442–50.
117. Michelakis ED, Wilkins MR, Rabinovitch M. Emerging concepts and translational priorities in pulmonary arterial hypertension. *Circulation* 2008; 118(14):1486–95.

9 Asymptomatic Carotid Artery Stenosis: Detection, Risk Stratification, and Management

ISSAM D. MOUSSA

OUTLINE

Physicians are often reluctant to intervene upon asymptomatic extracranial carotid artery stenosis (CAS). However, waiting for a first neurological event prior to identification and treatment of CAS is not an optimal strategy, particularly in high-risk patients. Data supporting the proven benefit of carotid revascularization over medical therapy, although modest, currently exists. Using a transient ischemic attack (TIA) as the only trigger for revascularization in these patients has several drawbacks:

1. Most strokes in patients with asymptomatic CAS occur without a preceding TIA (1).
2. A TIA cannot often be assessed objectively and may occur during sleep when it may not be recognized (2).
3. Even when a patient recognizes a TIA, the patient may not seek immediate medical attention increasing the risk of stroke to 5% to 8% during the first week (3).
4. Up to 22% of patients with TIA sustain brain parenchymal damage on CT scanning, suggesting that even a TIA can result in end organ damage (4).

Efforts directed at detection of CAS in asymptomatic patients have increased after the publication of studies demonstrating that carotid endarterectomy and carotid artery stenting can prevent stroke in these patients (5–7). The benefit of CAS detection, namely stroke prevention, depends on several factors:

1. The prevalence of asymptomatic CAS in specific populations
2. The natural history of carotid disease; the sensitivity and specificity of the screening method (most often, duplex ultrasonography)
3. The need to confirm the diagnosis—using methods such as magnetic resonance arteriography (MRA), computed tomographic arteriography (CTA), or contrast arteriography
4. The costs of screening
5. The cost-effectiveness of carotid revascularization (carotid endarterectomy [CEA] vs. carotid stenting)

DETECTION OF ASYMPTOMATIC CAROTID ARTERY DISEASE

Although carotid revascularization has been shown to confer benefit in reducing stroke risk over medical therapy in asymptomatic patients, the absolute benefit is small and, thus, does not justify the general population screening given the very low prevalence of significant asymptomatic CAS. The prevalence of asymptomatic CAS for stenosis >50% in the general population is from 2% to 8% (8). In a review of the published literature, Lee et al. (9) analyzed the cost-effectiveness of screening 65-year-old men for asymptomatic CAS to identify candidates for carotid endarterectomy. Screening this patient population was associated with a cost-effectiveness rate of $120,000 per quality-adjusted life-year, that is, less cost-effective than most accepted health interventions. Therefore, a more selective approach to screening for asymptomatic CAS is needed.

Screening for CAS in asymptomatic high-risk patients is more cost effective. Derdeyn and Powers (10) developed a computer model to evaluate the cost-effectiveness of screening 1,000 men over a 20-year period. A one-time screening program in an asymptomatic population with a high prevalence (20%) of >60% stenosis cost $35,130 per incremental quality-adjusted life-year, which is considered cost-effective. The greatest cost-effectiveness in this model was seen when the CAS produced a peak systolic velocity of 230 cm/sec. Neither one-time screening of a low-prevalence population nor annual screening was considered cost-effective in their analysis. Although medical societies have yet to endorse specific guidelines recommending screening certain patient subsets for asymptomatic CAS, data support consideration of screening in some types of patients.

■ WHO SHOULD BE CONSIDERED FOR SCREENING FOR ASYMPTOMATIC CAS?

Patients with Carotid Bruits

The prevalence of carotid bruits in asymptomatic individuals varies according to age and other cardiovascular risk factors. Sandok and colleagues (11) evaluated the prevalence of cervical bruits in 509 asymptomatic individuals in Olmsted County, Minnesota. The prevalence of asymptomatic carotid arterial bruits increased with age: 0.9% at 45 to 54 years; 2.1% at 55 to 64 years; 3.8% at 65 to 74 years; and 5% at 75 years and older. The risk was higher in females (4.4%) than in males (1.6%). The prevalence of carotid bruits is significantly higher in patients with established atherosclerotic vascular disease. Gutierrez and colleagues (12) reported a prevalence of 24% among 300 neurologically asymptomatic patients prior to peripheral vascular surgery.

The prevalence of CAS in patients with carotid bruits is significantly higher than that in patients without carotid bruits. It is estimated that approximately 30% to 40% of asymptomatic patients with a carotid bruit will have an internal CAS >50% (13). However, these studies also demonstrate that many patients with asymptomatic bruits do not have significant carotid disease. Moreover, hemodynamically significant carotid stenotic lesions may exist in the absence of an audible bruit. Severe carotid stenoses (90–99%) that are associated with slow flow are often not associated with an audible bruit (14). Therefore, it is critical to remember that the absence of a carotid bruit does not rule out high-grade significant carotid stenosis and should not be used as a reason to deny screening, especially if other risk factors exist.

Elderly Patients with Severe Coronary or Peripheral Arterial Disease

The prevalence of asymptomatic CAS (50% or greater) in patients with systemic atherosclerotic vascular disease is significantly higher than that in the general population. Asymptomatic CAS has been reported to be present in 5% to 31% of patients with coronary artery disease, and in 13% to 50% of patients with peripheral arterial disease (8). Age, severity of atherosclerotic disease, diabetes, tobacco use, and hypertension have all been identified as additional risk factors associated with increased prevalence of asymptomatic CAS in this population. Furthermore, it has also been clearly established that these patients are also at high risk for future ischemic cardiovascular and cerebrovascular events. Therefore, screening for asymptomatic CAS should be strongly considered in elderly patients with coronary or peripheral artery disease, particularly in the presence of hypertension or smoking.

Asymptomatic CAS is prevalent among patients undergoing coronary artery bypass graft surgery (CABG). Screening patients prior to CABG for presence of asymptomatic CAS is attractive because carotid stenosis is a risk factor for stroke after CABG. In a recent review by Naylor and colleagues (15), the risk of perioperative stroke after CABG was <2% in patients without significant carotid disease, increasing to 3% in predominantly asymptomatic patients with a unilateral 50% to 99% stenosis, 5% in those with bilateral

50% to 99% stenoses, and 7% to 11% in patients with carotid occlusion. In a case-control study (16), Hill and colleagues demonstrated that while a carotid stenosis of 50% to 90% increases the risk of ipsilateral stroke 5.2-fold, a carotid stenosis of 80% to 90% increases the risk of ipsilateral stroke by 24.3-fold. Although a properly conducted prospective natural history study is still needed for confirmation, the available evidence certainly supports an association between asymptomatic CAS and post CABG ipsilateral neurological events.

Whether all patients undergoing CABG should be screened is debatable; prevalence of asymptomatic CAS in patients undergoing CABG increases with age, left main coronary artery involvement, concomitant peripheral arterial disease, diabetes, tobacco use, and the presence of carotid bruits (17,18). In a study by Durand and colleagues (19) designed to evaluate the merits of selective versus systematic screening in CABG patients, the authors found that selectively screening only patients with either an age >65 or the presence of a carotid bruit could significantly reduce the screening load with negligible impact on neurologic outcomes.

Table 9.1 The number of patien tomatic CAS who need to be treated (I endarterectomy to prevent one stroke

NNT to Prevent One Stroke	
At 2 years [19]	67 patients
At 3 years [20]	53 patients
At 5 years [19]	16–20 patients 40 patients (for disabling or fatal stroke)

Table 9.2 The number of patients with asymptomatic CAS who need to be treated (NNT) with carotid endarterectomy, statins, or aspirin to prevent one stroke at 5 years

Treatment	Study (Ref.)	NNT to Prevent One Stroke at 5 Years
CEA + usual medical care	ACST (6)	16–20 patients
Statins	Primary prevention trials (28)	200 patients
Aspirin*	Primary prevention trials (29)	500 patients

*Follow-up 6.4 years; no stroke reduction in men.

CAROTID REVASCULARIZATION FOR PATIENTS WITH ASYMPTOMATIC CAROTID ARTERY STENOSIS: THE CONTROVERSY

Critics of carotid revascularization for asymptomatic CAS advance two arguments against the routine use of carotid revascularization to treat moderate to severe asymptomatic CAS (20,21). First, they propose that the number of patients with asymptomatic CAS who need to be treated with CEA (number needed to treat, NNT) to prevent one stroke is too high (Table 9.1). Proponents of this view also insist that stand-alone medical therapy is sufficient for stroke reduction. Although medical therapy should always be the cornerstone of any treatment strategy for patients with asymptomatic CAS, declaring stand-alone medical therapy as the optimal therapeutic strategy remains to be proven in clinical trials. Although medical therapy undoubtedly reduces the incidence of stroke, the number of neurologically asymptomatic patients who need to be treated to prevent one stroke is very high. Table 9.2 lists the number of neurologically asymptomatic patients who need to be treated with statins or aspirin to prevent one stroke at 5 years. It is clear from these data that although primary prevention with medical therapy is efficacious, a significantly larger number of patients will need to be treated to prevent a single event.

Second, opponents of revascularizing asymptomatic CAS lack confidence in the generalizability of the CEA trials. The complication rate after CEA in clinical trials has not been reproduced in the community. Rothwell et al. (22) compared the operative risks in ACAS with the results of a meta-analysis of 46 surgical case series that published operative risks for asymptomatic CAS during ACAS and the five years after publication (23). The operative mortality rate was eight times higher than in ACAS (1.11% versus 0.14%; *P* <0.01), and the risk of stroke and death was approximately three times higher among comparable studies in which outcome was assessed by a neurologist (4.3% versus 1.5%; *P* <0.001). Both original p values were correct. The higher perioperative complication rate after CEA in the community significantly diminish the long-term efficacy of this operation.

This concern extends to carotid artery stenting. Although carotid artery stenting in patients with asymptomatic CAS can be performed by experienced operators with a low complication rate, the procedure can be associated with high complication rate if performed by inexperienced operators, particularly in older patients with complex anatomy (24). In any case, institution-specific assessment of the risk of carotid intervention, endarterectomy, or stenting should be a prime consideration in clinical decision making regarding carotid revascularization in patients with asymptomatic CAS.

■ RISK STRATIFICATION OF PATIENTS WITH ASYMPTOMATIC CAS

Most experts agree that certain patients with asymptomatic CAS are at high risk for stroke and may derive significant benefit from carotid revascularization. Identification of those patients, however, has been elusive in clinical trials. Risk stratification of patients with asymptomatic CAS is particularly important among patients with 60% to 79% stenosis, in whom the appropriate management is more uncertain. Identifying high-risk patients will certainly lead to better resource utilization for both medical and revascularization therapies for patients with asymptomatic CAS.

In current clinical practice, deciding who should be revascularized is often based solely on stenosis severity at the time of patient encounter (>70% for low-surgical risk patients and >80% for high-surgical risk patients). Simplification of clinical decision-making certainly has advantages, but the available data clearly indicate that stenosis severity is only one of many other parameters that determine future stroke risk in these patients.

Demographic and Clinical Parameters

Age

Patients older than 80 years are at higher risk of stroke from carotid disease, as well as from other causes (25). These patients are also at higher risk of complications after carotid revascularization (24,26). The decision to proceed with carotid revascularization in octogenarians should be made on a case-by-case basis by implementing a strict risk stratification process to select those at highest risk for ischemic stroke, those at lowest risk for overall mortality, and those at manageable risk for the carotid revascularization procedure under consideration (CAS versus CEA). Other factors, such as mental health, functional capacity, and the extent of other comorbidities, should also be considered. Age alone should not exclude otherwise-qualified candidates from consideration for carotid revascularization.

Gender

The effect of gender on outcome of patients undergoing carotid revascularization (CEA in particular) for asymptomatic CAS remains controversial despite numerous studies that addressed this topic. In the ACAS trial (25) the incidence of perioperative stroke or death was nearly twice as high for women than for men (3.6% versus 1.7%, $P = 0.12$). Subsequently, the 5-year relative stroke risk reduction was only 17% for women versus 66% for men ($P = 0.10$). In the ACST trial (6), the largest prospective randomized clinical trial comparing CEA to medical therapy in asymptomatic CAS, women (one third of patients) had slightly higher rate of perioperative complications (3.6% versus 2.5%, P = ns), however, they did realize net benefit from CEA at 5-year follow-up. Nonetheless, the absolute risk reduction of 5-year risk of nonopertive ischemic stroke was twice as high in men (8.21%, 95% CI 5.64–10.78, $P < 0.0001$) than women (4.08%, 95% CI 0.74–7.41, $P = 0.02$). Therefore, it is reasonable to state that properly selected women with asymptomatic CAS may benefit from CEA; however, the magnitude of benefit is less than that in men.

The underlying cause of this benefit differential from CEA between men and women, aside from the higher perioperative risk in women, is probably the more favorable natural history of asymptomatic CAS in women who are treated conservatively (27). The lower rate of ischemic stroke in women versus men with asymptomatic CAS was also apparent in the medical treatment arms of both the ACAS and ACST trials. The 5-year risk of ipsilateral ischemic stroke was lower for women than men in ACAS (8.7% versus 12.1%) (5) and ACST (7.5% versus 10.6%) (6).

Whether the differential in the risk to benefit ratio between men and women after CEA is also applicable to carotid artery stenting remains a subject of investigation. Convincing data will need to await the results of the ongoing prospective randomized clinical trials comparing carotid stenting to CEA in patients with asymptomatic CAS (CREST and ACT 1 trials).

Therefore, until further evidence is available, selected women with asymptomatic CAS should be considered for carotid revascularization; however, with two caveats: the threshold for carotid revascularization should be higher in women than that in men and patients are counseled that there is more pronounced benefit for men compared with women undergoing CEA.

Comorbid Conditions

Among patients with severe asymptomatic CAS, the presence of renal insufficiency and a history of contralateral neurological symptoms significantly increase the risk of future stroke. These patients should be considered for carotid revascularization (28).

Carotid Stenosis Parameters

The higher the degree of carotid stenosis in neurologically asymptomatic individuals the higher the risk of stroke and TIA (28,31). Most experts agree that a critical threshold of >80% stenosis is associated with a rise of ipsilateral ischemic neurological events and should trigger an evaluation for carotid revascularization. Nonetheless, it should be clear that lesion severity is only one of many variables that have an impact on future stroke risk.

Among patients with asymptomatic CAS, the risk of stroke and TIA is three times greater in those with carotid stenosis progression to 80% stenosis or more compared to those without such progression (31,32).

Data on the prognostic significance of carotid plaque qualitative parameters in neurologically asymptomatic patients are either lacking (plaque ulceration) or conflicting (plaque echogeneccity). Some studies have shown that echolucent carotid plaques are associated with a two- to fivefold increased risk for stroke. However, the clinical utility of these observations for triaging patients to carotid revascularization awaits prospective confirmation (33).

End-Organ (Brain) Parameters

Silent Brain Infarcts

The prognostic value of silent cerebral infarcts in patients with asymptomatic CAS is an open question. Tegos and colleagues (34) demonstrated that the presence of discrete cortical or subcortical silent cerebral infarcts on brain CT in patients with carotid disease increases their risk of future stroke by approximately fourfold. These findings have been corroborated by magnetic resonance diffusion-weighted imaging (35).

Therefore, it is possible that the presence of ipsilateral silent cerebral infarcts in patients with asymptomatic CAS, particularly when discrete and cortical, may be indicative of higher risk for future stroke.

Cerebral Microembolic Signals

Cerebral microembolic signals are detected by transcranial Doppler in 1% to 23% of patients with asymptomatic CAS (36–38). The prevalence of cerebral microembolic signals in patients with asymptomatic CAS varies with the severity of the carotid stenosis, the morphology of the carotid plaque, and the frequency and duration of transcranial Doppler monitoring. The presence of cerebral microembolic signals in patients with asymptomatic CAS has been associated with a risk of stroke increased four to five times (38). However, the clinical utility of this technique to discriminate among patients who will benefit from carotid revascularization versus those who would not awaits confirmation in prospective trials.

Cerebral Vascular Reserve

Cerebral vascular reserve is the capacity of the brain to maintain a constant cerebral blood flow during a wide range of changes of mean arterial blood pressure. Cerebral vascular reserve can be tested by increasing passive CO_2 or by altering mean arterial blood pressure. Techniques to accomplish this include breath holding (passive CO_2 accumulation), acetazolamide challenge, inhaled CO_2, valsalva maneuver, and other methods (39–41). Changes in cerebral blood flow during the cerebral vascular reserve testing may be measured by transcranial Doppler, positive emission tomography, mRI-based techniques, single photon emission computed tomography, and xenon CT (42,43). Patients with asymptomatic CAS and impaired cerebral vasoreactivity are at higher risk of ischemic neurological events, and they can be considered for carotid revascularization (44).

■ CAROTID ARTERY STENTING FOR ASYMPTOMATIC CAROTID ARTERY DISEASE

While there are several single and multicenter reports of outcomes following carotid artery stenting, both before and after the advent of embolic protection devices (45–48), this discussion will focus on pivotal multicenter trials with neurologically audited results. Such individual pivotal trials performed for device approval have generally been underpowered for subset analysis, each typically having 300 to 500 patients with approximately 70% to 75% of them asymptomatic. In the interim, attention has been focused primarily on the larger data sets available from the FDA-mandated postmarket approval surveillance registries with 90% asymptomatic patients (49,50), along with the CREST lead-in phase registry (51), both of which have neurologically audited outcomes reporting and robust enough numbers to allow some subset analysis and conclusions.

Carotid Artery Stenting with Embolic Protection in Asymptomatic Carotid Artery Disease

High-Surgical-Risk Patients

There have been several device approval trials in high-surgical risk patients. Detailed outcomes data are available for the ARCHeR and SAPPHIRE trials. SAPPHIRE randomized patients between CEA and stenting with the Precise stent and Angioguard filter (Johnson & Johnson/Cordis); the trial cohort included 72% of patients who were asymptomatic (7). In this noninferiority trial, a prespecified analysis in the asymptomatic subset demonstrated no difference between CAS and CEA in both the 30-day periprocedural and one-year outcomes, with trends favoring stenting in each case. Specifically, carotid stenting in asymptomatic patients resulted in 6.0% 30-day MAE rate versus 9.2% in the CEA cohort. These results were further supported by data generated from the ARCHeR studies (52). Of the 581 high surgical risk patients treated with the Acculink stent and Accunet embolic filter system in this nonrandomized registry, 76% were asymptomatic. While the overall rate of periprocedural adverse events (death, stroke, and mychardial infarction) was 8.3% (95% CI 6.2–10.8%), asymptomatic patients experienced less events (6.8%, 95% CI 4.6–9.5%). Further, at 2.5 years, 95.7% of asymptomatic patients were free from periprocedural death/major stroke and major ipsilateral stroke. It is important to note that in the CEA trials previously detailed, the 30-day endpoints did not include MI. If the results from ARCHeR exclude MI, the 30-day periprocedural event rate falls to 5.4% (95% CI 3.5–8.0%).

The results of these trials suggest rates of adverse outcomes in high-surgical risk patients which approach those from the normal-risk CEA landmark trials, but are underpowered to draw significant conclusions. Subsequent studies that enrolled broader patient population with respect to surgical risk provide some of the additional numbers to aid in further comparisons with the CEA historical controls.

The primary intent of the FDA-mandated postmarket surveillance (PMS) registries was to both assess the transfer of stent technology into the clinical, nontrial, setting and to survey for any unanticipated device-related events. On both counts, data from the Carotid RX ACCULINK® /RX ACCUNET™ Post-Approval Trial to Uncover Unanticipated or Rare Events (CAPTURE; Guidant Corporation) (49) and Carotid Artery Stenting With Emboli Protection Surveillance (CASES, Johnson & Johnson/Cordis) (50) demonstrate no device-related issues and successful outcomes across operator experience. These registries also represent the largest neurologically audited outcomes databases available in stenting or surgical carotid intervention and allow subset analyses with a reasonably robust statistical power. The only drawback to using data from these two registries is that they include, in part, learning curves of multiple operators.

CAPTURE has reported outcomes on 2,500 high-surgical-risk patients treated using the Guidant filter and stent system at 137 centers across the United States, 90.7% of whom were asymptomatic (49). The 30-day major adverse event rate (death, stroke, myocardial infarction) for asymptomatic patients (n = 2268) was 4.9% and for asymptomatic patients under the age of 80 years (n = 1741) was 4.2%. Moreover, if only the 30-day rate of stroke and death is considered the event rate fell to 3.6% in asymptomatic patients under the age of 80 years. Lastly, CASES-PMS enrolled 974 asymptomatic high-surgical risk patients who were treated with Cordis/Johnson & Johnson stent and filter system (50). The 30-day risk of stroke and death in the entire asymptomatic group was 4.2% (the breakout for patients under 80 years of age is unavailable).

Low-Surgical-Risk Patients

Data regarding the role of CAS in low-surgical-risk patients with asymptomatic CAS are limited. The Carotid Revascularization Endarterectomy versus Stenting Trial (CREST) lead-in registry has reported data for investigators during the roll-in phase (51). The 30-day rate of stroke and death in the 960 asymptomatic patients was 4.0%, and if limited to only patients under the age of 80 years is 3.3%. The 30-day rate of death and major stroke in patients under the age of 80 years was 1.4%.

There are two ongoing prospective clinical randomized trials of CAS versus CEA in low-surgical risk patients in the United States (ACT 1, CREST). The Asymptomatic Carotid Stenosis Stenting versus Endarterectomy Trial (ACT 1, Abbott Vascular) is in the enrollment phase and it will randomize up to 1658 patients to CAS with the Abbott system or CEA in a 3:1 scheme. The Carotid Revascularization Endarterectomy versus Stenting Trial (CREST) has already finished enrollment and one-year follow-up data will be available shortly.

The Carotid Artery Stenting Procedure

Patient Selection

Once a decision has been made to proceed with carotid revascularization, institution specific risk assessment for appropriateness of CEA and carotid artery stenting should be performed and the patient triaged accordingly (Figure 9.1). Currently, stenting is accessible to asymptomatic high-surgical risk patients under the post marketing surveillance registries, and to asymptomatic

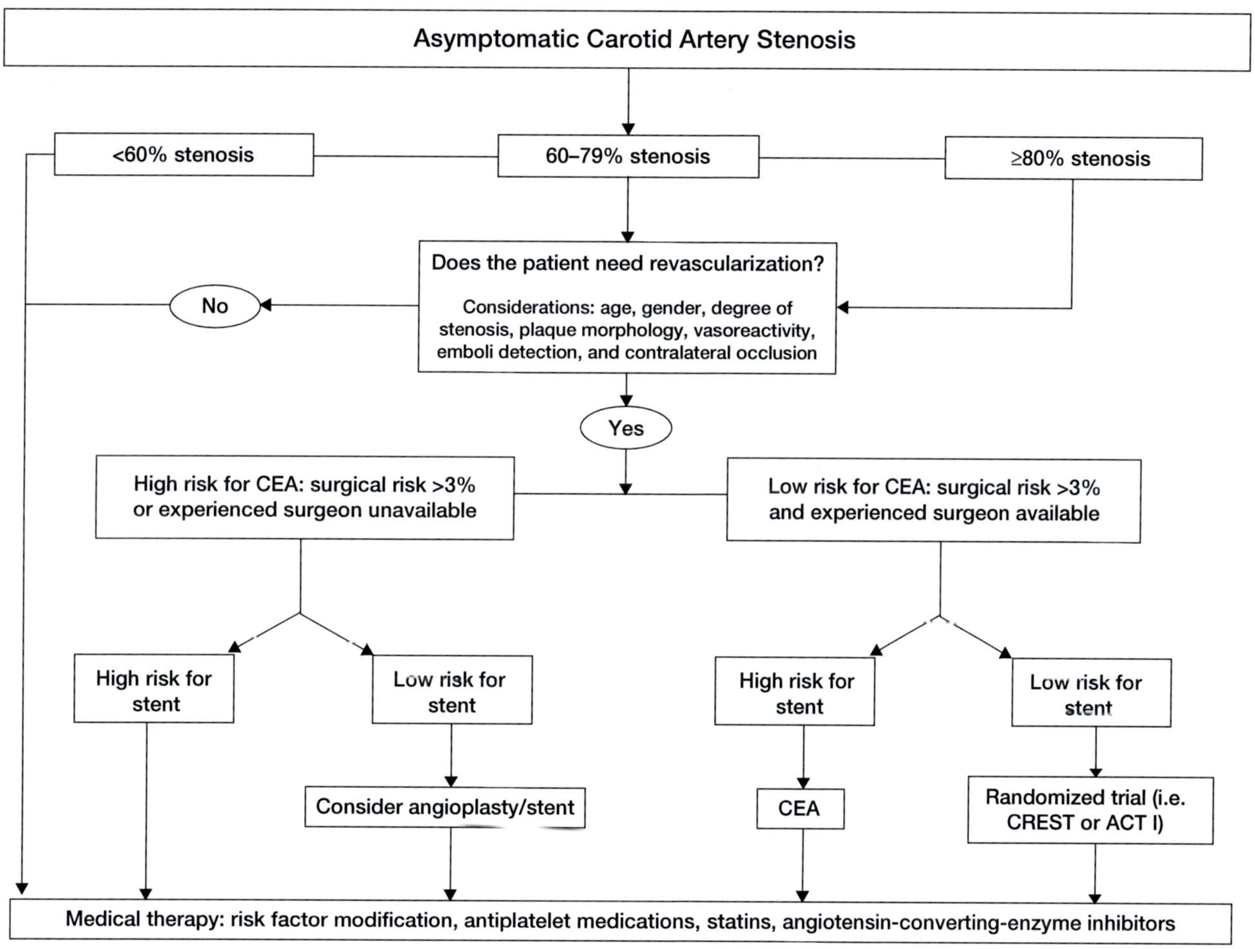

FIGURE 9.1 Triage of patients with asymptomatic carotid artery stenosis to carotid endarterectomy (CEA) versus carotid artery stenting. (Adapted from Ref. 8, with permission.)

low-surgical risk patients in the context of prospective randomized trials. To optimize patient selection for stenting, it is crucial to consider the clinical and anatomic features that may increase the risk of complications. As a rule of thumb, the higher the number of high-risk features, the higher the likelihood of stenting-related complications.

There are anatomic features that increase the risk of carotid artery stenting. The three most important anatomic high-risk features are: type 3 aortic arch, particularly in the presence of moderate to severe atherosclerosis; severe common or internal carotid artery tortuosity; and severe lesion calcifications. A type 3 aortic arch may lead to prolonged catheter manipulation and difficulty in accessing the common carotid artery with potentially higher risk of aortic arch plaque embolization (Figure 9.2). Excessive vessel tortuosity proximal or distal to the carotid stenosis increases the difficulty of EPD delivery and potentially deployment, and it increases the likelihood of vascular spasm. Occasionally, extreme tortuosity may even preclude a patient from undergoing intervention (Figure 9.3). Finally, severe calcification, particularly in combination with tortuosity, can cause difficulties in device delivery, lesion dilation, and stent expansion (Figure 9.4).

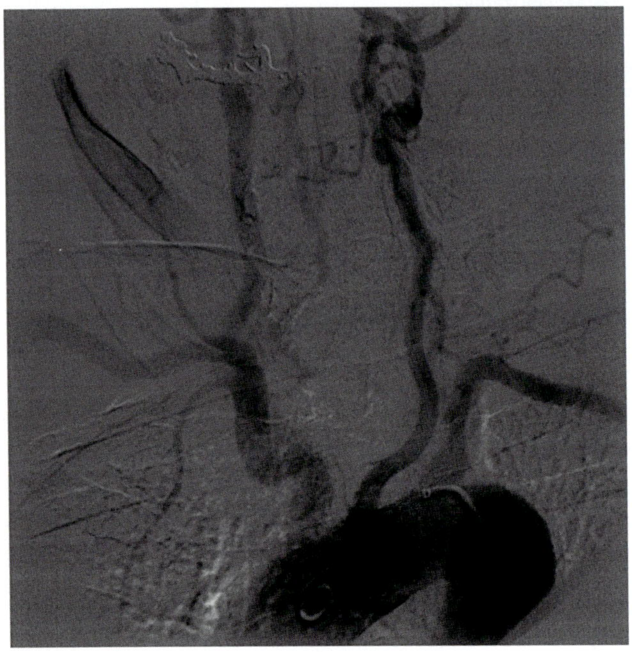

FIGURE 9.2 Type 3 aortic arch in a high-surgical-risk patient with asymptomatic severe left internal carotid artery stenosis.

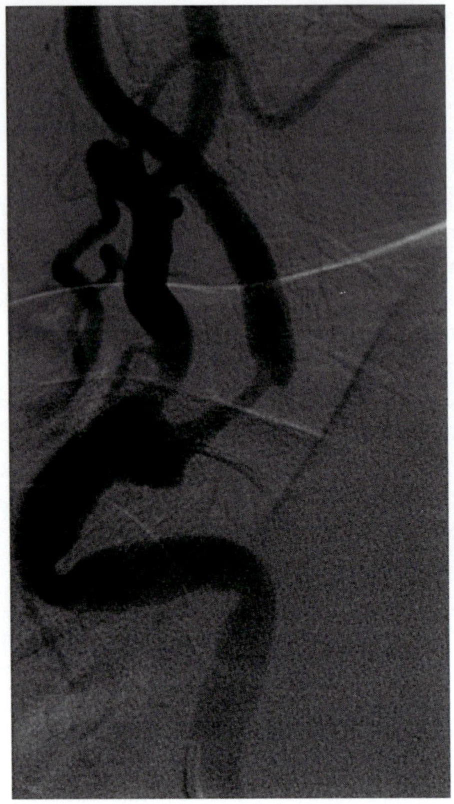

FIGURE 9.3 Severe tortuosity of the right distal common carotid artery in a high-surgical-risk patient with asymptomatic right internal carotid artery stenosis.

Preprocedure Patient Preparation

The standard antiplatelet regimen for patients undergoing carotid artery stenting include aspirin 325 mg a day and clopidogrel 75 mg a day for at least one week prior to the procedure. Currently, there is no role for elective use of glycoprotein IIb–IIIa receptor antagonists. All patients should be adequately hydrated to reduce the incidence and severity of intraprocedural hypotension. Traditionally, all antihypertensive medications are withheld on the day of the procedure. This is done to avoid excessive hypotension after CAS, particularly in patients with known severe coronary artery disease or critical aortic stenosis.

Procedure Execution

In the absence of preprocedure anatomic imaging (MRA or CTA), aortic arch angiography is essential for proper procedural planning. This information

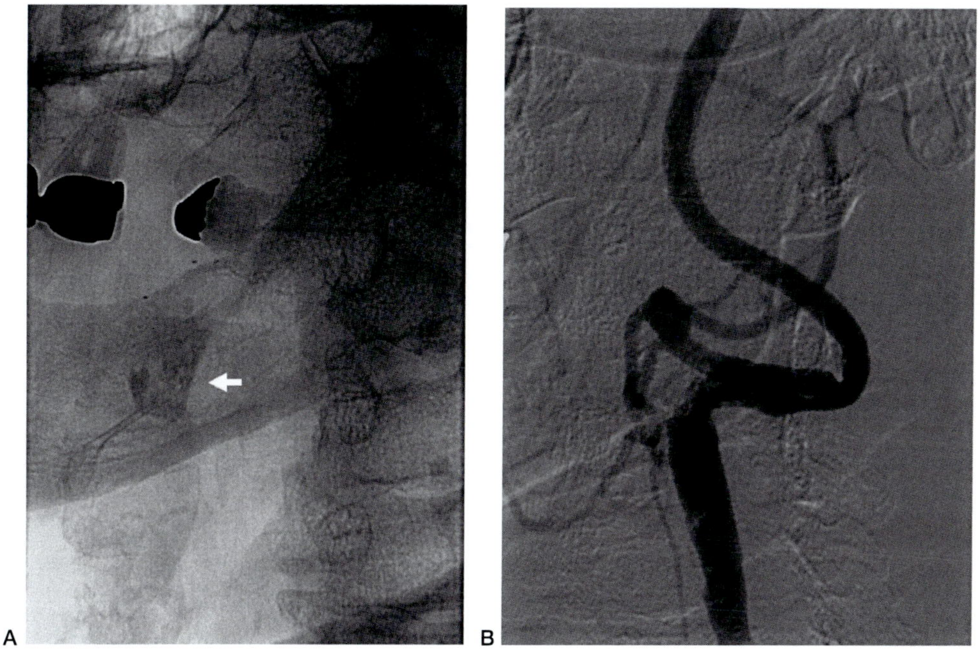

FIGURE 9.4 Severely calcified left carotid bulb stenosis (A, white arrow) with 90 degrees bend distal to the stenosis (B).

helps the operator choose the most appropriate diagnostic cerebral angiography catheter, plan and anticipate the level of difficulty in accessing the common carotid artery. Carotid and intracerebral angiography should define lesion severity, the degree of tortuosity and calcification, presence or absence of tandem extra or intracranial atherosclerotic disease, the extent and source of collateral circulation, and the presence or absence of large intracranial aneurysms or AV malformations. Neurological events associated with carotid angiography are often due to excessive and prolonged manipulation of the diagnostic catheter in the aortic arch. Operator experience and proper choice of diagnostic catheters are paramount in reducing these complications.

Embolic Protection Devices

Embolic protection devices (EPDs) are beneficial in reducing cerebral embolic complications with stenting. There are three categories of EPDs: distal occlusion balloons, distal filter devices (Figure 9.5), and flow-reversal devices. Although there are clear differences among these devices in design, profile, deployment method, and technical performance, once an EPD is deployed there is no proof of differences in clinical outcome. The choice of one category of EPDs versus the other depends on the particular anatomy. The anatomic features that need to be considered when choosing an EPD include the following:

1. Angle of origin of the internal carotid artery (ICA)
2. Degree of ICA tortuosity distal to the lesion particularly at the exit point
3. Adequacy of the landing zone
4. Adequacy of collateral circulation when distal balloon occlusion or flow-reversal is considered.

Self-Expanding Carotid Stents

Self-expandable stents are preferable to balloon expandable stents due to the risk of external compression of the latter. The nominal diameter of the self-expandable stent should be at least 1 to 2 mm larger than the distal reference of the lesion, but also large enough to provide good apposition to the common carotid artery. A wide variety of self-expandable open cell (Figure 9.6) and closed cell (Figure 9.7) carotid stents are available, each with its unique attributes. Although tailoring stent choice (in terms of conformability, lesion coverage and radial strength) to the specific anatomy makes intuitive sense, there is no proof that one stent is superior to others in terms of clinical outcome.

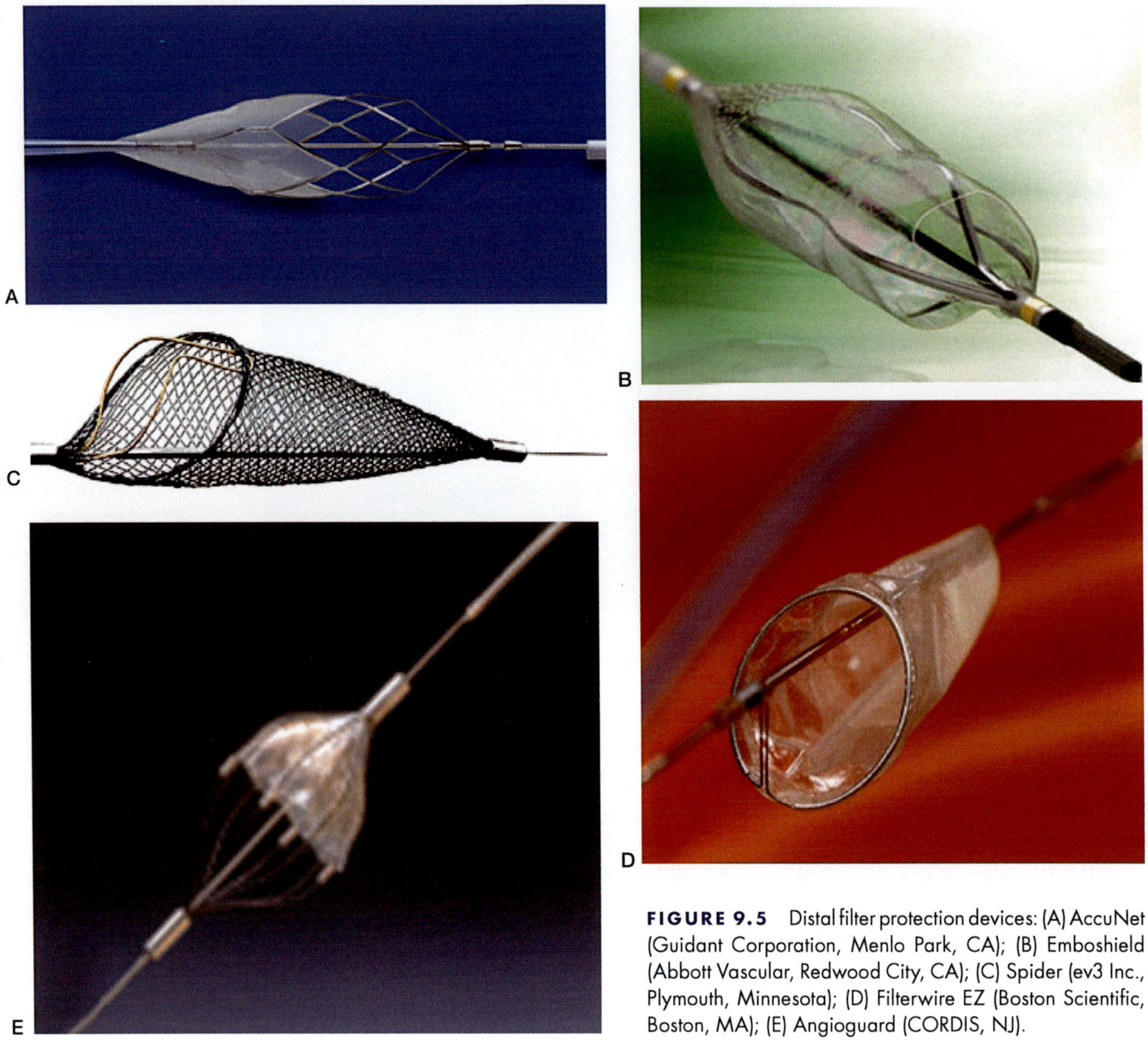

FIGURE 9.5 Distal filter protection devices: (A) AccuNet (Guidant Corporation, Menlo Park, CA); (B) Emboshield (Abbott Vascular, Redwood City, CA); (C) Spider (ev3 Inc., Plymouth, Minnesota); (D) Filterwire EZ (Boston Scientific, Boston, MA); (E) Angioguard (CORDIS, NJ).

■ SUMMARY

The decision to screen a patient for asymptomatic CAS requires individualized clinical judgment incorporating the current evidence with the particulars of that patient's condition. Although it is true that the incidence of stroke and death resulting from asymptomatic CAS is proportional to the prevalence and prognosis of untreated disease, the prevalence of asymptomatic CAS in the general population and the risk of subsequent ipsilateral stroke or death suggest that the yearly risk to any given individual is low. The number of patients who would require screening to prevent stroke or death in one patient makes general screening for asymptomatic CAS unjustified. However, limiting screening to patients at high risk for asymptomatic CAS such as those with carotid bruits and/or peripheral or coronary arterial disease improves the diagnostic yield and may improve clinical outcome with an appropriate management strategy.

Carotid artery stenting (CAS) with embolic protection in asymptomatic patients has demonstrated safety and long-term efficacy in multiple neurologically controlled settings including randomized trials, lead-in registries, and postmarketing surveillance registries in high-surgical risk patients. Specifically, in the cohort of

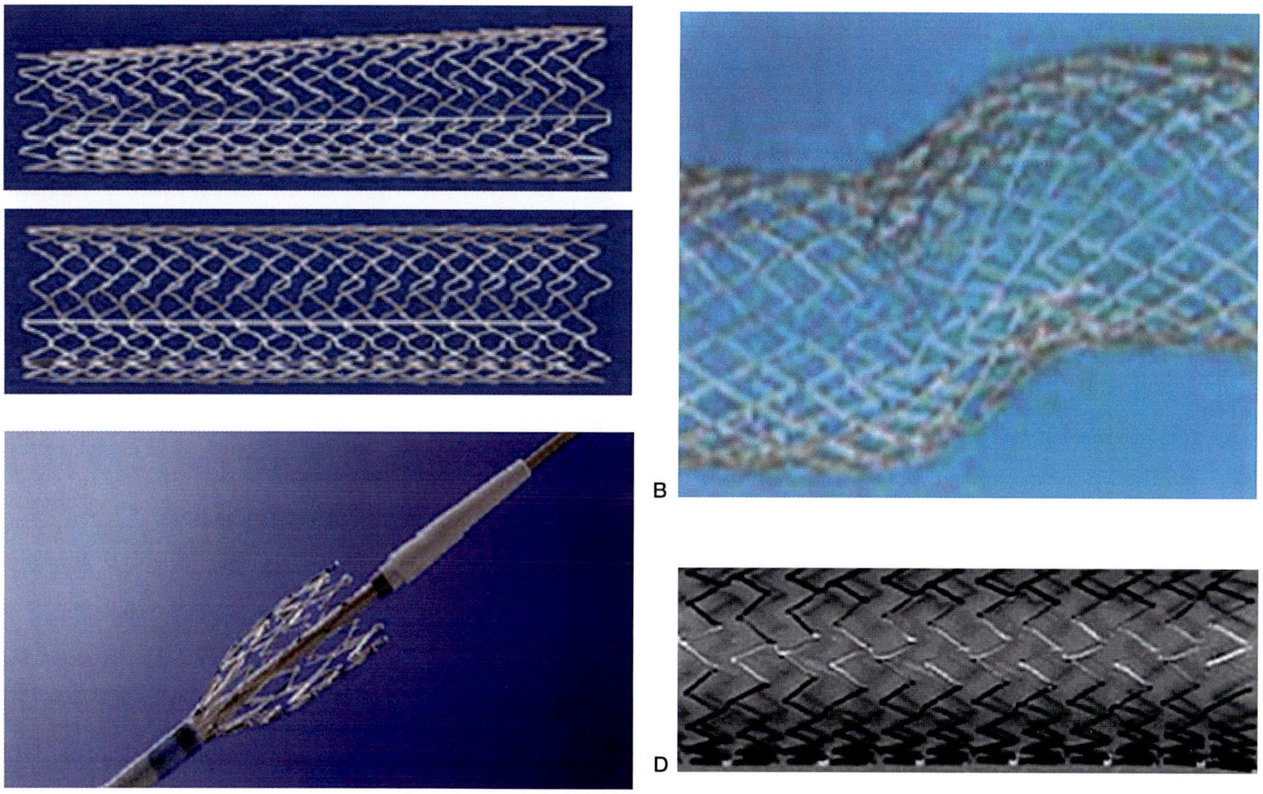

FIGURE 9.6 Self-expandable carotid stents (open cell). (A) Acculink (Guidant Corporation, Menlo Park, CA); (B) Exponent (Medtronic Vascular, Santa Rosa, CA); (C) Precise (CORDIS, NJ). (D) Protégé (ev3 Inc., Plymouth, Minnesota).

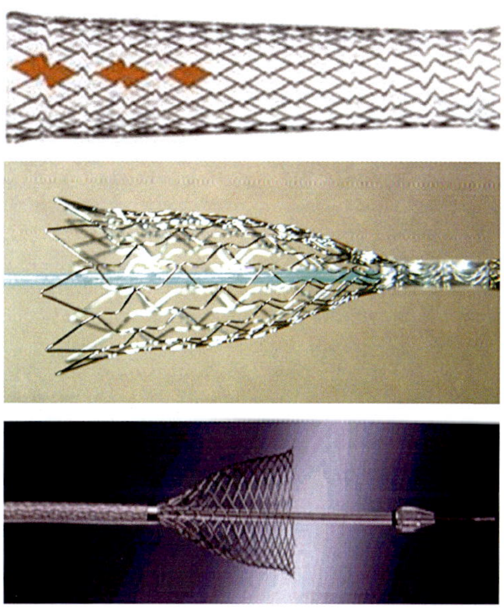

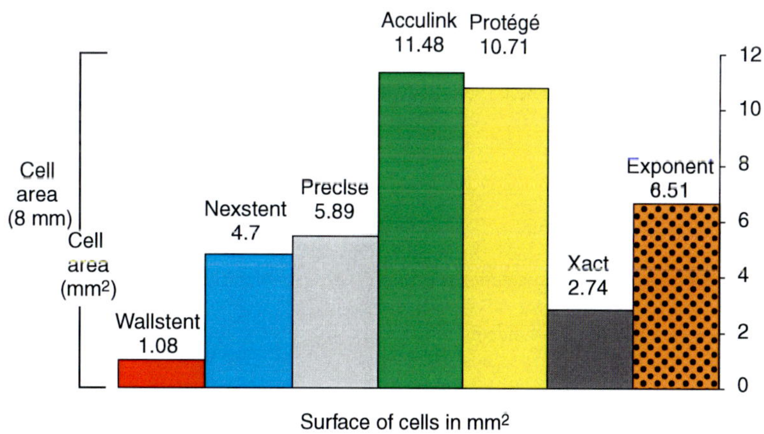

FIGURE 9.7 Self-expandable carotid stents (closed cell). (A) X-act (Abbott Vascular, Redwood City, CA); (B) NexStent (Boston Scientific, Boston, MA/EndoTex, Cupertino, CA); (C) Carotid Wallstent (Boston Scientific, Boston, MA).

patients under the age of 80 years, stroke and death rates approach normal-risk historical controls. Nevertheless at the time of this writing, Medicare only sanctions patients with symptomatic stenosis and high surgical risk. For standard-surgical-risk patients, the ongoing prospective randomized clinical trials comparing CAS with CEA will define the standard of care.

Most importantly, before considering any intervention asymptomatic patients with carotid artery disease need to undergo a rigorous risk stratification process to establish the need for carotid revascularization and to choose the optimal revascularization strategy (CAS versus CEA). Proper patient selection based on demographic, clinical and angiographic features, meticulous procedure planning and execution, and fastidious post procedural management are essential steps to insure a low complication rate with CAS.

REFERENCES

1. Mackey AE, Abrahamowicz M, Langlois Y, et al. Outcome of asymptomatic patients with carotid disease. *Neurology* 1997; 48:896–903.
2. Fisher CM. Transient ischemic attacks. Perspective. *N Engl J Med* 2002; 347:1642–3.
3. Eliasziw M, Kennedy J, Hill MD, Buchan AM, Barnett HJ. Early risk of stroke after a transient ischemic attack in patients with internal carotid artery disease. *CMAJ* 2004 Mar 30; 170(7):1105–9.
4. Taghavy A, Hamer H. Parenchymal "damage" in transient ischemic attacks (TIAs) and prolonged reversible ischemic neurologic deficits (PRINDs): the role of cranial CT and EEG. *Int J Neurosci* 1992 Oct; 66(3–4):251–61.
5. Executive Committee for the Asymptomatic Carotid Atherosclerosis Study. Endarterectomy for asymptomatic carotid stenosis. *JAMA* 1995; 273:1421–8.
6. MRC Asymptomatic Carotid Surgery Trial (ACST) Collaborative Group. Prevention of disabling and fatal strokes by successful carotid endarterectomy in patients without recent neurological symptoms: randomized controlled trial. *Lancet* 2004; 363:1491–1502.
7. Yadav JS, Wholey MH, Kuntz RE, et al. Protected carotid-artery stenting versus endarterectomy in high-risk patients. *N Engl J Med* 2004 Oct 7; 351(15):1493–501.
8. Moussa I, Mohr JP. Epidemiology and natural history of asymptomatic carotid artery stenosis. In Moussa I, Rundek T, Mohr JP, eds. *Asympomatic Carotid Artery Stenosis: Risk Stratification and Management.* London: Informa Healthcare, 2007.
9. Lee TT, Solomon NA, Heidenreich PA, Oehlert J, Garber AM. Cost-Effectiveness of Screening for Carotid Stenosis in Asymptomatic Persons. *Ann Int Med* 1997; 126(5):337–46.
10. Derdeyn CP, Powers WJ. Cost-effectiveness of screening for asymptomatic carotid atherosclerotic disease. *Stroke* 1996; 27:1944–50.
11. Sandok BA, Whisnant JP, Furlan AJ, Mickell JL. Carotid artery bruits: prevalence survey and differential diagnosis. *Mayo Clin Proc* 1982; 57(4):227–30.
12. Gutierrez IZ, Barone DL, Makula PA, Currier C. The risk of perioperative stroke in patients with asymptomatic carotid bruits undergoing peripheral vascular surgery. *Am Surg* 1987 Sep; 53(9):487–9.
13. Fell G, Breslau P, Knox RA, Phillips D, Thiele BL, Strandness DE Jr Importance of noninvasive ultrasonic Doppler testing in the evaluation of patients with asymptomatic carotid bruits. *Am Heart Journal* 1981; 102:221–6.
14. Sauve JS, Thorpe KE, Sackett DL, et al. Can Bruits Distinguish High-Grade from Moderate Symptomatic Carotid Stenosis? *Ann Int Med* 1994; 20(8): 633–7.
15. Naylor AR, Mehta Z, Rothwell PM, Bell PRF. Carotid Artery Disease and Stroke During Coronary Artery Bypass: a Critical Review of the Literature. *Eur J Vasc Endovasc Surg* 2002; 23:283–94.
16. Hill AB, Obrand D, O'Rourke K, Steinmetz OK, Miller N. Hemispheric stroke following cardiac surgery: A case-control estimate of the risk resulting from ipsilateral asymptomatic carotid artery stenosis. *Ann Vasc Surg* 2000 14:200–9.
17. Salasidis GC, Latter DA, Steinmetz OK, Blair JF, Graham AM. Carotid artery duplex scanning in preoperative assessment for coronary artery revascularization: the association between peripheral vascular disease, carotid artery stenosis, and stroke. *J Vasc Surg* 1995; 21(1):154–62.
18. Vigneswaran WT, Sapsford RN, Stanbridge RD. Disease of the left main coronary artery: early surgical results and their association with carotid artery stenosis. *Br Heart J* 1993 Oct; 70(4):342–5.
19. Durand DJ, Perler BA, Roseborough GS, et al. Mandatory versus selective preoperative carotid screening: a retrospective analysis. *Ann Thorac Surg* 2004; 78:159–66.
20. Barnett HJM, Meldrum HE, Eliasziw M. The appropriate use of carotid endarterectomy. *CMAJ* 2002; 166:1169–79.
21. Chambers BR, You RX, Donnan GA. Carotid endarterectomy for asymptomatic carotid stenosis. *Cochrane Database Syst Rev* 2003; 1:1–15.
22. Rothwell PM, Goldstein LB. Carotid endarterectomy for asymptomatic carotid stenosis. Asymptomatic Carotid Surgery Trial. *Stroke* 2004; 35:2425–7.
23. Bond R, Rerkasem K, Rothwell PM. High morbidity due to endarterectomy for asymptomatic carotid stenosis. *Cerebrovasc Dis* 2003; 16(Suppl.):65.
24. Howard G, Hobson RW, Brott T, et al. Does the stroke risk in stenting increase at older ages? Thirty-day stroke-death rates in the CREST lead-in phase. *Stroke* 2004; 35:258.
25. Manolio TA, Kronmal RA, Burke GL, et al. for the CHS Collaborative Research Group. The cardiovascular health study short-term predictors of incident stroke in older adults. *Stroke* 1996; 27:1479–86.
26. Rothwell PM, Slattery J, Warlow CP. Clinical and angiographic predictors of stroke and death from carotid endarterectomy: systematic review. *Br Med J* 1997; 315:1571–7.
27. Dick P, Sherif C, Sabeti S, et al. The role of gender is clearly illustrated by gender differences in outcome of conservatively treated patients with asymptomatic high-grade carotid stenosis. *Stroke* 2005; 36:1178–83.
28. Nicolaides AN, Kakkos S, Griffin M, et al. Severity of asymptomatic carotid stenosis and risk of ipsilateral hemispheric

ischaemic events: results from the ACSRS study. *Eur J Vasc Endovasc Surg* 2005; 30:275–84.
29. Baigent C, Keech A, Kearney PM, et al. Cholesterol Treatment Trialists' (CTT) collaborators. Efficacy and safety of cholesterol-lowering treatment: prospective meta-analysis of data from 90,056 participants in 14 randomised trials of statins. *Lancet* 2005; 366:1267–78.
30. Berger JS, Roncaglioni MC, Avanzini F, et al. Aspirin for the primary prevention of cardiovascular events in women and men: a sex-specific meta-analysis of randomized controlled trials. *JAMA* 2006; 295:306–13.
31. Lewis RF, Abrahamowicz M, Cote R, et al. Predictive power of duplex ultrasonography in asymptomatic carotid disease. *Ann Intern Med* 1997; 127:13–20.
32. Sabeti S, Exner M, Mlekusch W, et al. Prognostic impact of fibrinogen in carotid atherosclerosis: nonspecific indicator of inflammation or independent predictor of disease progression? *Stroke* 2005; 36:1400–4.
33. Mathiesen EB, Bonaa KH, Joakimsen O. Echolucent plaques are associated with high risk of ischemic cerebrovascular events in carotid stenosis: the Tromso study. *Circulation* 2001; 103:2171–5.
34. Tegos TJ, Kalodiki E, Nicolaides AN, et al. Brain CT infarction in patients with carotid atheroma. Does it predict a future event? *Int Angiol* 2001; 2:110–7.
35. Kang DW, Chalela JA, Ezzeddine MA, et al. Association of ischemic lesion patterns on early diffusion-weighted imaging with TOAST stroke subtypes. *Arch Neurol* 2003; 60:1730–4.
36. Siebler M, Nachtmann A, Sitzer M, et al. Cerebral microembolism and the risk of ischemia in asymptomatic high-grade internal carotid artery stenosis. *Stroke* 1995; 26:2184–6.
37. Abbott AL, Chambers BR, Stork JL, et al. Embolic signals and prediction of ipsilateral stroke or transient ischemic attack in asymptomatic carotid stenosis: a multicenter prospective cohort study. *Stroke* 2005; 36:1128–33.
38. Spence JD, Tamayo A, Lownie SP, et al. Absence of microemboli on transcranial Doppler identifies low-risk patients with asymptomatic carotid stenosis. *Stroke* 2005; 36:2373–8.
39. Kontos HA, Wei EP, Navari RM, et al. Responses of cerebral arteries and arterioles to acute hypotension and hypertension. *Am J Physiol* 1978; 234:H371–83.
40. Settakis G, Lengyel A, Molnar C, et al. Transcranial Doppler study of the cerebral hemodynamic changes during breath-holding and hyperventilation tests. *J Neuroimaging* 2002; 12:252–8.
41. Marshall RS, Rundek T, Sproule DM, et al. Monitoring of cerebral vasodilatory capacity with transcranial Doppler carbon dioxide inhalation in patients with severe carotid artery disease. *Stroke* 2003; 34:945–9.
42. Derdeyn CP, Videen TO, Simmons NR, et al. Count-based PET method for predicting ischemic stroke in patients with symptomatic carotid arterial occlusion. *Radiology* 1999; 212:499–506.
43. Carusone LM, Srinivasan J, Gitelman DR, Mesulam MM, Parrish TB. Hemodynamic response changes in cerebrovascular disease: implications for functional MR imaging. *AJNR Am J Neuroradiol* 2002; 23:1222–8.
44. Silvestrini M, Vernieri F, Pasqualetti P, et al. Impaired cerebral vasoreactivity and risk of stroke in patients with asymptomatic carotid artery stenosis. *JAMA* 2000; 283:2122–7.
45. Roubin GS, New G, Iyer SS et al. Immediate and late clinical outcomes of carotid artery stenting in patients with symptomatic and asymptomatic carotid artery stenosis: a 5-year prospective analysis. *Circulation* 2001 Jan 30; 103(4):532–7.
46. Wholey MH, Al-Mubarek N, Wholey MH. Updated review of the global carotid artery stent registry. *Catheter Cardiovasc Interv* 2003 Oct; 60(2):259–66.
47. Reimers B, Schluter M, Castriota F, et al. Routine use of cerebral protection during carotid artery stenting: results of a multicenter registry of 753 patients. *Am J Med* 2004 Feb 15; 116(4):217–22.
48. CaRESS Steering Committee. Carotid Revascularization Using Endarterectomy or Stenting Systems (CaRESS) phase I clinical trial: 1-year results. *J Vasc Surg* 2005; 42:213–9.
49. Gray WA for the CAPTURE investigators. Carotid RX ACCULINK®/RX ACCUNET™ Post-Approval Trial to Uncover Unanticipated or Rare Events. Presented at the ACC 2006.
50. CASES Steering Committee. Carotid Artery Stenting With Emboli Protection Surveillance (CASES Registry).
51. Roubin GS. CREST lead-in Phase Registry investigators. Presented at the ACC 2006.
52. Gray WA, Hopkins NL, Yadav S, et al. Protected carotid stenting in high-surgical-risk patients: The ARCHeR results. *J Vasc Surg* 2006; 44:258–69.

Index